Herbs and Nutrients
for the Mind

Herbs and Nutrients for the Mind

A Guide to Natural Brain Enhancers

Chris D. Meletis, N.D. and Jason E. Barker, N.D.

Complementary and Alternative Medicine
Chris D. Meletis and Margot Longenecker, Series Editors

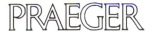

Westport, Connecticut
London

Library of Congress Cataloging-in-Publication Data

Meletis, Chris D.
  Herbs and nutrients for the mind : a guide to natural brain enhancers / Chris D.
Meletis and Jason E. Barker.
     p. cm. — (Complementary and alternative medicine, ISSN 1549–084X)
  ISBN 0–275–98394–3 (alk. paper)
  1. Herbs—Therapeutic use.   2. Dietary supplements.   3. Neurobehavioral
disorders—Alternative treatment.   I. Barker, Jason E.   II. Title.   III. Series.
RC350.H47M44   2004
616.8′04654—dc22   2004048057

British Library Cataloguing in Publication Data is available.

Library of Congress Catalog Card Number: 2004048057
ISBN: 0–275–98394–3
ISSN: 1549–084X

First published in 2004

Praeger Publishers, 88 Post Road West, Westport, CT 06881
An imprint of Greenwood Publishing Group, Inc.
www.praeger.com

Printed in the United States of America

The paper used in this book complies with the
Permanent Paper Standard issued by the National
Information Standards Organization (Z39.48–1984).

10 9 8 7 6 5 4 3 2 1

Contents

Series Foreword

The world of medicine has evolved with the changing needs and demands of the patient, the third-party payer, and a growing appreciation of the intimate relationship shared between the healthcare provider and patient. The evolution of medicine is not limited to these facets alone. An active reflection of the origins and heritage of medicine leads to a redefinition of medical care. Whether all forms of medicine must be compared to "Western-allopathic" medicine is now being overtly challenged by many patients and some conventional healthcare providers.

Many forms of medicine claim the Hippocratic model as their founding paradigm. However, the question could be raised as to whether Hippocrates would be accepted in the second millennium A.D. by his modern peers. Indeed, would his empirical approach to medicine stand up fully to the current medical model of scientific burden of proof?

Statistics show us that over 70 percent of the world's population uses something other than the Western-allopathic form of medicine as a primary source of medical care. This is not to dismiss the need for modern medicine, but rather to serve as a pivot for reflection of other forms of medicine that have sustained generations prior to our current era. In fact, some 25–33 percent of frequently used conventional prescription medicines originate from natural substances.

It is this new appreciation and objective perspective that has fostered the popularity of what is commonly called Complementary and Alternative Medicine or CAM. It is worthwhile to note that in order to have a complementary and alternative form of care, a single model must proclaim itself the primary form of care.

The goal of this series is to offer valuable insights into medical therapies currently categorized in the realm of CAM by Western-allopathic medicine. As more and more clinical trials are performed leading to scientific validation, current CAM therapies become embraced as mainstream treatment options. The intent of this series is to review healthcare therapies. The criteria for review are that the particular therapy has a foundation of clinical success, partial or full research validation, and/or rich historical use. The reviews of different therapies will provide critical insight into additional adjunctive therapies that might be incorporated in patient care. They will also provide a heighten appreciation of CAM as well as enhance the ability to converse about CAM therapies in an ever-evolving medical model.

Reflection on the present humbles all disciplines; for as we judge our predecessors, so shall we be judged by future generations for both current brilliance and shortcomings. Medicine is a part of an evolving reality. It is up to each provider to enrich history in the making.

Chris D. Meletis
Margot Longenecker

Introduction

The adage "The mind is a terrible thing to waste" truly lacks a depth of understanding and critical perspective essential to support foundational healing. When addressing brain-centered health promotion, patient and clinician alike must astutely appreciate that the "mind" is inseparable from the "body"; the brain, without question, is a physical structure that in its absence would eliminate any discussion of the concept of mind, psyche, or mental function. As an organ that influences the function of the entire being, the brain is central to both mental and physical health.

A simplistic illustration that compares the heart's function to that of the brain can be made to exemplify an appreciation of the brain and its function relative to mental and physical well-being. The heart beats over 100,000 times a day; it does so prior to our birth to the moment we die without exception, so we hope. This constant and reliable performance, giving blood throughout the body, serves as the cornerstone of the circulatory system and the flow of life. If the heart, which requires a constant source of energy, were to become inadequately fueled without the proper nourishment, it would begin to fail to maintain the very circulatory system that sustains our existence. Classically described conditions such as vitamin B-1 deficiency (known as wet beriberi) as well as recently discovered nutrient (Coenzyme Q10 and carnitine) deficiencies all contribute to the health of the cardiovascular system.

Such is the dilemma faced by the brain. Regardless of the brain's resilience, there is a time and a place in which inadequate intake can begin to yield the signs and symptoms of psychological or organic brain-altered function. Notable is that proper brain functioning is largely individual and can be affected by internal and external variables that may alter the needs of a given person's brain to function within normal expectations. Numerous nutrients must be present in sufficient levels, including B-1 as with the heart, to maintain brain function, yet variables and individual genetic signatures can change the required needs.

Whether it is heart or brain function as the center of discussion, both function as a result of a complex series of biochemical reactions, yielding nerve impulses and chemical reactions that maintain function. Notable in both circumstances is that the difference between the adequate and optimal functions of each can make the difference between surviving and thriving. The presentation of the clinical and germane medical research relative to supporting brain function targets the augmentation of function, with the goal of shifting away from surviving and becoming closer to thriving within the confines of human understanding of the miraculous creation of the central processor, the brain, which governs the human body's entire operating system.

Indeed the concepts of mind, mental and psychological attributes are all dependent upon a very real and physical component of the body, that being the human brain. Often, the terms "mental" or "psychological" are attributed to the mind portion of the mind-body connection.

Throughout this work, it is our hope that the reader does not look at the mind as separate from the body. Realize that the physical presence of a properly functioning brain is the requisite for mental health, accepted psychological presentation, and healthy functioning of the central nervous system. We have thus intentionally included such conditions as Parkinson's and multiple sclerosis in the list of health conditions addressed. Though Parkinson's and multiple sclerosis reflect a well-delineated spectrum of organic brain-altered function, they are in many ways no more organic than the patient with depression.

This book offers a select view of natural medicine interventions, focusing on nutritional and botanical treatments, referred to within the confines of these covers as "Nutra-botanical" therapies, evidenced by clinical practice and research findings. The individual sections of this work are intended as springboards for further investigation by the reader. Often, the human dilemma arises from accepting limits when perceptions of confining factors seem to have been reached even though a new perspective may be just a glimpse away over the walls of our personal reality's boundaries.

It is not the intent of this book to advocate for the replacement of standard drug therapy.

However, individuals suffering from a health condition affecting brain performance should not limit their options to drug therapy when other biochemical interventions could perpetuate heightened function and the ever-important quality-of-life issue. A concerted effort for the integration of natural medicine approaches alongside standard drug therapy should be pursued in every patient-doctor relationship. The sharing of all therapeutic interventions being pursued with all clinical providers is of paramount importance in order to avoid unnecessary potential drug–natural medicine interactions. Tell your medical doctor if you are on any medication and use—or plan to use—natural treatments.

By supporting health through the use of optimal nutrition, people are placed in a decision-making role regarding their health. Previously, health was attributed to nothing more than luck and the use of medicines designed to treat the symptoms of the disease itself. With today's new focus on prevention of disease by fueling the body and its systems correctly, people can now make a decision to pursue health rather than simply react once a disease manifests.

May all that read the following pages do so with an open mind and—equally important—a healthy brain.

PART I

Brain Ailments and Nutra-Botanical Interventions

ADD/ADHD

Attention deficit disorder (ADD), formerly known as attention deficit/hyperactivity disorder (ADHD), is one of the most common mental disorders among children today. It is estimated that approximately 3 percent to 5 percent of all children (two to three times as many boys are affected than girls) or nearly 2 million American children (which correlates to one child in each classroom in the United States) have ADHD according to the National Institute of Mental Health.[1] ADHD does not only affect children, as symptoms can progress into adulthood as well.

The specific causes of ADHD are currently unknown, with several factors being responsible in different people. No solitary causative factor has been identified as being responsible for the different behavior patterns observed in ADHD. ADHD is only diagnosed by certain characteristic behavior patterns that are observed over time; no other clear physical signs can be seen. Common behavioral pattern categories in ADHD include inattention, impulsivity, and hyperactivity.

- Inattention: This is marked by difficulty in keeping the mind focused on any one subject and a short attention span. People with ADHD often become bored after only a few minutes at work on a subject, and placing focused attention on new or unfamiliar topics can be challenging.
- Impulsivity: This is marked by an inability to refrain from immediate reactions, making it difficult to wait and first think before speaking or acting.
- Hyperactivity: This is marked by constant perpetual motion; staying in one place and sitting still can be difficult. Adults may feel quite restless and may start several projects and have a difficult time finishing them.

Diagnosis of ADHD is based upon an analysis of the person's behavioral patterns, which are compared to established criteria. These criteria are defined in the *Diagnostic and Statistical Manual of Mental Disorders* (*DSM-IV*). The manual outlines the three previously mentioned behavior patterns, and people may display varying amounts of each pattern or only one. Because nearly everyone displays some of these symptoms at some time in their life, certain criteria, including age of onset (early in life, before age seven), duration of symptoms (continuous for at least six months), frequency (occurring more often in themselves than others of similar age), and most importantly, behavior(s), must occur in at least two different areas of the person's life, namely, school, home, work, or social settings.

A recent report issued by the Centers for Disease Control and Prevention claimed that nearly 1.6 million elementary school–aged children have a diagnosis of ADHD, and a national survey revealed that the parents of 7 percent of children ages 6–11 years old were told by a healthcare professional that their child had ADHD.[2] The report also included the following demographic information: boys are nearly three times as likely to have ADHD than girls; white children are twice as likely than Hispanic and black children to have a diagnosis of ADHD; children with health insurance are diagnosed with ADHD more often than children without health insurance; and children with ADHD use more healthcare services, including mental health services, than those without ADHD. This report went on to propose that ADHD is probably overdiagnosed in those with regular access and may be underdiagnosed in those with limited healthcare access.

A common neurodevelopmental disorder, ADHD results in impaired educational processes, social growth, and adaptation that lead to increasing rates of behavioral difficulty, depression, school dropouts, and substance abuse,[3] which have lead to the mass prescription of stimulant psychotropic medications in children affected with this disorder. With no fully established biological causes recognized, ADHD does display prominent heritability. Mainstream treatment focuses on the use of mainly stimulant drugs, and because of the perceived relative success of these drugs in alleviating ADHD symptoms, many studies have focused mainly on genes that are responsible for the development and regulation of brain neurotransmitter systems, specifically that of dopamine, wherein the physiologic basis for the action of these drugs exists.

Genetic factors do play a role in the genesis of ADHD; estimates of heritability are greater than those of nearly every other child and adolescent psychiatric disorder and first-degree relatives have increased rates of ADHD, including conduct and affective disorders as well as substance abuse and dependency. Additionally, the subtypes of ADHD (impulsivity, hyperactivity, inattention) do not correlate with that of additional family members, leading researchers to conclude that nongenetic factors are responsible for intrafamilial variability.[4] Factors other than genetics have been implicated in the development of ADHD prior to birth. Prenatal exposure to nicotine and psychosocial adversity have been identified as risk factors for ADHD; a review of the studies in ADHD literature exploring the relationship between prenatal exposure to these factors and the risk of developing ADHD revealed that smoking (specifically nicotine exposure) and exposure to psychosocial stress during pregnancy indicated greater and modest risk, respectively, in contributing to the development of ADHD.[5] Other causes/contributors of ADHD that have been implicated in the literature include food sensitivities and allergies, food additive intolerance, imbalance and deficiency of nutrients, environmental toxicity (including heavy metal poisoning, thyroid irregularities, and other toxic pollutants).[6]

NUTRITIONAL FACTORS

The role of vitamins and minerals in brain function is equally important to their contribution to other organ systems. Just as organs and tissue systems may be compromised by inadequate or imbalanced nutrients, the functioning of the brain is easily affected by these imbalances or lack thereof; research points to the benefits of supplementation for nutrient deficiencies that resulted in improved academic and behavioral performance in ADHD children.[7] One hallmark study followed the effects of vitamin and mineral supplementation in healthy schoolchildren over 18 years old. Researchers found that supplementation with vitamins and minerals resulted in significantly less antisocial behavior and improved cognitive performance in children taking the supplements when compared to those taking a placebo.[8] However, improvement was not noted unless a frank nutrient deficiency of at least one nutrient (most often folic acid, thiamine, pyridoxine, vitamin C, or niacin) was found in blood testing. Because of findings such as these, the importance of multivitamin and mineral supplementation comes into play. It is interesting to note that these children had actual blood-level deficiencies; this comes at quite a nutritional cost with the wide food availability seen in modern times in the United States. Multinutrient dosing provides a backup strategy in the event of inadequate intake, or more commonly, inefficient absorption and utilization of these nutrients. A body that does not receive or is unable to fully utilize the nutrients necessary for optimal functioning will exhibit symptoms of dysfunction at its weakest areas. Studies investigating the use of B vitamins have yielded interesting results as well. One investigator employed varying combinations of B vitamins to successfully treat hyperactive children (more properly known as hyperkinesis) who did not respond to treatment with Feingold's diet (a diet espousing the removal of food additives and salicylate-containing foods).[9]

One B vitamin in particular, vitamin B-6 (pyridoxine) has been shown to be an effective treatment for hyperactive children; a double-blind study comparing the use of vitamin B-6 to methylphenidate (also known as Ritalin—the most commonly prescribed drug for ADHD) revealed a slightly greater effectiveness of B-6.[10] What is even more interesting in this study is that the researchers based their idea for the study on the observation noted by other doctors that hyperactive children tended to have lower blood levels of a specific neurotransmitter (serotonin) and that supplementing with large amounts of B-6 normalized the levels of serotonin and subsequently improved the children's behavior. B-6 serves as an enzymatic cofactor in the metabolism of several neurotransmitters, including serotonin, dopamine, and histidine.[11] The use of B-6 among physicians for the treatment of ADHD symptoms is widespread; it enjoys a positive reputation among clinicians treating these patients.

Phosphatidylserine is a biological molecule known as a "phospholipid." Phospholipids are one of the main components of cellular membranes in the human body and serve to stabilize the other constituents of which the cellular membranes are composed. Phosphatidylserine is the main phospholipid of human brain cells, and it serves to regulate cellular functions such as controlling the internal environment of the cell, communication between cells, signal transduction (communication from outside the cell to within), release of secretory vesicles (another mode of cellular communication), and regulation of cell growth and division.[12] Phosphatidylserine is beneficial to several different brain functions and also contributes to nerve cell synaptic membranes, a key anatomical aspect of nerve signal production and transmission. As a supplement, its benefits include increased neurologic energy via facilitated synaptic communication and increased production, release, and effectiveness of the neurotransmitter dopamine.[13] One study investigating the use of phosphatidylserine supplementation in ADHD patients resulted in a slightly greater than 90 percent improvement in these cases, with doses of 200 to 300 milligrams per day for up to four months providing the greatest absolution of symptoms.[14] Supplemental administration of phosphatidylserine is thought to normalize brain lipid content, thereby assisting the return of normalized function of neuronal cells.[15]

OTHER NUTRIENTS

Iron: Insufficient iron is one of the most common nutrient deficiencies among children in the United States,[16] and it is known to contribute to decreased attention span, activity, and persistence. Supplementation of nonanemic children with ADHD resulted in fewer symptoms of ADHD (marked by a 30 percent improvement).[17] Interestingly, iron serves as an essential cofactor in the synthesis of the brain neurotransmitters dopamine, norepinephrine, and serotonin, and deficiency in the early years of life can negatively affect neural and behavioral development.[18] It is essential to note that iron poisoning is the leading cause of accidental poisoning, thus guidance by a skilled healthcare provider is essential and close monitoring is a must.

Magnesium: Magnesium is another commonly deficient nutritional mineral. Magnesium supplementation can be helpful in alleviating some symptoms of ADHD. In one study, one group of children with ADHD was treated for six months with supplemental magnesium and changes in ADHD symptoms were compared to another group of ADHD children who did not take the supplement. Investigators noted a "significant" decrease in hyperactivity symptoms in the treatment group.[19] Another study demonstrated actual deficiencies of magnesium in 95 percent of ADHD children studied, leading the researchers to conclude that magnesium deficiency in children with ADHD occurs more often than in healthy children without ADHD.[20]

Zinc: A collection of studies reveal that the level of this mineral is low in people with ADHD,[21] and lower serum zinc levels are found in children with ADHD in comparison to children without.[22] A relationship exists between levels of free fatty acids in the blood and zinc in children with ADHD; these children, when compared to controls without ADHD, were found to have low blood levels of zinc and free fatty acids.[23] This indicates that a deficiency of zinc may contribute to the development of ADHD; the study hypothesized that the low levels of free fatty acids may be a result of the decreased zinc levels. Another interesting study revealed a relationship between the responsiveness to standard stimulant pharmacotherapy and zinc levels in the body: low zinc levels equated to poor treatment response from the medication.[24] Zinc serves as a cofactor in the synthesis of neurotransmitters and indirectly affects dopamine metabolism, a neurotransmitter that is believed to be involved in ADHD (low levels of dopamine are associated with ADHD, and supplementation of dopamine has alleviated some ADHD symptoms).[25] As the principal investigator of the ZAD (zinc–attention deficit) study, one of the authors of this book, Chris D. Meletis, has noted, through the course of reviewing the scientific literature and clinical findings over the last decade, a clear relationship between low levels of zinc in relation to copper stores and notable signs and symptoms of attention dysfunctions and cognitive deficits.

Because solitary nutrient deficiencies have been implicated in ADHD, it stands to reason that inadequate doses of the earlier mentioned nutrients in combination may act synergistically to cause ADHD. A group of researchers determined that the most common nutrient deficiencies among children with ADHD were magnesium, copper, zinc, calcium, and iron, and these deficiencies occur more often among hyperactive children than healthy children; these deficiencies were determined by measuring their levels in blood serum, red blood cells, and in the hair.[26] Of the implicated nutrients, magnesium was the most frequently deficient. Additionally, when the researchers supplemented the ADHD children with magnesium, zinc, and calcium, hyperactivity was decreased; and when a group of these children was treated with standard therapy minus magnesium, symptoms of hyperactivity actually increased.

These studies underscore an important revelation in ADHD in that the cause of these symptoms seems to be related to one or more types of suboptimal nutrient levels. A common theme carried throughout this book and noted in medicinal literature is that each individual has a unique weakness that becomes more manifest when certain environmental influences are exerted (in this case inadequate levels of micronutrients). When adequately supplied with correct nutrition, symptoms are often diminished and can be attenuated with time. In the treatment of the person with ADHD, it may not be as important to discover the exact nutrient or nutrients that are lacking in order to alleviate symptoms. By prescribing a full-spectrum nutritional plan (that may or may not include dietary alterations and supplements), people with ADHD receive the nutritional factors that are needed to avert the manifestation of their symptoms. Patients' individual nutritional needs should be taken into account prior to prescribing a nutritional treatment plan. An individualized approach is important; each person with ADHD may react differently to various nutritional factors. Both current and past dietary practices and habits are important to consider; the development of physiologic systems depend on varying levels and types of nutrients at different periods during the course of development.

Nutritional factors other than deficiency play a large role in the symptomology of ADHD. Food additives, refined sugars, food sensitivities, and food allergies have been linked to ADHD; mounting evidence has shown that children with ADHD will react to more than one food and or its components, leading to negative behaviors.[27] Dietary modification plays an equally important role to ensuring adequate nutritional supplementation; both treatments should be part of the ADHD treatment regimen. One of the most influential dietary approaches in the treatment of ADHD is the Feingold diet. Starting in the1970s, Feingold claimed that the cause of up to 50 percent of hyperactivity in children was attributable to food additives, including artificial colorings, flavors, and preservatives as well as naturally occurring salicylates.[28] Feingold arrived at this conclusion by investigating 1,200 cases of food additive–linked behavioral and learning disorders in patients; he implicated more than 3,000 different food additives in these cases. A large body of research is dedicated to negating this relationship, however Murray and Pizzorno, in reviewing the outcome data from theses studies, report that 50 percent of the children in these studies actually improved (experienced less hyperactivity) when on the Feingold diet.[17]

There are approximately 5,000 food additives in use today, most of which are used to preserve and enhance the appearance of food; Americans consume nearly 15 grams per day on a per capita basis (nearly 100 million pounds of food coloring alone is ingested on a yearly basis in the United States).[14] A study of 78 children with hyperactivity were placed on an elimination diet designed to remove offending foods that may cause hyperactive symptoms and 59 of these children experienced less hyperactivity while on the diet.[29] In a crossover portion of the study, the researchers were able to disguise previously established offending foods by mixing them in foods that were tolerated. This resulted in worsened behavior and impaired psychological test performance, demonstrating that observable changes in behavior associated with diet are reproducible using double-blind methods. The investigators used this point to emphasize the ability of the parent/teacher/caretaker's ability to note the relationship between food ingestion and behavior outcomes and to consider these observations as valid when they present this association to the family physician.

A review of 23 double-blind studies investigating the roles of food dyes versus ordinary foods as the cause of worsened ADHD behavior revealed a worsening of symptoms following dye consumption in eight of nine studies using ADHD children. There was improvement when a food additive–free diet was consumed. In 10 of the other 14 studies, children with ADHD and asthma, food allergies, and/or eczema saw their symptoms improve when additive-free foods were consumed.[30] Other subjects in these studies experienced a worsening of symptoms when they consumed food dyes, corn, wheat, dairy products, soy, oranges, and chocolate. Another study demonstrated that 73 percent of ADHD children responded favorably to a food additive elimination diet and also worsened when certain foods, dyes, and additives were reintroduced into their diet.[31] Another study employed the use of a diet consisting of rice, turkey, pear, and lettuce in the treatment of ADHD symptoms. Of the children studied, 62 percent demonstrated an improvement of symptoms of 50 percent or greater on the Connors list and the ADHD Rating Scale at the end of the study period, leading the researchers to conclude that ADHD children can experience statistically significant symptom improvement when placed on an elimination diet.[32] These studies demonstrate the benefits of removing certain foods that may be suspect in causing ADHD symptoms; foods containing additives and those that may be allergenic should be among the first to eliminate from the diets of patients with ADHD—they more than likely play a significant role in the etiology of ADHD. Dietary modification should be attempted prior to treating symptoms with pharmaceuticals.

CONCLUSION

With no specific etiology, ADHD is a perplexing condition that continues to increase in incidence. This chapter includes only a sampling of the studies demonstrating various links between ADHD and nutritional factors. In addition to micronutrient deficiencies, food additives and allergenic foods play a large role in the treatment of ADHD. Although it is difficult to imply that these are the causes of ADHD, research does show a causal relationship: when such foods are removed, patients have fewer symptoms, and when patients are supplemented with the correct amount of nutrients, negative symptoms decrease. Readers of this chapter are strongly encouraged to investigate the pharmaceuticals that are prescribed for ADHD; a large amount of data regarding their toxicity and effects on the developing nervous system are a must-know.

The question that must be posed is whether all the millions of children diagnosed with ADD/ADHD were born drug deficient or whether a deeper fundamental cause needs to be addressed. An analogy may be drawn between the performance and potential of a large eight-cylinder Corvette sports car and the health of a newborn: regardless of the inherent potential of such a high-performance vehicle, if it is operated with suboptimal fuel, then the full horse-power and drivability of such an amazing creation will not be realized, just as the human body's complex fuel needs are essential for peak performance.

NUTRIENTS

- Diet
  A diet that includes carbohydrates, proteins, and fats in a ratio of 40:30:30 percent three times per day
- Multivitamin/mineral
  A suitable age-specific supplement should be taken twice per day with meals
- B vitamin complex
  One capsule of B complex twice per day with meals.
- Phosphatidylserine
  200–300 milligrams per day
- Iron
  Must establish the presence of a deficiency prior to supplementing this nutrient*
- Magnesium
  5 milligrams per kilogram body weight per day
- Zinc
  25 milligrams per day

*Testing for food allergies and food sensitivities is imperative.

Alcoholism (Alcohol Abuse/ Dependence)

DEFINITION

Although alcoholism, or alcohol abuse or dependence, is not necessarily caused by deficiencies of nutritional factors, it may be propagated by and definitively leads to frank nutrient deficiencies with startling health effects. Alcoholism, or alcohol dependence, is by definition a disease. Alcohol dependence has a chronic, progressive course, follows a predictable course, and has symptoms; and the risk of developing alcohol dependence is influenced by a person's genes and lifestyle. Cravings can be a strong as the need for food or water, and a person who is alcohol dependent will continue to drink despite its negative effect on family, career, and health. The four most common symptoms of alcohol dependence are:

- Cravings
- Loss of control (unable to stop drinking once drinking has begun)
- Physical dependence manifested by nausea, sweating, tremors, and anxiety when alcohol is withdrawn
- Tolerance, manifested by the need for increasing amounts of alcohol in order to feel the effects of alcohol

More expansive definitions of alcohol dependence and abuse have been developed for clinical and research purposes; this criteria is included in volumes such as *Diagnostic and Statistical Manual of Mental Disorders*, fourth edition, published by the American Psychiatric Association, as well as in the *International Classification Diseases*, published by the World Health Organization.

STATISTICS (PREVALENCE AND ETIOLOGY)

The most recent statistics surrounding alcoholism places the lifetime prevalence of the disease in the United States at 20 percent (9.8 million) in men and 8 percent (3.9 million) in women, with a heritability (attribute to both genetic and lifestyle influences) for both sexes at 50–60 percent.[1] Afflicting more than 14 million Americans (1 out of every 13), alcoholism is often associated with several other predisposing disorders such as antisocial personality, depression, anxiety, and tobacco addiction (nearly 80 percent of alcoholics are cigarette smokers). Recent evidence classifies alcoholics into two broad categories: Type 1 alcoholics begin drinking later in life in response to feelings of anxiety, guilt, and avoidance of harm. Type 2 alcoholics are more often men with decreased levels of the neurotransmitter serotonin in their brain and who act impulsively and antisocially.

Recent statistics reveal nearly 20,000 people died from alcohol-induced deaths, excluding motor vehicle fatalities in one year in the United States, 62 percent of 18-year-old and older Americans drank alcohol in the past year, 32 percent of drinkers had five or more drinks on one occasion at least once in the past year, and 61 percent of men 18–24 years and 42 percent of women had five or more drinks on the same occasion.[2] The toll of alcoholism and drunk driving has been well publicized in the last two decades, with social and judicial tolerance decreasing substantially. The disease of alcoholism itself is lesser appreciated; as like many people with varying types of chronic disease, alcoholics are at some point along their disease continuum able to maintain outward appearances of normalcy.

Causes of alcoholism vary between genetic and lifestyle influences. As stated earlier, a large percentage (50–60 percent) of children of alcoholics will be alcohol dependent themselves. Additionally, researchers have been searching for a definitive genetic link that explains the origins of alcoholic behavior. A recent ongoing study, "The Collaborative Study on the Genetics of Alcoholism (COGA)," is searching for the genes that may contribute to alcoholism and some of its related traits (phenotypes) that include depression. The study so far has revealed a positive link between depressive syndrome (depression that may or may not occur in concert with increased alcohol intake) and alcoholic subjects. Further, this study has linked alcohol dependency and depression to specific chromosomal regions, namely on chromosome #1, suggesting that a solitary gene or genes on chromosome #1 may predispose people to depression and/or alcoholism, which may be induced by depression.[3]

Specific nutritional deficiencies have not yet been elucidated in the cause of alcoholism itself. However, the progression of the disease is definitively marked by specific conditions resulting from specific nutrient deficiencies and their effects on the human body. As alcoholism progresses, the brain, liver, gastrointestinal tract, and pancreas are severely affected. Nutrient deficiency in alcoholism is attributed by decreased intake (chronic progressive alcoholics derive more and more calories from alcohol rather than food), reduced storage as a result of decreased food intake and nutrient replacement, and impaired utilization due to the effects of alcohol on the gastrointestinal tract.

BOTANICAL MEDICINES IN THE TREATMENT OF ALCOHOLISM

The effects of botanical medicines on alcoholism are providing interesting results. Several herbs demonstrate a reducing effect on voluntary alcohol intake in animal models of alcoholism, suggesting interesting new forms of therapy for alcoholism, and therefore may also demonstrate a preventative effect in individuals prone to this disease. Among the herbs with these effects are Hypericum perforatum (St. John's Wort), Peuraria lobata (kudzu), *Salvia miltiorrhiza* (Dan Shen), and Tabernanthe iboga (Iboga). Additionally, these plants demonstrate an ability to reduce alcohol absorption from the gastrointestinal tract.[4]

Salvia miltiorrhiza

The use of this herb in reducing alcohol intake in laboratory animals has been demonstrated in several recent studies. *Salvia* is a botanical medicine with a long history of use in China. Administration of a standardized extract of *Salvia* dose dependently delayed alcohol drinking in ethanol-preferring animals and was compensated by increased water intake.[5] Another study demonstrated the ability of the standardized extract of the herb to reduce alcohol intake by 40 percent in animals that were conditioned to prefer alcohol; this effect is attributed to the ability of the extract to alter ethanol absorption from the gastrointestinal tract: 200 milligrams per kilogram of *Salvia miltiorrhiza* decreased blood alcohol levels by up to 60 percent compared to control animals. Furthermore, alcohol-dependent animals dosed with *Salvia* extract were less able to discern the effects of alcohol-laden water from plain water than other animals trained to do so; the authors of the study conclude that the reducing effect of *Salvia miltiorrhiza* extract on ethanol absorption in animals may have caused a decreased perception of the psychoactive effects of ethanol.[6]

Additionally, *Salvia* also demonstrates antirelapse effects.[7] Alcohol-dependent animals demonstrate a transient increased rate of alcohol consumption in comparison to previous levels after a period of deprivation. Considered to model alcohol relapse in human alcoholics, alcohol-dependent animals treated with *Salvia* extract exhibited a complete suppression of extra alcohol consumed following deprivation. Because of these findings, *Salvia* may possess antirelapse properties in addition to its alcohol-curbing properties and may constitute a novel strategy for reducing and controlling alcohol consumption in human alcoholics.

Hypericum Perforatum

Hypericum, also known as St. John's Wort, has been established as an effective treatment for mild to moderate depression. Both depression and alcoholism share similar nuerochemical weaknesses, such as decreased brain serotonin levels. In one study, a standardized extract of St. John's Wort was shown to be significantly effective in decreasing alcohol intake, and these effects did not decrease due to tolerance after consecutive doses.[8] In another experiment, alcohol-preferring animals were given a dry extract of Hypericum and a 30–40 percent reduction in alcohol intake was noted.[9] It was noted in this study that the effects of Hypericum were selective in that food or water intake was unmodified, and further examination revealed that the decreased alcohol-ingesting effects were not attributable to the antidepressant effects of the herb (decreased alcohol consumption was noted after a single administration of the medicine, whereas antidepressant effects were only noted after repeated doses), and the effects were not related to altered pharmacokinetics of alcohol either. Hypericum has been demonstrated repeatedly to inhibit alcohol intake in alcohol-dependent animals, yet a clear mechanism has not been established. Further studies are needed to identify the exact mechanism for St. John's Wort on alcohol intake; however, the existing findings demonstrate St. John's Wort as a potential therapuetic agent in the treatment of alcoholism.

Pueraria Lobata

Kudzu (Pueraria lobata) exerts several profound pharmacological actions including antidipsotropic (antialcohol abuse) activity. Pueraria has a history of use in treating the symptoms of alcohol overdose (hangover), including stomach upset, headache, nausea, vomiting, and dizziness. In traditional Chinese medicine, kudzu was used for managing alcoholism and drunkenness and other disease conditions. An extract of kudzu, known as daidzein, can decrease alcohol consumption and blood-alcohol levels, as well as decrease the duration of alcohol-induced sleep in animal models; and the ability of kudzu to lower blood-alcohol levels is attributed to its ability to delay gastric emptying, slowing the entrance of alcohol into the bloodstream.[10] Other affects of kudzu on the body, which may contribute to its use in treating excessive alcohol intake, include its ability to decrease platelt aggregation; its antioxidant ability; the ability to dilate heart and brain blood vessels, increasing flow to these areas; and increased blood oxygen levels.[11]

An extract of the plant was shown to suppress the alcohol intake of alcohol-dependent animals when given a choice between water and alcohol.[12] Researchers attribute two isoflavone constituents of the plant, daidzin and daidzein, for this action. Additionally, other studies have repeated and confirmed the suppressant effect of this plant on both genetically alcohol-dependent animals and on animals that were trained to crave large amounts of alcohol. Earlier research suspected that daidzin was capable of inhibiting an enzyme known to detoxify alcohol known as aldehyde dehydrogenase. Disulfiram, otherwise known as antabuse, is a pharmaceutical medication used by some patients incapable of stopping alcohol intake that operates on this mechanism. When a person consumes alcohol while taking this medication, only small amounts of alcohol will cause tremendous nausea and physical suffering, acting as a deterrent to continued alcohol intake. However, newer research reveals that inhibition of aldehyde dehydrogenase is not the mechanism that inhibits drinking behavior, and it is suspected that daidzin operates in a different biochemical pathway. Newer research has revealed that daidzin inhibits a second step of a pathway known as MAO/ALDH-2 (monoamine oxidase/aldehyde dehyrdogenase-2), a pathway of alcohol detoxification in the body, leading to its suppressive effect on alcohol-craving animals.[13]

Tabernanthe Iboga (Iboga)

Native to Africa, Iboga has been used ceremonially as a hallucinogen. A powerful medicinal plant, Iboga has several pharmacological effects that have led it to be employed in the use of breaking addictive cycles, including tobacco and alcohol addiction. An extract of this plant (Ibogaine) can cause stimulation of the brain (central nervous system) ranging from mild excitation to euphoria and hallucinations.[14] Additionally, iboaine exerts serotonergic effects, meaning that it can mimic the effects of this neurotransmitter, which is often found in low amounts in alcoholics. Animal studies have shown that these effects may exert some value in the treatment of human addiction, including alcoholism.[15] Ibogaine administered to animals exerts short-lived decreases in alcohol intake, and it is suspected that longer term effects may be mediated over long-term treatment periods with this plant extract as the extract is stored in fatty tissues, allowing for a sort of time release effect.[16] Iboga and its constituent iboaine have been used successfully in breaking cycles of addiction; further studies of the plant medicine may reveal greater understanding of its use in breaking alcohol dependency.

NUTRIENTS AND ALCOHOLISM

Thaimine

The most well-known vitamin deficiency associated with alcoholism is that of thiamine (B-1) deficiency. Classically, long-term deprivation of this vitamin leads to Wernicke-Korsakoff syndrome and features neurologic symptoms such as confusion, memory loss, impaired movements, and peripheral neuropathy. Wernicke-Korsakoff syndrome is actually two disorders that can occur independently or together. Wernicke's disease involves damage to the central and peripheral nervous systems, and can include alcohol withdrawal symptoms.

Korsakoff syndrome involves impairment of memory and intellectual skills. The most distinctive symptom is confabulation, or fabrication of facts as the person tries to fill in gaps in memory when recounting experiences. Depending on time of treatment and how long the patient has been deprived of thiamine, this condition may or may not be reversible. Treatment of this condition involves the administration of thiamine intravenously and in repeated doses over a period of days to weeks.

Zinc

Zinc is required for several biological functions including DNA synthesis, cell division, and expression of genes. Additionally, zinc is required for the functioning of numerous enzymes in biologic systems and immune system function. Alcoholism is a predisposing factor for zinc deficiency due to the effects of alcohol on nutrient absorption. Zinc can positively affect the metabolism of alcohol in the body and can reinforce the functioning of both stomach and liver alcohol dehydrogenase enzymes.[17] These effects can lead to increased metabolism of alcohol in the body, thereby negating some of its negative side effects, especially in the liver and brain.

The development of alcohol dependence is accompanied by a decrease in zinc content in an area of the brain known as the hippocampus, and supplementation of zinc may prevent this deficiency.[18] In another interesting study demonstrating the importance of zinc and alcoholism, alcohol-dependent animals were shown to have deficient zinc brain levels, and when supplemented with zinc, alcohol consumption was reduced.[19] These studies demonstrate a link between zinc and healthy brain functioning; supplementation of zinc in chronic alcoholics may serve to improve treatment and prevent some negative long-term effects of deficiency.

Niacin

Deficiency of niacin (vitamin B-3) is known to occur in alcoholics as well. Frank deficiency of niacin leads to a disease known as pellagra. Pellagra leads to the triad: dermatitis, diarrhea, and dementia, eventually followed by death; skin changes are characteristic and define the condition by themselves. Often masked by other alcohol-related nutritional deficiencies, pellagra can coexist with other vitamin deficiency diseases in chronic alcoholics. Because of this, supplementation with a multivitamin and mineral is imperative in the treatment of chronic alcoholic disease, although pellagra by itself is responsive to niacin therapy.

Considered a mainly psychiatric disease, the known familial and genetic influences on this disease have become increasingly well defined. Indeed, the adage that genetics may load the gun, but diet and lifestyle pull the trigger rings true when it comes to alcoholism. Not everyone with a family history of alcoholism becomes an alcoholic. Nutritional, botanical, and lifestyle can all help ward off the consequences of alcoholism. A preemptive strategy for individuals with family histories of alcohol abuse should at a very young age (at least age 12) take a multivitamin that has abundant sources of chromium and zinc in balance with other nutrients. Taking these nutrients in the form of a high-quality multivitamin is better than individual dosing, since these and most nutrients are dependent on the synergy of other vitamins and minerals. Another important consideration is to look for early signs of hypoglycemia that clinically appear to present in some, but not all, alcoholics. Thus the presentation of fluctuations of blood sugar after eating or if a meal is missed may be a warning sign indicating that working with a nutritionally oriented physician could be helpful.

BOTANICALS*

- Hypericum perforatum (St. John's Wort)
  300 milligrams (standardized to 0.3 percent hypericin or 4 percent hyperforin content), three times daily
- Pueraria lobata (Kudzu)
  1,500 milligrams root extract, twice daily
- *Salvia miltiorrhiza* (Dan Shen)
  2,000–3,000 milligrams, twice daily
- Tabernanthe iboga (Iboga)

The standardized extract Ibogaine is efficacious at 200–300 milligrams twice daily. However, this herb is hallucinogenic and should only be used under close medical supervision.

NUTRIENTS**

- B-1 (Thiamine)
  Doses of 5 to 300 milligrams have been used depending on state of deficiency. A good starting dose is 10 milligrams twice per day.
- B-3 (Niacin)
  100 milligrams three times per day
- Chromium
  200 micrograms twice per day
- Zinc
  40 milligrams per day, divided doses with food

*It is important to consume these doses with a multivitamin/mineral supplement, as many nutrients are dependent on each other for proper assimilation and physiologic synergy.

**All herbs should be taken in capsule or tablet form or as a tea; liquid extracts should be avoided due to potential alcohol content that can be as high as 50 percent (100 proof).

Alzheimer's Disease

Alzheimer's disease (AD) is a progressive degenerative disease of the brain and is the most common form of dementia among older people. Typically, it affects the part of the brain that controls thoughts, memory, and language skills. Alzheimer's disease is physically manifested inside the brain by amyloid plaques and tangled neuronal fibers that replace normal brain cell organization. Additionally, nerve cells die in vital areas of the brain responsible for memory and other cognitive abilities, and some brain chemicals responsible for cell-to-cell communication are found in lower levels, disrupting the thinking process. At this point in time, no definitive cause or cure is known for Alzheimer's disease; rather there are probably numerous causes that affect each person differently. The diagnosis of AD is made on a presumptive basis; after interviewing and testing a patient, and speaking with the people with whom the patient is closest, a probable diagnosis can be made. However, a definitive diagnosis cannot be positively established until an autopsy is performed, when a pathologist can confirm the existence of the previously mentioned anatomical changes (neurofibrillary tangles and plaques). The clinical course of AD is fairly well established at this point in time; mortality rates increase with greater levels of cognitive disabilities.

It is estimated that approximately 4.5 million Americans have Alzheimer's disease. Symptoms typically begin after the age of 60, although rarely younger people can also develop Alzheimer's disease. Close to 5 percent of men and women ages 65 to 74 have Alzheimer's disease, and the numbers increase to nearly 50 percent in those age 85 and older; the number of people in this age group will grow to 8.5 million by 2030. Despite these numbers, it is important to note that Alzheimer's disease is not a normal part of aging; rather it is a disease process related to the continuous effects of external and internal events in the environment and body. At the current rate of disease incidence, 14 million Americans will have AD in the next 50 years. From the time of initial symptom presentation, a person with AD will live an average of eight years; however, some will live up to 20 years with AD. In the United States, $100 billion is spent on AD; the majority of health insurance plans, including Medicare, do not cover the long-term care that many AD patients require. Perhaps related to this, 70 percent of people with AD live at home, and immediate family and friends provide nearly 75 percent of their care. The rest of the care provided for AD patients costs an average of $12,500 per year per family, which is paid almost entirely out of pocket. For families who have the means to provide nursing home care, the average cost for this is $42,000 per year and can cost up to $70,000 in some parts of the country. Average lifetime cost per AD patient is $174,000; AD is ranked as the third most costly disease to have, after heart disease and cancer. Finding a cure for AD is costly as well; the U.S. government spent close to $349.2 million for Alzheimer's disease research in 1998 alone.[1]

In addition to these costs, it is widely stated that there are always two patients in AD, the person with AD and his or her caregiver, often a spouse. Caregivers bear a huge burden in caring for the person with AD; large amounts of physical, emotional, and financial stress are often the result. Support is crucial for the caregiver in these situations; caring for a patient with AD has been compared to caring for an infant, a task that is not commonly endured by most seniors. Depression is quite common in caregivers of AD patients, as well in the patients themselves.[2]

ETIOLOGY

Although a complete understanding of the origins of AD are not firmly established at this time, conclusions can be drawn from epidemiologic studies (studies of specific populations of people) hinting at possible disease initiators. Presently, four specific risk factors for AD have been identified: increasing age, familial clustering of the disease, the presence of the apolipoprotein E variation, (epsilon 4 allele), and Down's syndrome (a type of mental retardation). The following are associations that have been fairly well established, although not all of them hold true in every population study. For instance, more women suffer from AD than men; people with lower levels of education have more AD; history of depression and past head injury are risk factors; and aluminum exposure (occupational and food/waterborne sources) add excess risk, as do high blood pressure and other vascular diseases. Aluminum exposure is a particularly troubling association, especially because, as Americans consume more and more soda out of aluminum cans (despite their being "sealed" on the inside), our exposure to aluminum continues to increase. Also, the popular fad of using aluminum foil on the barbecue grill and in the oven add extra risk as well. Population studies have also revealed protective factors for AD as well, including: estrogen use by postmenopausal women; use of nonsteroidal antiinflammatory drugs in arthritis;

exercise and active lifestyles; moderate amounts of red wine; and a diet high in vitamins B-6, B-12, and folate.[3] The use of lifestyle and nutritional therapies as preventative medicines will be covered in greater detail later in this chapter.

GENES

Family history is an important factor in the development of Alzheimer's disease. Familial Alzheimer's occurs in much younger people (age 30 to 60) and is inherited through genetic transmission. The more common form of Alzheimer's disease is known as late-onset and displays no obvious inheritable pattern; not everyone with a family history of AD will end up getting the disease. So far, the only identifiable genetic risk factor in the development of AD is a gene that produces a variation in a common protein that all people manufacture. This protein, known as apolipoprotein E (apoE), is produced under normal circumstances and serves the function of transporting cholesterol in the blood stream. The variant version of this gene has been found in people with AD. Much needs to be learned about Alzheimer's disease in addition to genetic causes. Increasing evidence is mounting in discovering the factors that precipitate the disease and factors that may provide some type of relief for disease symptoms.

DIET

Recent research findings suggest a probable role of the diet in age-related cognitive decline and dementia, including Alzheimer's disease. Senior populations consuming a diet high in monounsaturated fatty acids (Mediterranean diet) display protection against age-related cognitive decline, whereas fish consumption and fortified cereals seem to reduce the prevalence of AD in Europe and North America. In addition, aluminum consumption, whether in foods or water, may increase the risk of developing AD, and deficiencies of the vitamins B-6, B-12, E, C, and folate can negatively affect memory capability and cognitive decline. These findings demonstrate that the use of antioxidants and dietary macronutrients in the form of beneficial fatty acids and grains may act as preventative factors in the development of dementia and other conditions of cognitive decline.[4]

AD is becoming more common in Western societies due to both longer life and most probably increasing incidence. There are numerous hints that AD may be linked to the typical Western diet (characterized by excessive intakes of sugar, refined carbohydrates with a high glycemic index, high saturated fats, and decreased consumption of unrefined seeds, nuts, and vegetables, with high amounts of fiber, vitamins, and antioxidants) as well as seafood (containing omega-3 fatty acids).[5] Because it is has been hypothesized that AD may be promoted by the side effects of the aforementioned dietary trends, it stands to reason that this disease may be prevented or attenuated by adhering to simple dietary measures with effects that include increasing insulin sensitivity (by decreasing refined sugars and saturated fats), improving the intake ratio of omega-3 to omega-6 fatty acids (by increasing fish and seed oil consumption), and by increasing intake of antioxidants such as folic acid, vitamins B-6 and B-12, and flavonoid food compounds. Currently, studies are underway to determine the effects of such preventive measures.

HOMOCYSTEINE

Homocysteine is an amino acid metabolite of another vital amino acid in the body, methionine. Homocysteine is produced through a process in which methionine donates a part of its chemical structure to other metabolic reactions in the body; the end result produces homocysteine. Homocysteine does have uses in the body; however, large amounts of research now implicate this amino acid as a critical risk factor in the pathogenesis of both heart disease and AD. Additionally, it is also well known that the vitamins B-12 and folate directly reduce levels of homocysteine in the blood, and lower levels of homocysteine are related to decreased amounts of cardiovascular disease. New research now implicates homocysteine in the development of cognitive function decline, including age-related memory loss and AD. When present in large amounts, homocysteine is known to inflict vascular damage throughout the body, including the blood vessels in the brain. This amino acid causes vascular damage that compromises brain functioning, leading to areas of damaged brain (infarcts) and resultant dementia. Elevated levels of homocysteine (hyperhomocysteinemia) have been shown to be an independent risk factor for cognitive decline, and a correlation exists between hyperhomocysteinemia and AD, including low levels of folate and the vitamins B-6 and B-12.[6] More recently, Seshadri and colleagues have shown hyperhomocysteinemia to be a significant, independent risk factor for dementia and AD; they found a graduated increase in risk of both dementia and AD that directly correlated with homocysteine concentration after controlling for established AD risk factors.[7]

Additionally, these researchers noted that homocysteine levels decreased in conjunction with increased B vitamin levels, leading to the hypothesis that dementia and AD may possibly be circumvented by an alteration in dietary habits that include fortification and or consumption of B vitamins in greater amounts.

ANTIOXIDANTS

The oxidative process, evidenced by protein, lipid, and DNA oxidation, plays a major role in the initiation and propagation of several human disease conditions, including AD.[8] Reactive oxygen species (ROS; otherwise known as free radicals) extol neurologic damage via direct oxidative destruction or through secondary events that initiate programmed cell death (apoptosis). Excessive production of ROS is known to contribute to degenerative brain conditions, propagating several detrimental effects on the brain tissue. Experimental evidence demonstrates a neuroprotective role of direct application of antioxidants, and studies are underway to establish antioxidant compounds as clinically protective agents.[9]

Measurements of lipid and protein oxidative processes along with total antioxidative capacity have been taken from patients with both the familial and late-onset forms of AD, as well as from similarly aged healthy control subjects. Samples from the AD patients exhibited a profound increase in biologic products of pro-oxidative processes, whereas the antioxidant potential of these same samples were lower than those of the control subjects. Additionally, when intentionally exposed to oxidative agents, the cellular samples of the familial AD patients exhibited greater oxidative damage than those from controls. These results demonstrate the role of oxidation as a significant early event in the development of AD.[10]

New evidence continues to mount in the role of oxidation and the development of AD; some of this evidence points to oxidative damage prior to the formation of both beta-amyloid-containing plaques and neurofibrillary tangles (disease-defining physical signs in the brain tissue). In a review of studies that explored the use of antioxidants as a preventative medicine in AD, a positive relationship has been identified between dietary intake of antioxidants and a decreased association with AD.[11] Such evidence is highly suggestive of the possibility of using antioxidants as an early preventative and treatment strategy in AD. At this time, studies have not established a directly measurable answer that antioxidants can completely protect against AD. Because of the multifactorial contributions to the development of this disease, and the evidence provided so far detailing the link between oxidative damage and AD, it is highly suggested that antioxidant therapy be considered among the key treatment and prevention strategies for AD.

STANDARD MEDICATIONS AND AD

At this time, AD is considered largely a disease caused by numerous insults. Current drug therapy has not proven to be successful in the treatment of AD; it aims to control symptoms of the disease, rather than prevent it. However, newer therapies are being directed at manipulation of the development of aberrant proteins that appear in people with AD. Standard therapy primarily involves the use of drugs known as acetycholinesterase inhibitors that allow the neurotransmitter acetylcholine to stay present in the brain for longer periods of time, producing a stronger effect. Only used in mild to moderate AD, patients with advanced disease are not as readily helped. Treatment for dementia is mainly focused on attempts at preserving and or improving the patients and their family's quality of life; this includes treatment of the concomitant medical and emotional issues facing these patients and their family.

BOTANICAL MEDICINES AND ALZHEIMER'S DISEASE

The use of botanical medicines in AD is providing new therapies that are comparable to some standard pharmaceutical medications, but without the side effects. Botanical medicines including Ginkgo biloba, Rosmarinus officinalis, Salvia officinalis (sage), and Melissa officinalis (balm) have positive effects on the clinical course of AD and have been scrutinized in modern efficacy studies.

Ginkgo biloba

Ginkgo is perhaps best known for its memory-enhancing qualities in healthy people. These effects carry over into AD, a disease with obvious severe memory impairment. The active constituents of ginkgo, known as ginkgolides, have antioxidant, neuroprotective, and cholinergic activities that are relevant to the disease mechanisms in AD. The therapuetic efficacy of standardized ginkgo extracts in comparison to placebo is similar to the most currently prescribed cholinesterase inhibitors pharmaceuticals including tacrine, donepezil, rivastigmine, and metrifonate and has few if any side effects.[12] Because of ginkgo's effectiveness at treating dementia, it is registered as a drug of choice for treating AD in Europe.[13] Ginkgo has been shown to have similar pharmacologic effect and clinical efficacy to prescription medications used to treat reduced cerebral performance. The principal actions of ginkgo include improved blood flow properties; protective effects against ischemia and hypoxia in the brain; improvements in nerve cell energy metabolism, antiswelling and myelin (the insulating layer surrounding nerve cells that allows for nerve transmission) protecting effects; and antioxidant and free radical scavenging activity, as well as nonspecific effects on neurotransmitters and their receptors.[14] Furthermore, clinical trails have demonstrated the beneficial effects of ginkgo on cognitive performance, global functioning, and activities of daily living.

The most recent evidence for the effectiveness of ginkgo extract indicates a protective effect against neuronal damage from several sources; however, the exact cellular and molecular mechanisms of action are unknown at this time. In experimental cell lines that produce AD-causing amyloid-beta neurofibrillary tangles (a key diagnostic finding in AD), formation of the tangles was inhibited along with cell-specific self-destruction (apoptosis), prompting investigators to conclude that prevention of apoptosis and inhibition of amyloid-beta accumulation underscore the neuroprotective effects of Ginkgo biloba.[15]

When combined with the phospholipid molecule phosphatidylcholine, ginkgo is better absorbed by the tissues in which it has an affect. Phosphatidylcholine acts as a "waterproof" carrier of the herb, assisting its delivery to the brain tissues and resulting in greater efficacy of the herb.

Rosmarinus officinalis

This herb is often listed among herbal treatment recommendations for AD and dementia. Similar to ginkgo, rosemary purportedly improves blood flow to certain areas of the body and has been used historically as an aid for improving cerebral function, specifically with memory loss and dementia. Rosemary posses fairly strong antioxidant capacity,[16] and therefore may be useful in the treatment and prevention of AD. More research is needed exploring the use of this herb and its applications in AD. The German Commission E monograph suggests a dose of 4–6 grams (3/4 to 1 1/4 teaspoons) of rosemary leaf per day.[17] This amount can be incorporated into a tea taken several times a day. No known drug-rosemary interactions are recognized, and no negative side effects are associated with moderate use of the above dose. Large amounts should be avoided in pregnant women, as the oil contained in the leaf may act to disrupt preganancy.[18]

Salvia officinalis (Sage) and Melissa officinalis (Balm)

Historic medical reference books from Europe document the effects and use of the herbs sage and balm as having memory-enhancing properties and were used for this purpose among others. Interestingly, modern discoveries of clinically relevant pharmacologic actions in plant medicines with historic applications have revealed strong links tying historic use with modern scientific explanations. It has been revealed that sage and balm both exhibit cholinergic activities, meaning they have similar effects to the neurotransmitter acetylcholine (specific neurons that utilize this neurotransmitter degenerate in AD—thus the use of cholinergic pharmaceuticals).

The use of Melissa officinalis in treating the symptoms of mild to moderate AD was recently shown to produce a "significantly better" outcome in alleviating AD symptoms when compared to a placebo medication.[19] Additionally, the AD patients treated with Melissa exhibited less agitation, a common occurrence in people with AD. The treatment dose in this study was only 60 drops a day of extract. Both behavior and psychological symptoms can be extremely problematic in this population of patients, and management is difficult for both the patient and caregiver. Another study using an essential oil derived from Melissa was tested to determine its use in alleviating symptoms of agitation in patients with advanced cognitive impairment and AD. In this study, the oil of balm was incorporated into lotions that were applied to the patient's face and arms twice a day for four weeks, and its effects were compared to a placebo oil-lotion base. Sixty percent of the treatment group experienced a reduction of roughly 30 percent in agitation symptoms as determined by the Cohen-Mansfield Agitation Inventory (CMAI) and quality of life indices (percentage of time spent socially withdrawn and percentage of time engaged in constructive activities, measured with Dementia Care Mapping).[20]

Salvia officinalis, more popularly known as sage, has been tested in studies to determine its effectiveness in treating AD symptoms. These studies were based on the knowledge of the cholinergic binding properties of sage as well as its betterment of mood and cognitive performance in humans. One study used a dose of 60 drops sage extract in patients with mild to moderate AD over four months. According the researchers, the herb created a "significant better outcome" on cognitive function when compared to placebo, and patients taking the active medicine exhibited less agitation than those taking placebo.[21] The use of sage as a medication in AD is supported by further research; extracts of sage have been shown to possess cholinergic (via anticholinesterase), antioxidant, anti-inflammatory, and sedative effects, all of which are clinically relevant in the treatment of AD.[22] *Salvia* can reduce the neuropsychiatric symptoms experienced by people suffering from AD, making the use of this herb a suitable choice in the treatment of AD.

Acetyl-L-carnitine

This nutrient has been shown to be helpful in some aspects of AD as well. Acetyl-L-carnitine (Alc) occurs naturally in the body and is somewhat structurally related to acetylcholine, the neurotransmitter and may contribute toward its formation.[23] Taken as a supplement, Alc is useful in AD, age-related memory deficits, and senile depression. On the cellular level, Alc assists in transporting acetyl groups (portions of fatty acid molecules) into the power generator (mitochondria) of the cell and promotes the manufacture and release of acetylcholine.[24] This is important in AD because part of the disease process involves loss of the neurons that respond to the acetylcholine neurotransmitter, and acetylcholine in the brain is easily depleted.[25] Used therapeutically, Alc has demonstrated neuroprotective actions, improves neurotransmitter pathways, enhances synthesis of acetylcholine, enhances synaptic transmission, and increases blood flow to the brain in people with cerebrovascular disease.[26]

OTHER INFORMATION FOR PREDICTION

Prediction of disease is becoming more and more of a focus in medicine today using the best of technology. However, one interesting aspect of AD is that one's fingerprints may yield relatively significant information about their risk of developing AD. There are several types of fingerprint patterns that all humans share; this does not mean that they are all alike, but rather that we all share certain fingerprint features (so much so that each pattern has a name) much like we all have two eyes, yet none are alike. The frequency of the major fingerprint patterns (ulnar loops, radial loops, arches, and whorls) was studied in a group of men with early and late-onset degenerative dementia in comparison to healthy control subjects.[27] The people with early onset disease had a significantly larger amount of ulnar loops than the late-onset and control groups. Similar findings have been discovered in similar studies,[28] indicating that there is a deeper biologic basis for the occurrence of early onset dementia. In this type of disease occurrence, it is noted that these people are "prone" to getting the disease. Predicting the possibility of disease occurrence may be possible utilizing fingerprint analysis. More studies are needed to absolutely correlate these finding with early onset disease, however.

CONCLUSION

Treatment of AD and its symptoms is a challenge. Standard medications offer some relief of symptoms; however, these medications are not free from side effects, and almost more importantly, few if any medical treatments are geared toward preventing AD prior to the appearance of symptoms. New research is exploring gene alteration and reversal of the pathologic disease changes in the brain; however, a greater emphasis must be placed on preventing this disease through the use of nutritional and herbal medications, the most promising of which have been reviewed in this chapter. As medical science continues to learn more about the disease process involved, greater emphasis will be placed on preventing the organ damage that serves as a precursor to Alzheimer's disease.

Alzheimer's by some patients is feared even more than heart disease or cancer, for the concept of being trapped within one's body without the according mental connectivity with the outside world is terrifying. There are now medications that can assist many patients in their battle with this dreaded condition. Likewise aggressive and consistent use of select natural medicines can augment brain function by supporting normal biochemical pathways.

NUTRIENTS

- Dietary
  The anti-AD diet should include healthy portions of complex carbohydrates in the form of fruits and vegetables, grains, nuts, and seeds, as well as essential fatty acid-rich sources such as cold-water fish and seed oils (flax, borage)
- Multivitamin/mineral
  Two tablets, twice per day with food or as directed
- Antioxidants
  A rich antioxidant supplement should be taken twice per day

BOTANICALS

- Ginkgo
  60 milligrams twice per day (24% standardized)
- Rosemary
  Crude herb (leaf): 1–2 grams in a tea twice per day

Liquid extract (1:1 in 45 percent alcohol) 2–4 milliliters three times per day
- *Salvia officinalis* (sage)
  1–2 grams twice per day
- *Melissa officinalis* (balm)
  Liquid extract (1:1 in 45 percent alcohol) twice per day

Anorexia

Anorexia nervosa (AN) is a severe psychiatric disorder characterized by a combination of abnormal eating behavior and weight regulation with disturbances of attitudes toward body weight and shape. It is a condition worthy of great respect and, if not treated properly by skilled specialized healthcare providers, can lead to death or serious lifelong consequences. Anorexia nervosa has been defined as the relentless pursuit of a thin physique, in which a person does not maintain normal body weight that is appropriate for his or her age and weight. Often, people with anorexia weigh 85 percent or less of the norm for their height and age group. These people are terrified of becoming fat, continuously deny the dangers of their own low weight, and will feel as if they are overweight despite their thinness. Additional symptoms include depression, social withdrawal, irritability, and sometimes compulsive food habits and rituals. Some people may experience problems such as assumption of adolescent roles or fears of adult responsibilities and have ineffective coping skills with life problems.

Estimates of the prevalence of these disease range from 0.5 percent to 2 percent of the female adolescent population with an average age of onset between 14 and 18 years. Another way of looking at these numbers reveals that approximately 1 percent of all female adolescents have anorexia nervosa. However, it must be recognized that accurate data is difficult to obtain due to the secretive nature of the disorder and the fact that a large majority of those affected do not seek treatment. The large majority of the populations suffering from anorexia nervosa are adolescents, although this disease can affect young adults and other age groups. Anorexia nervosa is uncommon among males; however, it is estimated that 5–10 percent of diagnosed cases are males younger than 14 years of age. In older adolescents, however, 10–30 percent of those with anorexia are males.

Among the diagnostic criteria are a refusal to maintain body weight at or above a minimally normal weight for age and height (less than 85 percent of expected weight); an intense fear of gaining weight; a disturbed view of one's physical status; denial of the danger associated with low weight; and, in menstruating females, the absence of at least three consecutive menstrual cycles (amenorrhea). In addition, a full physical exam is required to rule out other physical disorders manifested by mental states, and a full diagnostic interview performed by a licensed mental health professional must be made before an official diagnosis can be made.

There is no solitary cause of eating disorders such as anorexia. Causes are multifactorial and may vary from person to person. Despite the difficulty in isolating the exact causes of anorexia, research is discovering pertinent information relating to biologic, societal-cultural, and psychological factors. Biologically related issues include genetic influences that predispose certain people to different types of behaviors that may lead to the development of eating disorders. There is a large body of research pointing to this possibility. Twin studies (studies of twins and their health) and family studies indicated that sisters of anorexics have a higher incidence of anorexia than those in the general population, and twin studies demonstrate a similar pattern, with even higher concordant rates.

In fact, one study estimated the influence of heritability, or the influence that genes have on physical manifestations of a particular disease or condition, of anorexia nervosa as 50–80 percent.[1] A search for a definitive gene or gene mutation as the cause of anorexia has been unrewarding, despite the strong familial link that exists. Researchers are in agreement that further large-scale prospective (will an anorexic woman more often have anorexic children than a nonanorexic woman?) and adoption (is anorexia related to family dynamics?) studies are needed. A better understanding of the heritability of anorexia will, of course, allow for greater understanding of its causes and therefore better treatment and preventions.

Similar to other psychiatric conditions, hormones play an important role. Some older research defined a link between anorexia and hormonal dysregulation, specifically in the hypothalamus and pituitary gland. Not definitely linked as causes of anorexia, perturbations in hormone levels are the result of chronic and recurrent starvation. Loss of adipose (fat) tissue and starvation has an effect on mental states, producing anxiety, depression, and personality changes.[2] Another aspect of anorexia nervosa may be anorexia athletica, or compulsive exercise. Intense and excessive exercise will produce endorphins, the opioid-like brain chemical that allows us to feel good and masks pain. Coupled with muscle breakdown (starvation causes the muscles to be broken down for fuel) from starvation and intense exercise, this phenomenon may produce a high feeling, creating another addictive component in the already addictive pattern.

Another component of anorexia nervosa includes sociocultural effects. A commonly discussed problem is the image of women that is projected in popular media, which portray a body image that is difficult for the large majority of women to obtain. Anorexia and eating disorders are more common in the in-dustrialized countries, although as other countries in the world become more modernized, their rates of anorexia also increase. It is thought that anorexics are sensitive to disapproval and approval, and the media is often blamed for pro-jecting that self-worth is to be equated with a lean physique. Indeed a powerful effector, media and its many outlets may very well play a role in the develop-ment of eating disorders in all age groups, particularly adolescents, the most impressionable of all age groups. Anorexia nervosa is supported by an interest-ing paradox in that incredible amounts of food are widely available and much of modern life is centered on obtaining and consuming "fun" and "extreme" foods, yet a slender physique is highly praised throughout the popular media. As for male anorexics, an emphasis on a muscular build leads to fanatical attempts to build a similar physique that leads young men to exercise to the point of physi-cal exhaustion.

Psychological states play a large role in the etiology of anorexia, and the de-velopment of psychological factors are often linked to familial status, wherein both influence each other. The interaction of anorexic behavior and family en-vironment are intertwined, and factors such as family dysfunction, sexual abuse, excessively strict parenting, and self-esteem issues are often linked to anorexic behaviors. People with anorexia exhibit low self-esteem, inadequacy, fear of grow-ing up, poor conflict resolution, and separation issues from parents. Families with anorexics have been described as too closely intertwined, and overprotective; often there are issues between the two parents and triangulation is a common occurrence. This is not to say that the problem is the fault of the parents, yet the proverbial straw that breaks the camel's back may be, in part, due to family dynamics.

The consideration of all factors in the development of anorexia nervosa must be considered when attempts at prevention and treatment are being made. Socio-cultural and psychological origins may at first look to be more difficult to treat than biological factors; however, by acknowledging the role of biology and the effects that a well-nurtured organism has on psychologic outcomes and responses to sociocultural influences, one may be better equipped to deal with and respond to these external influences. Because all factors are interrelated, considering individual biology is the first place to begin treating and preventing anorexia nervosa.

NUTRITIONAL FACTORS

A large area of research into nutritional causes of anorexia has been dedicated to the effects of the mineral zinc and its role in the development of anorexia and other eating disorders. Although many anorexics exhibit the signs and symp-toms of zinc deficiency (loss of appetite, dermatitis, depression, diarrhea, and weight loss), it is difficult to postulate whether a deficiency in zinc leads to more intense manifestations of the disease or whether progression of the disease and resultant malnutrition causes zinc deficiency, manifesting these symptoms. However, as it is true for many diseases, causes and symptoms are often difficult to separate into definitive categories of cause and effect. The premise of this book is to provide the facts and research demonstrating that proper health factors (nutrition) allow the body and brain to function correctly, negating the development of diseases. Therefore, it is logical to reason that a person with suboptimal levels of nutritional factors may be biologically prone, or more susceptible, to a condition when deprived of adequate resources. The role of zinc and its effects on proper biologic functioning has been revealed in a number of areas pertaining to the development and treatment of anorexia.

Clinical effects of suboptimal zinc levels include emotional disorders, weight loss, and biochemical and hormonal endocrine organ function (production of estrogen, thymopoietin, and prolactin), all of which are observed in anorexics and those with other eating disorders.[3] Several studies involving zinc supplementation and weight gain have provided interesting results in this area. These studies were designed to explore the relationship between zinc supplementation and weight gain in anorexic females, as measured by rate of increase of the body mass index (BMI), which is a measurement derived by calculating a person's height and weight to determine appropriate weight. When anorexics were supplemented with 100 milligrams of zinc until they acquired a 10 percent increase in BMI, the rate of weight gain was twice that of anorexics who were not treated in this particular study.[4] In another study utilizing 50 milligrams of zinc one time per day, 17 of the 20 women participants were able to increase their weight by 15 percent, one patient increased her weight by 57 percent in two years, and another had an increase of 24 percent in only three months.[5] Additionally, after starting on the zinc therapy, no weight loss was recorded in any of the patients.

In addition to assisting with weight gain and preventing weight loss, zinc plays an important role in treating some of the psychological aspects of anorexia nervosa. After comparing mean urinary zinc excretion in a group of female adolescents with anorexia compared to a group of nonanorexics, it was concluded in one study that the zinc status of these patients was compromised due to inadequate intake of zinc.[6] The patients were treated with 50 milligrams of zinc for six months; after which they exhibited decreased levels of depression and anxiety (assessed by the Zung Depression Scale and the State-Trait Anxiety Inventory), leading researchers to suggest that anorexics with low levels of zinc may benefit from zinc supplementation. In addition, these women also experienced gains in height and weight, clearing of skin abnormalities, improved taste, and acceleration of sexual maturation in comparison to controls not treated with zinc. The outcomes from this study underlie the premise that fueling the body correctly with the appropriate nutrients assists the mind in functioning at optimal levels. Many other examples of mood and nutritional supplementation exist in the literature that will be highlighted in subsequent chapters.

In addition to zinc deficiency and its benefits on weight and mood, other vitamins play an important role as well. Calcium, magnesium, vitamin D, vitamin B-1 (thiamine), vitamin B-12, folate, and copper, as well as essential fatty acid deficiencies have been reported in women with anorexia symptoms.[7] A stark example of the effects of generalized vitamin supplementation was recently outlined in a study in which women with mild to moderate symptoms of depression who were not taking any other medications were instructed to take a multivitamin and mineral and to walk outdoors at a level of 60 percent of maximum heart rate. In comparison to the control/placebo group, the women on the multivitamin regimen experienced improvement in their overall mood, self-esteem, and general sense of well-being, and they experienced decreased depressive symptoms.[8]

Essential fatty acid status is, of course, greatly altered in anorexics, following a period of food restriction. A study that examined the levels of essential fatty acids in anorexics revealed fatty acid deficiencies that were different from those seen in simple fatty acid deficiencies as well as that of chronic malnutrition. Researchers noted significant changes in the structure of the fatty acids present in anorexics, implying that this was the effect of the body synthesizing its own type of replacement fatty acid, which did not appear to be a suitable alternative to the typical fatty acid found in cellular membranes, allowing for their normally optimal fluidlike function.[9] The significance of these altered fatty acids is a decrease in membrane fluidity (a physiologic state that allows for greater communication between cells throughout the body). Decreased levels of essential fatty acids have numerous health implications and have been associated with conditions such as coronary artery disease, depression, cancer, arthritis, Crohn's disease, ulcerative colitis, and lupus.[10] Another group of researchers has advanced the theory that inappropriate utilization and deficiency of essential fatty acids may precipitate anorexia nervosa.[11] Combined with metabolic abnormalities of hormone systems, a cascade of irregularities (which are far beyond the scope of this chapter) of fatty acid metabolism culminates in an impairment of the endocrine system causing sensations of fullness (satiety) and alterations in body image perception by the individual affected. New theories that provide a role for nutritional factors in the development of diseases such as anorexia provide greater insight into the treatment and prevention of these diseases with proper use of nutritional cofactors.

CONCLUSION

Nutrition can play an important role in the prevention of symptoms of depression, especially in those prone to these feelings. By supplementing the brain with adequate levels of nutritional cofactors, one may prevent metabolic dysregulation that so often accompanies anorexia nervosa and other eating disorders. Nutritional deficiencies may contribute to the cycle of decreased nutritional status followed by less-than-optimal neurologic and physiologic functions, driving the symptoms of this disease. Anorexia nervosa is a complex disease with many contributing factors that all may have beginnings in less-than-adequate nutrition. One of the chief initial occurrences in this disease is a decrease in food intake. Diets in the United States, and for that matter the rest of the modernized world, do not provide optimal amounts of the vitamins, minerals, and trace mineral cofactors that play vital roles in hormonal regulation and carbohydrate and protein metabolism. When a person with anorexia begins to decrease their food intake, they may be propagating the symptoms of this disease by further tipping the scales in favor of nutrient deficiency.

We live in a society that sends so many cues to our children via advertising, with print and nonprint marketing both reflecting overly thin models, that for those who biochemically predisposed to undereating, the maladies of anorexia are all too often triggered to manifest. Indeed, if as a society we are to curb such unnecessary health trials, we must be more careful in our selection of our models who end up being role models for mind, body, and spirit.

NUTRIENTS

- Zinc
  50 milligrams per day
- Calcium
  500 milligrams per day
- Magnesium
  300–400 milligrams per day
- Vitamin D
  400 International Units per day
- B-1
  20–30 milligrams per day
- B-12
  1,000 micrograms per day
- Folate
  1–2 milligrams per day
- Copper
  1–2 milligrams per day
- Essential Fatty Acids
  2–3 grams per day

Anxiety

Anxiety seems to becoming more and more prevalent today. Anxiety has become a permanent fixture in many people's lives, affecting not only the mind, but also the body and day-to-day living as well. This chapter will address anxiety not only in the sense of an officially diagnosed psychological disorder, but also as a generalized state that so many people find themselves in from a variety of causes. Anxiety can be defined in two different ways: the first defines anxiety as an apprehensive, uneasy state of mind, typically due to an anticipated event (i.e., life stressors), and the second, more clinical definition defines anxiety as an abnormal, overwhelming feeling of apprehension or fear that is punctuated by physiologic reactions such as tension, sweating, and rapid pulse. This picture of anxiety more often involves extreme self-doubt over one's ability to cope with the stressor. Regardless of definition, anxiety affects both the mind and the body to varying degrees, and more people find their lives full of these feelings.

The prevalence of anxiety in the population today is undoubtedly on the rise. Americans in particular continue to work longer hours, all the while balancing relationships, family, and home responsibilities. Because of this, it is no wonder that more people experience stress and anxiety today than ever before. However, it is an arguable point whether more people are experiencing pathologic anxiety, or what would be considered a true anxiety disorder as diagnosed by the *Diagnostic and Statistical Manual of Mental Disorders* (*DSM-IV*). (This publication describes the diagnostic criteria for the most common mental disorders including diagnois, treatment, and research findings. It is published by the American Psychiatric Association and is the main diagnostic reference for Mental Health professionals in the United States.) Regardless, anxiety is an ever-increasing problem among people today, with more and more of them seeking treatment options to relieve their suffering.

DSM-IV diagnosed anxiety disorders are the most common psychiatric illnesses affecting both adults and children today. Anxiety disorders may spring
from a set of complex risk factors including genetic predisposition, alterations
in neurochemicals, personality traits, and life events. Anxiety disorders can be
grouped into the following general categories.

- Generalized Anxiety Disorder: This is characterized by excessive, un-
  realistic worries that last beyond six months. This form of anxiety can
  be accompanied by physical symptoms associated with stress such as insomnia, gastrointestinal upset, and headaches.
- Obsessive-Compulsive Disorder: People suffering form this form of anxiety often experience persistent, recurring thoughts that are caused by
  exaggerated fears or anxiety. These obsessive thoughts may cause the
  person to perform ritualized routines in an attempt to absolve their
  anxieties.
- Panic Disorder: People with panic disorder suffer from debilitating attacks of panic that are often accompanied by symptoms such as heart
  palpitations, chest tightness, difficulty breathing, and overwhelming
  fear.
- Post-Traumatic Stress Disorder (PTSD): This type of stress becomes
  manifested following an extremely traumatic event. People with PTSD
  generally experience flashbacks, avoidance behaviors, emotional numb-
  ing, and physiologic symptoms such as insomnia and poor concentration.
- Social Anxiety Disorder: Characterized by an extreme fear of being
  judged by others or becoming embarrassed typically leads people with
  this type of anxiety to avoid situations involving other people.
- Specific Phobias: People with phobias will react with an intense level
  of fear to a specific situation or object that can lead to avoidance of the
  most common everyday situations.

It is estimated that 19 million adults in the United States suffer from anxiety
disorders. The cost of anxiety disorders is estimated to be nearly $42 billion a
year; nearly $23 billion is associated with the cost of repeated medical visits for
the relief of symptoms caused by anxiety that appear to be physical illnesses, and
people with anxiety are three to five times more likely to see a doctor and are
six times more likely to be hospitalized for these disorders than those without.[1]
The economic and individual burdens of anxiety disorders are high as these conditions can be chronic and quite disabling. People with anxiety disorders utilize
primary healthcare providers more often than psychiatric medical personnel,
exerting a large cost on the healthcare system itself. Costs are incurred in the
psychiatric, emergency care, hospital, medication, and primary-care sectors of
the healthcare system; costs also include decreased productivity and work ab-
senteeism. Only 30 percent of individuals afflicted with anxiety disorders seek

treatment for their condition, and 30 million people will experience some type of anxiety disorder at apoint in their lives.[2] Affixing a specific number to the prevalence of anxiety is difficult because small changes in diagnostic criteria, interviewing, and study methods can greatly affect the results.

As mentioned previously, the etiology of anxiety disorders is multifactorial. The likelihood of developing anxiety involves a combination of life experiences, genes, and personality/psychological traits. The individual effects of these influences differ from person to person and between types of anxiety. The roles of some influences weigh differently in each type of anxiety as well, such as the familial pattern in panic disorder, despite the fact that no genes have been found that directly link the two. It is, however, generally accepted that the large majority of anxiety is rooted in stressful lifestyles and events; most anxiety disorders share a state of increased arousal and fear.[3] It is important to note, however, that in many classic anxiety states there is no immediate external stressful event occurring. Science continues to attempt to uncover a complete understanding of the neurobiology of anxiety.

DIETARY FACTORS

Diet in itself is a major contributor to anxiety states and may also serve to inhibit the onset of anxiety. Perhaps one of the most important contributors to the perpetuation of anxiety is hypoglycemia, or lowered blood sugar levels due to infrequent eating or inadequate dietary choices. Symptoms of hypoglycemia have been traced to the deprivation of glucose in neurons themselves, and symptoms of low blood sugar include effects that are the result of the autonomic nervous system's perception of the physiologic changes caused by hypoglycemia, which can include anxiety, sweating, hunger, tremors, and palpitations.[4] People who do not consume the proper nutritional fuels to sustain blood sugar are at risk from this physiological phenomenon. Nearly everyone can associate with the aforementioned symptoms occurring in the late afternoon following no lunch or very little lunch with inadequate caloric value. Infrequent and/or poor food choices with a high glycemic index (foods that greatly raise one's blood sugar leading to a drastic, reflexive lowering of blood glucose levels) are the most frequent causes of this syndrome. Other symptoms might include irritability, poor concentration, and fatigue. In one study, patients demonstrating anxiety in the form of obsessive behavior secondary to hypoglycemia (confirmed by glucose tolerance test) were treated with dietary therapy intended to avert hypoglycemic states.[5] One of the subjects demonstrated a complete recovery following the dietary therapy and the other subject has made improvements comparable to his level of compliance to the therapy. Although small in nature, this study provides insight into origins and treatments for anxiety syndromes; maintaining adequate blood sugar levels (90–110 milligrams per deciliter) may serve as a key factor in preventing episodes of anxiety. One of the most interesting studies investigating the link between diet and anxiety looked at the relationship between type of diet (vegetarian versus omnivorous) and levels of anxiety and depression. In a group of 80 subjects, significant differences in anxiety and depression levels existed between the two groups, with increased anxiety and depression in the omnivore group.[6] The reasons for this are at this time undetermined; however, increased regulation of blood sugar levels may be one of the reasons for the outcome of this study.

Other precipitating causes of anxiety include dietary influences such as alcohol and caffeine. Although alcohol does exert a calming effect on the brain via its depressant effects (alcohol targets gamma-aminobutyric acid receptor [GABA(A)]–neurons; potentiation of the response of these inhibitory neurotransmitter receptors results in anxiolytic, sedative, and anesthetic activities in the human brain), it also may be responsible for increased feelings of anxiety. Subjects in one study given ethanol or a placebo were evaluated for anxiety using the Spielberger State Anxiety Inventory, a measuring device for anxiety. Subjects who received the ethanol experienced significant increases in anxiety compared to the placebo group, which actually reported decreased feelings of tension following administration of the placebo.[7] As a drug that primarily exerts negative effects on brain function, alcohol should be avoided in people with increased feelings of anxiety. This is not to say, however, that alcohol should be entirely avoided by all people who at times feel anxious, but people who choose to drink and have elevated levels of anxiety should use extreme caution. Moderation, of course, is always recommended, especially in the case of anxiety.

Caffeine, on the other hand is a well-known stimulant drug, causing excitatory neurotransmission. The effects of caffeine were studied in a group of patients with agoraphobia and panic disorder; caffeine consumption produced significant increases in anxiety, nervousness, fear, nauseas, heart palpitations, restlessness, and tremors compared to the group of patients taking a placebo.[8] Additionally, 71 percent of the patients taking caffeine in this study reported that the effects of caffeine were very much like the symptoms experienced during a panic attack. Another study demonstrated that patients with anxiety had anxiety levels that directly correlated with their level of caffeine consumption.[9] The results of this study also suggested that people with anxiety had an increased sensitivity to the effects of only one cup of coffee; this sensitivity was reinforced by the observation that more patients with panic disorder were more likely to discontinue coffee because of its negative side effects compared to controls. Caffeine overdose may also mimic anxiety disorders, and increased sensitivity to caffeine may contribute to these patients' symptoms; some cases of anxiety were improved for the duration of a six-month follow-up period after the discontinuation of caffeine.[10] Because of these findings, it is important that patients with anxiety disorders avoid caffeine-containing foods and beverages as this may prove to be beneficial for them.

INTERVENTIONS IN ANXIETY

Treatments for anxiety disorders themselves include psychological therapies (psychotherapy and others), medication, and a combination of both. Typical medications employed in the treatment of anxiety include selective serotonin reuptake inhibitors (SSRIs), tricyclic antidepressants, benzodiazepines, beta-blockers, and monoamine oxidase inhibitors (MAOIs). These medications can be helpful to some patients; however, a large majority of people on these medications report negative side effects and discomfort with these therapies.

Several nonpharmacologic treatments for anxiety exist and have been backed by appropriate research trials. Attempts at treating anxiety without the use of pharmaceutical drugs can exist on two levels. The first is to medicate (palliate) the patient with a treatment that acts similarly to accepted pharmaceuticals or one that elicits a calming/sedative effect on the patient. The second therapeutic approach involves the use of medicines that serve to prevent the initiation of anxiety in the first place; this involves various nutritional and/or botanical therapies that work to alter a patient's susceptibility to anxiety (prevention). The use of counseling and other forms of psychotherapy should always be considered in the treatment of a person with anxiety; a review of these therapies are not included in the scope of this book. Instead, the authors are attempting to highlight biochemical interventions (not that psychotherapy does not alter brain biochemistry itself). The complexity of anxiety warrants that several therapies be used; however, a change in treatments, whether pharmaceutical or naturally derived, demands strict attention to side effects and interactions that may occur as a side effect of using these treatments.

VITAMIN AND MINERAL DEFICIENCIES

Niacin

The basis for health functioning of any organism is complete nutrition. Yes, it is often argued that an organism, or a person for that matter, can get by on less-than-optimal amounts of the basic nutritional necessities. Getting by is, however, a less-than-optimal state of being. Several vitamin and mineral nutrients and their lack in certain people may contribute to the occurrence of anxiety. Nicotinamide, a form of the B vitamin niacin, is known to have similar effects to benzodiazepines on the brain.[11] Nicotinamide acts to stimulate the GABA-benzodiazepine receptor complex, an inhibitory neuron grouping, thereby exerting a calming effect through modulation of these specific neurons.[12] Other experiments designed to test the efficacy of nicotinamide and brain function revealed that GABA nerve receptors were under less control (meaning that because they are inhibitory in nature, when they are not engaged the brain is more excitable—which in theory may lead to more anxiety) when nicotinamide was lacking in the test subject, and reintroduction of nicotinamide lead to a calming effect on the GABA receptors.[13] Supplementation with adequate amounts of niacin may contribute to fewer anxiety symptoms.

Pyridoxine

Pyridoxine, otherwise known as vitamin B-6, is an important coenzyme in the biosynthesis of the neurotransmitters GABA, dopamine, and serotonin, all of which are affected in anxiety, as well as depression and perception of pain. Additionally, deficiency of pyridoxine causes an increased sympathetic discharge (increased excitatory nerve impulses) and hypertension in animals that has been hypothesized to reflect a decrease in production of the previously mentioned neurotransmitters. Further, adding pyridoxine to the diets of these animals will lower their blood pressure.[14] In a separate study investigating the use of magnesium and pyridoxine on anxiety-related premenstrual symptoms, investigators found that women who were supplemented with 200 milligrams of magnesium and 50 milligrams of pyridoxine each day experienced a significant reduction in anxiety-related PMS symptoms such as nervous tension, irritability, and generalized anxiety.[15] Although magnesium could be considered a confounding variable in relation to the complete anxiolytic effects of pyridoxine, the information contained in this study is relevant in reference to the effects of vitamin B-6 on resolving anxiety and related symptoms.

Magnesium

Magnesium supplementation enjoys a broad reputation as having a calmative effect on anxiety symptoms and stress levels. Only a few indirect studies of magnesium's effect on anxiety exist; however, these studies demonstrate interesting results. Daro observed decreased levels of nervousness as well as insomnia in patients supplemented with 200 milligrams of magnesium in combination with 400 milligrams calcium,[16] and Seelig noted an association between magnesium deficiency and anxiety symptoms.[17] A separate study investigated the use of magnesium in postsurgical patients and its effectiveness in alleviating pain. Patients were infused with magnesium both during and following surgery and were evaluated for anxiety levels. Patients receiving the magnesium infusion required significantly less pain medication (morphine and fentanyl) in comparison to the control group that received no magnesium, and the magnesium group reported less anxiety as well.[18] Magnesium deficiency is common in the typical American diet, with one major survey determining that adequate magnesium is lacking in nearly 72 percent of people's diets. It also found that 50 percent of people consume less than three-quarters of the Recommended Daily Allowance (RDA) of magnesium and 30 percent of these people ate less than half of the RDA for magnesium.[19] People taking oral contraceptives–diuretic medicines (medicine that is designed to increase water loss from the body through urination) or large amounts of laxatives may be at risk of magnesium deficiency. In addition, deficiency of magnesium has been linked to conditions such as cardio-vascular diseases, alcoholism, kidney diseases, premenstrual syndrome, and cramping.[20]

CONCLUSION

These studies endorse the idea that adequate levels of nutrition are essential in both the prevention and treatment of anxiety symptoms. With multiple causes, anxiety is a condition that more than likely has multiple treatments in different individuals. Treating the person who has anxiety with adequate nutritional sources may possibly alter anxiety levels and offer the patient a greater quality of life.

To be human is to be anxious at some point in one's existence. Yet, when anxiety becomes a fixture in one's life, it is time to preemptively seek a way to intervene in order to redirect one's life back onto a more calm, relaxed, and enjoyable road. It is not surprising to many to see more and more advertisements for anxiety medications and national talk shows discussing how to cope with the trials and tribulations of life that seem to more often than ever throw us into tailspins. By far, the best defense is a good offense, and nourishing one's body is a great way to start. Also, the proper use of relaxing and stress-reducing exercise, mental exercises, and even prayer can all play a very important role in maintaining that inner peace that we all desire to not only achieve but to maintain at least most of the time.

NUTRIENTS

- Dietary
  Maintaining recommended blood sugar levels (90–110) throughout the day
- Niacin
  25 milligrams per day
- Pyridoxine
  25 milligrams per day
- Magnesium
  300–400 milligrams per day

Autism

Autism is a highly complex developmental disability that can become manifest within the first three years of life. A neurological disorder that adversely affects brain function, autism affects mainly communication and social interaction areas, leaving the child with difficulties in both verbal and nonverbal communications. One of five related disorders among the Pervasive Developmental Disorders grouping, autism has a specific set of diagnostic criteria that is defined in the *Diagnostic and Statistical Manual of Mental Disorders* (DSM-IV). Autism affects each individual differently and with varying severity. Overall, autism incidence is fairly consistent around the globe and displays no racial or ethnic trends. The following statistical information reveals the most current statistics surrounding autism[1]:

- 1 to 1.5 million Americans have autism, affecting 2–6 per 1,000 individuals.
- It is the fastest growing developmental disability, affecting 1 out of every 250 children born.
- It is four times more common in boys than girls.
- Incidence is currently growing at 10–17 percent annually.
- Ninety percent of care costs are directed at autistic adults, costing $90 billion per year.

Autism affects each individual differently; those afflicted with autism process the world differently, leading to abnormal behaviors in comparison to other people in their age grouping. A person with autism may perceive certain normal sounds or sensations differently, and communication can be limited to repeated phrases or words or the use of gestures and pointing. Autistic people may laugh, cry, or be upset for reasons that others are unaware of; they may appear aloof and prefer solitude, refusing to be touched. They may appear to have a hearing problem, not responding to any sounds or words despite normal audiologic testing. Some of these behaviors are thought to be the result of an inability of the autistic person to integrate sensory information.

No specific cause of autism is known at this time; however, it is widely thought that an alteration in brain structure and function cause the symptoms of autism (autistic brains are of different size and shape than a person without autism). Currently, researchers are investigating the link between genes and autism, as many families display patterns among their members with autism or other related disorders. An autism gene or grouping of genes has not yet been isolated, nor has a single weak link or trigger that results in the development of autism. Other research is investigating events during pregnancy and delivery, environmental factors, metabolic diseases, and toxic exposures as other possible causes of autism.

Other considerations of causative factors in autism include the occurrence of the disorder in greater frequency with other medical conditions such as Fragile X syndrome, tuberous sclerosis, untreated phenylketonuria (PKU), and congenital rubella. One of the most debated causative factors for autism is that of mercury-containing vaccines, a theory with much plausible weight despite widespread refutation of this theory by the medical establishment. Because of the absence of one specific causative factor, autism is considered a condition that people are born with or have the potential to develop if exposed to a certain factor. Autism is not due to bad parenting or poorly disciplined children, and it is not caused by any known psychological factors that may affect the child.

Not diagnosable using standard medical testing, autism is diagnosed wholly on observing the patient's behavior, especially the communicative and developmental aspects. Autism does share some of the same characteristics as the other previously mentioned Pervasive Developmental Disorders, and other tests may be necessary to differentiate autism from one of these other conditions, including metabolic testing. Early diagnosis is considered essential, because the sooner treatment and education is initiated, the better the outcomes that are achieved.[2] Autism is detectable at the very earliest by 18 to 24 months and can become fully obvious by 24 months to 6 years of age. Some of the earliest signs a physician will screen for include: absence of babbling or cooing and gestures by 12 months, absence of speech by 16 months, absence of two-word phrases by 24 months, and a reversion or loss of language or social skills at any age thereon. Any one of these symptoms does not confirm a diagnosis; however, further testing by a physician is warranted. Several screening behavioral and communications tests are used to diagnose autism, including the Childhood Autism Rating Scale, Checklist for Autism in Toddlers (CHAT), Autism Screening Questionnaire, and the Screening Test for Autism in Two-Year Olds, all of which feature objective observational approaches to evaluating a child suspected of having autism.

In perhaps one of the most comprehensive pieces written on the various causes of autism, Kidd explores the link between numerous causative factors and their roles in the development of autism.[3] Among the causes investigated in that text are congenital factors such as inborn errors of metabolism, prenatal susceptibilities and the genetic interplay between the two; biochemical imperfections such as impaired hepatic detoxification abilities and nutritional deficits; central nervous system factors such as imbalances and abnormalities of neurotransmitters; gastrointestinal tract dysfunction including impaired digestion and food intolerances; and immune system dysregulation including hypersensitivity and abnormalities in antibody- and cell-mediated functions.

NUTRITIONAL FACTORS

The vitamin and mineral status of children with autism is a subject that requires much attention. Although not implicated in the causation of autism, vitamin and mineral therapy may be beneficial for these people, due to their often less-than-optimal eating and resultant nutritional status. Feeding dysfunction, wherein the autistic child will only consume certain foods for lengthy durations, can set the autistic person up for stark nutritional deficiencies.[4] An evaluation of autistic children's nutrient status in one study revealed that greater than 50 percent of the subjects had insufficient levels of vitamins A, thiamine (B-1), niacin (B-3), pantothenic acid (B-5), and biotin as well as the minerals magnesium, selenium, and zinc.[5] In addition to these nutrient deficiencies, the subjects had less-than-optimal levels of essential fatty acids (omega-3 eicosapentaenoic acid [EPA] and the omega-6 dihomogammalinolenic acid [DGLA] fatty acids) and essential amino acids. A study that investigated the supplementation of autistic children with a multivitamin and mineral over a three-month period resulted in improvements in bowel pattern symptoms and sleep quality, in addition to elevations in blood levels of vitamins C and B-6, revealing some of the benefits of nutritional supplementation for these childen.[6]

Other research on nutrient-focused deficiencies and treatment of autistic symptoms has provided interesting results in this area. The use of folic acid as a treatment for people with autism was begun with the use of this vitamin in large doses (250 mcg of folic acid per pound of body weight per day) in the treatment of Fragile X syndrome (a common familial form of mental retardation with behaviors similar to autism) as well as children with autsim.[7] In addition, the Autism Research Institute (ARI) proclaims a strongly positive effect from folic acid supplementation according to their "better:worse" scale, a collection and average of comments from thousands of parents who treat their children with various therapies.[8]

Vitamin C (ascorbic acid) use in autism was tested in a 30-week trial in which the vitamin was supplemented at a dose of 8 grams per 70-kilogram body weight per day; a reduction in symptom severity was noted among the group supplemented with vitamin C.[9] The Autism Research Institute scores vitamin C as highly favorable, with a better:worse ratio of 16:1.[8] An essential nutrient not manufactured by the human body, ascorbic acid plays an integral role in the functioning of several metabolic pathways, namely that of neurotransmitter production. More studies are needed in order to determine the full efficacy of vitamin C in autism therapy.

Zinc is also given a very favorable better:worse ratio from the Autism Research Institute, with a ratio of 17:1.[8] One study of zinc in autism revealed that nearly 90 percent of autistic cases in the study were deficient in zinc, while at the same time 90 percent of the subjects had excessive copper levels.[10] A normal biologic occurrence, zinc and copper levels are intimately linked wherein levels of one nutrient will rise resulting in corresponding decrease in the other nutrient, and vise versa. However, low levels of zinc are not favorable in any condition, especially those affecting the brain, because of zinc's importance in neurologic tissue function and synthesis of the brain neurotransmitter serotonin, which is dependent on zinc-driven enzyme systems. Another study again found elevated copper:zinc levels in 85 percent of the autistic children enrolled.[11] It is difficult to analyze the role of zinc in particular in autism from these studies; however, the importance of zinc in proper biologic function cannot be understated. The second most abundant trace element in the human body, zinc totals nearly 2 grams.[12] Several of the proteins involved in gene regulation (and therefore biologic function) contain varying amounts of zinc, and it is found in approximately 300 enzymes, 100 of which depend on zinc as a catalyst.[13] Additionally, zinc plays a large role in growth, development, behavior, and learning.[14] Zinc is highly important in the normal and healthy function of the individual, and plays an important role in the autistic patient.

The role of essential fatty acids (EFAs) (omega-3 and omega-6 fatty acids) is integral to proper health and proper metabolic functioning. The clinical effects associated with disproportionate intake and metabolism of the two main EFAs, linoleic and alpha-linolenic acids, are most readily apparent in their metabolic byproduct concentrations in the membrane phospholipid layer, the fat-and-protein-composed cellular coat that is directly responsible for correct cellular function. Cellular fatty acid content can be manipulated by dietary intake and disease processes, thereby altering the severity, character, and intensity of pathologies.[15]

EFAs allow for both inter- and intracellular communication, providing the substrate for signal messengers between cells. The longest of the biologically active fatty acids plays a highly important role in the neurological development of both fetal and postnatal stages.[16] Additionally, infants have a limited ability to synthesize the longer chain fatty acids (that can serve as building blocks for EFAs) from shorter chain fatty acids typically found in the Western diet. Perhaps because of this, nature has done its part in assuring that infants receive these essential fats in breast milk, which contains the longer chain omega-3 and omega-6 fatty acids docosahexaenoic acid (DHA) and arachidonic acid (AA).[17]

Richardson and Ross have proposed that abnormalities in fatty acid distribution in membrane phospholipid metabolism may play a significant role in the development of several neurodevelopmental and psychiatric disorders including ADHD, dyslexia, coordination disorders (dyspraxia), and autism.[18] These researchers explain that the aforementioned disorders may have causation in disorders of phospholipid dysfunction, explaining the high amount of similar symptomology between those conditions and their familial grouping. Omega-3 fatty acids were found to be nearly 100 percent deficient in a population of autistic cases studied,[10] whereas another study determined that blood plasma levels of omega-3 fatty acids were decreased by 20 percent in comparison to control subjects in another study.[19] As reported by the Autism Research Index, essential fatty acid supplementation retains a better:worse ratio of 12:1 among people that care for autistic persons.[8] Theory dictates that humans probably evolved on a diet containing a 1:1 ratio of omega-6 to omega-3 fatty acids, yet modern times have produced typical Western diets that consist of a ratio between 10:1 and 25:1, and in some cases it may be as high as 40:1. Undoubtedly, this imbalance has definitely contributed to several chronic health conditions, and newer research is elucidating the role of proper fatty acid balance and intake in autism.

A large amount of research focused on vitamin B-6 (pyridoxine) and the mineral magnesium provide very interesting results in the treatment of autism. Pyridoxine is required for the metabolism of amino acids (the building blocks of protein), carbohydrates, and lipids (fats). Pyridoxine is converted to two different coenzymes, pyridoxal phosphate and pyridoxamine phosphate, both of which play a major role in numerous metabolic reactions in the body, such as synthesis of the neurotransmitters gamma-aminobutyric acid (GABA) and the metabolism of serotonin, norepinephrine, epinephrine, and dopamine, as well as the metabolism of polyunsaturated fatty acids and phospholipids.[20] As one of the most abundant minerals in the body, magnesium plays an integral role in upwards of 300 different cellular reactions and is required for the formation of cyclic AMP, an internal cellular signaling molecule.[21] Additionally, magnesium shepards ion movements across the cellular membranes and is critical to proper muscular and nervous electrical impulses.[22]

A series of trials using both combination therapy (pyridoxine and magnesium) and solitary administration of pyridoxine and magnesium produced positive results in autistic children only when the combination therapy was administered.[23] Improvements in behavior were noted along with measurements of improved biochemical markers in relation to autistic biology (Urinary homovanillic acid excretion decreased—a measurement of improved dopamine utilization in the body) as well as improved electrophysiological measurements (improved neurologic nerve transmission). The results from another study utilizing large doses of pyridoxine in autistic children yielded significant benefits from the treatment including increased eye contact, greater interest in the surrounding environment, decreased tantrums and self-stimulatory behaviors, and improved speech.[24] In a review of 18 different studies utilizing magnesium and pyridoxine to treat autism, Rimland summarized that each study led to some type of positive results among the autistic subjects, and no significantly untoward side effects were noted in each study.[25] Galand writes in a review of magnesium and its use in stress and neuropsychiatric disorders that neuronal hyperexcitability is one manifestation of low magnesium stores, and supplementation with magnesium in conjunction with pyridoxine benefits approximately 40 percent of autistic patients, perhaps due to magnesium's effect on dopamine metabolism.[26]

Dimethylglycine

A form of the amino acid glycine, dimethylglycine (DMG) exists in foods as well as transiently in the body for small amounts of time in small quantities as a result of rapid metabolism.[27] It has been used recently to improve neurological function, prevent epileptic seizures (one-third of people with autism will have seizures,[28] although they do not have epilepsy), reduce the effects of stress (internally and externally), and as an anti-inflammatory agent. Having received a mildly favorable rating by the Autism Research Index,[8] DMG is used in the treatment of autism symptoms despite relatively little research into this molecule. However, the studies that exist present favorable results. In a double-blind study comparing DMG to a placebo, 37 autistic children were treated with DMG for four weeks.[29] Improvement in behavior was noted among both the placebo and DMG group; however, the difference was not statistically significant. Some of the children responded favorably to the DMG supplementation, and a smaller percentage of negative changes were noted in the DMG group. In his report on autism and its treatment using magnesium, B-6, and DMG, Rimland cites a trial of DMG use in Korea by a Lee Dae Kun, director of the Pusan Research Center on Child Problems, in which DMG was shown to provide beneficial effects on 80 percent of the supplemented autistic children.[25] Rimland recommends that the initial starting dose of DMG be approximately 60 milligrams per day with a morning meal, and then slowly increased to 500 milligrams per day; effects may become noticeable within one to four weeks, although sometimes they are evident sooner.[25]

CONCLUSION

A highly challenging condition to treat, autism is becoming more common in our society. The causes of autism remain highly elusive today; and yet similar to several other "disorder-type" conditions affecting the brain, autism more than likely has multiple contributing factors. Supplying the autistic person with early and continuous nutritional treatment provides an effective, safe way to augment standard treatment and supplies a much-needed boost to current pharmaceutical therapeutics. Because autism is a highly individualized condition and improvements are gained after large amounts of effort, caregivers and physicians are encouraged to explore the most effective nutritional therapies that the individual autistic derives the most benefit from, even if only minimal improvements are noted.

Clinically, there is no greater single privilege than helping unlock the world of an individual suffering from autism. Indeed the untapped potential of all of us is amazing, and to work with the wonderfully dynamic individuals with autism provides the opportunity to help solve each unique biochemical, environmental, and genetic riddle relative to the proper and most effective intervention. The previously approaches shed light on a select few therapies, and one should allow adequate time with any given series of treatments so that the support of the body's biochemical and psychological pathways have time to respond. Yet, the key, as with most health conditions, is to never stop knocking on the door of invention. After all, necessity is the mother of invention and many talented clinicians and researchers are seeking the answers to this and other puzzling health concerns.

NUTRIENTS

- Folic acid
  1–2 grams per day, divided doses
- Vitamin C
  3–4 grams per 70 kilograms body weight
- Zinc
  40 milligrams per day
- Essential Fatty Acids (EPA/DHA)
  2–3 grams per day
- Pyridoxine
  50–100 milligrams per day
- Magnesium
  5 milligrams per kilogram body weight per day in divided doses
- Dimethylglycine
  60–500 milligrams per day; this dose should be worked up to slowly

Bipolar Disorder

Bipolar disorder, also known as manic depression, is a condition that is punctuated by wide changes in mood, thought, energy levels, and behavior. A person with bipolar disorder may witness his or her moods alternating between excessive highs (mania) and excessive lows (depression). Changes can be apparent for as little as a couple of hours to days, weeks, and even months. The cyclical or episodic occurrences of depression and mania can be solitary in nature, and episodes of mixed mania and depression can appear as well, becoming increasingly frequent leading to disruptions in all aspects of the person's life.

Affecting approximately 2.3 million adults in the United States,[1] or nearly 1.2 percent of the population age 18 years and older in any given year,[2] bipolar disorder typically begins in late adolescence. Bipolar disorder can occur in younger people and may be masked as depression during teenage years; however, it can begin in young children and in older adults as well. The average age at onset of the first episode of mania is in the early 20s.[3] Bipolar disorder is not a personality flaw or character weakness, and it affects men and women equally and shows no preferential distribution among age groups, race, ethnicity, and social class.

Although different from clinical depression, the depressive episodes in bipolar disorder are similar. The following are standard attributes of a depressive episode (not all people with bipolar disorder will experience the range of symptoms listed):

- Loss of energy, persistent lethargy
- Prolonged sadness or unexplained crying spells
- Irritability, anger, worry, agitation, anxiety
- Inability to take pleasure in former interests, social withdrawal

- Pessimism, indifference
- Feelings of guilt, worthlessness
- Inability to concentrate, indecisiveness
- Significant changes in appetite and sleep patterns
- Unexplained aches and pains
- Recurring thoughts of death or suicide

Mania symptoms are exhibited by the following behaviors and feelings (not all people with bipolar disorder will experience the range of symptoms listed):

- Racing speech, racing thoughts, flight of ideas
- Increased physical and mental activity and energy
- Excessive irritability, aggressive behavior
- Decreased need for sleep without experiencing fatigue
- Heightened mood, exaggerated optimism and self-confidence
- Grandiose delusions, inflated sense of self-importance
- Impulsiveness, poor judgment, distractibility
- Reckless behavior
- In the most severe cases, delusions and hallucinations

Another phase of bipolar disorder known as the "mixed" state includes symptoms from both the manic and depressive phases. During the mixed state, symptoms may include agitation, changes in appetite, psychosis, insomnia, and suicidal ideation. People can have a depressed mood while being manically activated.

Early bipolar disorder may be marked by intervals between manic and depressive episodes during which the person experiences periods of wellness, with few or no symptoms. If a person experiences four or more episodes of illness during the course of one year, they are said to have *rapid cycling*. In the more severe cases, a person may have difficulties with alcohol and/or substance abuse,[4] and the mania or depression may be accompanied by psychosis that includes symptoms of hallucinations and delusions reflecting the mood state at that time.

There are several types of bipolar disorder; each is divided into types that reflect timing of symptomology. *Bipolar I disorder* is characterized by one or more manic or mixed episodes nearly every day for at least one week and one or more major depressive episodes. This is the most severe form of the disorder. *Bipolar II disorder* is marked by one or more depressive episodes accompanied by at least one hypomanic episode (a manic episode that is less severe than a typical manic state—these may not be severe enough to disrupt life, although they may in some people). *Cyclothymic disorder* is charachterized by constant mood fluctuations involving hypomanic and depressive episodes. These episodes are shorter and less severe than typical manic-depressive episodes and do not occur with the same frequency as in bipolar I and II. A final classification, known as *bipolar disorder not otherwise specified (NOS)* has similarities to the other classifications; however, its symptom patterns do not fit into any one of them.

CAUSATION

Bipolar disorder is a familial disease; two-thirds of people with bipolar disorder have one close relative with bipolar or depression, proving that bipolar disorder has a genetic component.[5] In fact, studies investigating the genetic basis of bipolar disease indicate that multiple genes are involved in bipolar disorder.[5] Studies of twins have indicated that if one twin has the mood disorder, the chances of an identical twin having it are three times higher than that of a fraternal twin; the concordance rate (the occurrence of the disorder among both twins) among identical twins is 80 percent, whereas it is only 16 percent for fraternal twins.[6] Evidence of this caliber directly suggests that mood disorders, including bipolar, are partially the result of an underlying genetic susceptibility.

Uncovering the correct genetic contribution to bipolar disorder will allow for improved treatments and preventative interventions designed to target the causative factors of this illness. The cause of bipolar disorder is not only genetically linked however. The approach to this and other psychopathologic diseases is that multiple biologic and psychological factors interact to create the condition. Said otherwise, there are physical, mental, environmental, and emotional causes that when combined in certain patterns in different individuals may result in mental illnesses in susceptible people.

Unfortunately, ascribing the occurrence of bipolar disorder to genetics does not provide much information in the treatment and prevention for persons living with this disease. Whatever the exact causative factors may be, they may all interact in such a way that a person with a genetic susceptibility for bipolar disorder will manifest imperfections in the brain neurotransmitter system. Current theories hypothesize that either too high or too low of levels of neurotransmitters such as serotonin, norepinephrine, or dopamine will cause the symptoms seen in bipolar disorder, and other theories hypothesize that despite adequate levels of neurotransmitters, an imbalance exists between them, and the ratio between them is most important. Another theory suggests that differences in the sensitivity of the neurotransmitter receptors on nerve cells may lead to symptoms. All of these theories are borne out by interesting research, and chances are that each theory explains a probable role in bipolar disorder.

NUTRIENTS

One of the most popularly prescribed pharmaceuticals for the treatment of bipolar disorder is lithium. Known by many other trade names, lithium is primarily one of the basic elements and is classified in the same chemical grouping as sodium and potassium. Primarily a naturally derived substance, lithium is used to control manic episodes and is not generally sedative. The precise mechanism by which lithium works to control mania is unknown; however, it is suspected that lithium affects nerve conduction in the brain and reduces the action of the neurotransmitters norepinephrine and serotonin, thereby altering brain chemistry. Although lithium can be considered a "natural" medicine (30 percent of all pharmaceutical drugs today are naturally derived), it is used to treat the symptoms of bipolar mania and does not necessarily contribute to resolving the cause of the symptoms. That being said, the authors acknowledge the usefulness of this medication in the treatment of bipolar disorder.

Folic Acid in Mania and Depression

Folic acid, one of the B vitamins (rarely known as vitamin B-9), is intimately linked to proper brain functioning, especially in the areas of mania and depression. Several studies linking suboptimal folate levels and manic as well as depressive symptoms appear throughout the literature. A survey of 45 patients diagnosed with mania had red blood cell folate levels that were slightly less than 20 percent in comparison to those in a healthy control group.[7] Serum folate in both groups were similar, however; and both groups were derived from the same socioeconomic class, demonstrating that the reduction in red cell folate in people with mania is associated with the illness and possibly related to dietary deficiency.

The roles of folic acid in psychiatric conditions have been relatively well researched, and many interesting conclusions can be drawn between this essential nutrient and bipolar disorder. A review of folic acid and its role in neurobiology by Young and Ghadirian reveals the following information: Folic acid deficiency is quite common among people with various psychiatric disorders, absorption of folate is inhibited by anticonvulsant medications (which are employed in the standard treatment of bipolar disorder), and these patients' psychiatric symptoms are associated with folate deficiency; several studies have displayed the effectiveness of folate in the treatment of psychiatric symptoms in folate-deficient patients; folic acid deficiency will lower brain levels of two chemicals (S-adenosylmethionine [SAMe] and 5-hydroxytryptamine [5HT]) intimately involved in proper brain function.[8] S-adenosylmethionine is known to have antidepressant properties and will elevate levels of 5-hydroxytryptamine in the brain, leading researchers to conclude that deficiency of folate is related to decreased levels of brain 5HT. SAMe is involved in chemical reactions known as methylation, which contribute to the healthy function of membrane phospholipids, influencing nerve transmission. In addition, another study involving folate suggested that a deficient amount of this nutrient in the body might inhibit the formation of a molecule known as tetrahydrobiopterin (BH4), which is essential in the formation of 5HT and other monoamine neurotransmitters involved in bipolar and other affective disorders.[9] A study investigating the therapuetic application of folic acid in patients on lithium therapy revealed that during the course of the trial, patients who were supplemented with 200 micrograms of folic acid and had the highest blood (plasma) levels of folate experienced a 40 percent reduction in affective disorders morbidity (symptoms that affected their quality of life), leading these researchers to suggested a folic acid supplementation regimen of 300–400 micrograms daily would augment symptom control of patients on long-term lithium therapy.[10] These findings demonstrate the importance of folate in psychiatric disorders. The researchers in the cited study proclaimed that at least some of the patients with bipolar and other psychiatric disorders would respond favorably to folate supplementation.

Vitamin B-12

Vitamin B-12 is another well-known nutrient that when deficient can lead to psychiatric symptoms; this has been reported in the medical literature for several decades.[11] Among the symptoms caused by this vitamin deficiency are mental lassitude and depression, as well as acute psychotic episodes and mania, among others. Examples of this are highlighted in the following studies: One case of mania that was apparently due to B-12 deficiency became manifest in a patient without the telltale signs of deficiency, namely pernicious anemia.[12] Supplementation with B-12 over the course of six months resolved the patient's manic state, and continuous monthly injections of B-12 allowed the patient to maintain normal mentation. Another case report and study by Evans et al. describes the occurrence of manic psychosis that occurred in patients with no apparent hematological manifestations of B-12 deficiency that were accompanied by changes in the patients' electroencephalograms (EEG) along with other organic mental changes.[13] The authors of this study performed a review of the literature, again citing the causal link between B-12 deficiency and brain dysfunction, leading them to suggest that the manifestation of psychiatric symptoms may occur prior to other standard manifestations (macrocytic anemia and spinal cord disease) and that all patients with neuropsychiatric diseases be screened for B-12 deficiency. Several other investigations have produced similar findings of varied manifestations of depression, mania, and other neuropsychiatric symptoms, some of which included patients with blood studies that were reflective of B-12 deficiency (macrocytic anemia) and some in which the subjects had no such manifestations.[14] All of these studies recommended nutritional status screening of psychiatric patients and blood testing in order to evaluate for B-12 deficiency upon admission to care facilities.

Selenium

Minerals, in addition to vitamins, play a role in normalization of mood, including bipolar disorder. Evidence suggesting adequate intake and supply of selenium contributes to regularity in mood and exerts a positive effect on bipolar disorder (as an example of extreme mood dysregulation). A study of men utilizing the *Profile of Mood States—Bipolar Form* to evaluate mood in comparison to selenium levels and intake revealed that the men with initially low levels of selenium who were supplemented with a low-selenium diet scored lower on the mood scale than those who were supplemented at a higher level; investigators hypothesized that selenium may play a role in mood regulation in the brain and that low selenium status may result in a person experiencing relatively poorer moods.[15] The brain will preferentially store selenium during times of low supply, indicating an as of yet undetermined but still important role in brain function. In a review of studies involving selenium and psychological functioning, each instance revealed that low selenium intake was linked to poorer mood; selenium supplementation and mood is a clear example of a psychologic function modified by this trace mineral.[16] In this review, the investigators revealed that although the mechanism of action of selenium on mood is not known, selenium supplementation might further activate the selenium-linked antioxidant enzyme, glutathione peroxidase.

Vanadium

A trace mineral, vanadium plays numerous important roles in the body, including blood sugar regulation, proper bone growth, and as a cofactor in multiple enzymatic reactions. On the other hand, like all nutritional factors, vanadium has adverse effects when supplied or stored in excessive amounts in the human body, including kidney dysfunction, gastrointestinal upset, and central nervous system depression, to list only a few.[17] Additionally, excess amounts of vanadium may contribute to bipolar disorder, as elevated blood levels have been detected in patients with mania and depression, and elevated levels have also been found in the hair of people with mania.[18] Elevations in vanadium levels may cause bipolar disorder and depression by the way this trace mineral interacts with electrolyte-based nerve impulse generation systems (variations in Na-K-Mg ATPase and sodium pump activity) in the brain, which are known to be associated with bipolar disorder. Elevated blood levels of vanadium were negatively correlated with nerve cell electrolyte ratios (Na-K-Mg ATPase to Mg-ATPase) in patients with bipolar disorder, but not in healthy subjects, suggesting a relationship between vanadium and proper electrolyte-generated nerve cell transmission.[19] A study of bipolar patients and their intake of vanadium revealed that both manic and depressed patients felt better with a reduced dietary intake of vanadium, further suggesting the role that vanadium may contribute to bipolar disorder.[20] Although difficult to avoid, vanadium is found throughout the environment naturally and as a result of industrial processes. Decreasing vanadium levels in the diet may be difficult to achieve; however, by drinking only filtered water and avoiding excessive intake from large amounts of mineral supplements, blood levels of vanadium can be reduced by vitamin C and a compound known as EDTA (Ethylenediaminetetraacetic acid).[21] Known as a chelating agent, EDTA is a complex molecule that has the ability to bind certain metals in the blood stream, assisting the body's removal of them through the urine. Vitamin C may be helpful in the treatment of bipolar disorder through its mechanism by which it reduces the ability of vanadium to alter previously described nerve cell electrolyte systems.[22]

BOTANICAL MEDICINES

There are several botanical (herbal) medicines that may be helpful in normalizing moods, especially during times of mania. Valerian (*Valeriana officinalis*) is used as a sedative-hypnotic most successfully in insomnia and for reducing anxiety-induced restlessness and sleeping disorders, often seen in individuals suffering from both mania and depression. Valerian use on a daily basis has been shown to reduce sleep latency and to improve sleep quality as reported by patients taking the herb.[23] Described as having mildly sedative, anxiolytic, and antidepressant effects, the use of valerian in people with bipolar disorder may be helpful. Valerian works to relieve anxiety by the ability of its constituents (valepotriates) to prevent the breakdown of enzymes in the brain that are responsible for degrading inhibitory (GABA) neurotransmitters (allowing for greater sedation of the brain) and by another constituent known as hydroxy-pinoresinol to bind to the same brain receptors that the depressant drugs known as benzodiazapenes do.[24] Although valerian is considered a mildly sedative herb, it does not appear to slow important psychomotor functions such as reaction time, alertness, and concentration; however, it may cause morning sluggishness.[25] As a sedative, however, use of valerian with other "relaxing" drugs (i.e., benzodiazapenes) may cause additive effects, leading to too much sedation. This is, of course, a risk in patients with more than mild depression; patients should use caution when using this herb for bipolar disorder.

Lavender (*lavendula officinalis*) has mild relaxant effects and is used traditionally for restlessness, insomnia, depression, and nervousness. Lavender preparations are commonly derived from the plant oil; internal ingestion is contraindicated. However, plant oils do exert physiologic effects when inhaled, as the oil can penetrate mucous membranes lining the respiratory system. The constituents of lavender oil when inhaled lead to relaxation and decreased alertness.[26] Inhalation of lavender oil scents may serve to modulate feelings of anxiety in patients with mania.

Lemon balm (*Melissa officinalis*) is another botanical medicine with mild calming effects and the ability to reduce alertness,[27] which is useful in the treatment of nervous anxiety, as well as other nonrelated medical problems. The oils of this plant contain compounds known as terpenes, which have sedative effects are rapidly absorbed by the lungs, and can cross the blood-brain barrier, allowing them to directly affect brain function (terpenes are thought to act on some of the inhibitory neurons [GABA] in the brain, thereby eliciting their calmative effects).[28] A study utilizing both valerian and lemon balm demonstrated an improvement in the amount and quality of sleep in subjects taking this herbal combination.[29]

CONCLUSION

Bipolar disorder, or manic depression, is a condition with many possible causes; however, little is truly known about the origins of this disease. But science is beginning to uncover the link between nutritional elements that may contribute to the symptoms of bipolar disorder. Several vitamin and mineral deficiencies (Vitamin B-12, folic acid, and selenium), as well as excessive amounts of the trace mineral vanadium, may predispose certain individuals to this condition. The importance of nutrients in proper brain function and bipolar disorder is perhaps best demonstrated in the following study: A group of *DSM-IV*-diagnosed bipolar disorder patients aged 19 to 46 years were given a treatment of high-dose vitamin and mineral supplements.[30] After six months of this therapy, the patients experienced a decrease in symptoms by 55 percent to 66 percent and a reduction in the need for psychotropic medications by more than 50 percent; some patients were able to replace their pharmaceutical medication with the vitamin and mineral supplement, remaining well for the duration. This is an example that drives home the point that diseases are not the result of deficient pharmaceutical medications; rather they have definitive origins in nutritional deficiency. Additionally, the use of botanical medicine provides a more gentle approach to bipolar disorder and, when used properly, may serve to attenuate some of the extremes of moods with fewer side effects than those of pharmaceutical medications.

Life is full of ebb and flow, yet for patients with bipolar symptoms, the pendulum swings to the extremes and warrants concise intervention to assist them in maintaining their mental functioning between the proverbial yellow lines of the road of life. The condition we refer to as bipolar is no different then any other health concern in so much as the patient is manifesting with symptoms that need attention and a concerted effort to address the underlying cause of the problem at hand. Often patients will present with symptoms, whereas previously they were apparently symptom free. Thus the question must be asked, what was the trigger and how can it be best addressed?

NUTRIENTS

- Folate
  200–300 micrograms per day
- B-12
  2,000 micrograms per day
- Selenium
  200 micrograms per day

BOTANICALS (FOR EPISODES OF MANIA)

- Valerian
  300–400 milligrams twice per day

- Lavender
  Tincture (1:5 in 50 percent alcohol) 30 drops twice per day
- Lemon Balm
  80–100 milligrams twice per day

Bulimia Nervosa

Bulimia, in addition to anorexia nervosa, is a psychiatric disorder with severe health consequences. An eating disorder whose name literally means "nervous hunger," bulimia is characterized by cycles of binging on large amounts of food at one time followed by self-purging of the same food eaten in order to avoid weight gain. Diagnostic criteria[1] for bulimia include eating, in a specified period of time (i.e., in any two-hour period), an amount of food that far surpasses the amount of food that the majority of people would eat in the same period of time under similar circumstances (caloric intake typically ranges from 1,000 to as much as 20,000 calories during one such episode); a feeling of no control over the eating during the episode; compensatory behavior for the eating, including self-induction of vomiting, laxative abuse, enemas, fasting, excessive exercise, or other medications designed to hasten weight loss; episodes of binge eating and compensatory behaviors that both occur on an average of twice a week for three months; and self-esteem that is inordinately influenced by body weight and appearance. Additionally, these patterns do not occur exclusively during episodes of anorexia nervosa, although close to 50 percent of people who have been anorexic develop bulimia or bulimic patterns. Persons with bulimia begin the mentioned cycle because of the belief that this behavior will prevent them from gaining weight and will help them to lose weight as well. However, the opposite occurs, leading to more weight gain and more binging and purging that continually increase the illness's severity.

Millions of Americans are affected by eating disorders each year. Both bulimia and anorexia nervosa are estimated to affect 2 percent to 6 percent of the population, meaning that 5 million to 16 million people may be affected. Of these numbers, bulimia accounts for 1 percent to 4 percent of the population. Eighty-six percent of people with eating disorders report the onset of symptoms prior to age 20, and 90 percent of these people are women. In fact, the incidence of eating disorders among college women is considered near epidemic, as 19 percent to 30 percent of women in this age group exhibit bulimic behaviors; 11 percent of high school women may be affected.[2] Athletes in particular are most often affected, especially those who participate in sports in which success is dependent on thin body types, such as ballet, gymnastics, figure skating, track, and cross-country running. Sixty-two percent of women in these sports report eating disorders. However, like other eating disorders, obtaining truly accurate data is difficult due to the secretive nature of this disease, and many of those affected do not seek treatment until they are very ill. Moderate cases may go unnoticed and therefore unrecognized. And, like anorexia, only a small percentage (10 percent) of those affected by bulimia are males. Bulimia has serious medical side effects, as 10 percent of individuals suffering from bulimia will die from starvation, cardiac arrest, other medical complications, or suicide.[3] A complete physical exam is required to rule out other physical disorders manifested by mental states, and a full diagnostic interview performed by a licensed mental health professional must be made before an official diagnosis of bulimia can be made.

There is no solitary cause of eating disorders such as bulimia. The causes are numerous and vary from person to person. Despite the difficulty in isolating the exact causes of bulimia, research is discovering pertinent information relating to biologic, sociocultural, and psychological factors. Biologically related issues include genetic influences that predispose certain people to different types of behaviors that may lead to the development of eating disorders. Definitive, albeit partial, contributing factors to the development of bulimia include genetic inheritability,[4] sexual abuse,[5] strained parental relationship,[6] and even gastric dysfunction.[7] In addition to the multifactorial causes of bulimia, the role of nutrition in disease development and propagation has been insufficiently explored. The role of nutritional fueling of the body and its effect on health can be applied to a disorder such as bulimia as well, for it truly is a psychiatric symptom, beginning with alterations in a person's self-perception.

An interesting nutritionally related causative factor in the development of bulimia is the relationship between a brain neurotransmitter, serotonin, and its effect on appetite. Dysregulation of serotonin function in the brain is hypothesized to contribute to the main symptoms of bulimia and anorexia and is currently well researched in the literature.[8] This research demonstrates the effect of serotonin on regulation of food intake (suggesting that an impairment of this neurotransmitter system may contribute to patterns of recurrent binging on foods) and other symptoms commonly seen in people with eating disorders, including alterations in moods and behavior; the therapeutic ability of drugs that act to increase serotonin levels in the brain has also been demonstrated. It is thought that serotonin receptors in the brain are somehow altered initially in people with bulimia and that further dysregulation is caused by extremes in dieting, binge eating, purging, drug abuse, and other psychosocial stressors that work together to manifest bulimic symptoms and behaviors.[9]

Studies investigating the use of both 5-hydroxytryptophan (5-HTP) and L-tryptophan (amino acid precursors of serotonin) in the treatment of eating disorders have mainly focused on their effect on balancing the serotonin systems of the brain. When given intravenously (at a dose of 0.4mg/kg), 5-HTP caused a hormonal response (attenuated elevation of prolactin levels) that was consistent with the finding that bulimic patients have less serotonin in their brains compared to healthy people.[10] Additionally, this study demonstrated that bulimics are unable to utilize 5-HTP as well as normal healthy control subjects. Another study using L-tryptophan to treat bulimic patients reported "significant" improvements both in mood and in decreased bulimic behavioral symptoms after giving these patients 1 gram per day of L-tryptophan in addition to 45 milligrams vitamin B-6, three times a day.[11] This study also speaks to the benefit of supplemental pyridoxine (vitamin B-6) in the treatment of this eating disorder. As with other nutrients, pyridoxine is one that appears to be more readily deficient in more "selective" eaters. Another interesting study of tryptophan and bulimia involved giving women with bulimia a diet that contained no tryptophan, and observing them for seven hours afterward.[12] This study reported a significant decrease in mood, increased ratings of body image concern, and feelings of loss of control regarding food intake. These findings necessitate further research in supplemental serotonin precursors (L-tryptophan and 5-HTP) in the treatment of bulimia. Although not a complete curative, supplementing the brain with these important precursors to essential brain chemicals may alter a person's neurobiology just enough to help regulate any chemical imbalance that may lead to dysfunction. (*Author's note:* Although tryptophan was banned from sale several years ago due to a flaw in one manufacturer's process, tryptophan is available by prescription today and may be obtained in a compounding pharmacy.)

INOSITOL

Inositol is an important compound with many uses in the human body. Although not an essential nutrient (the body does make some inositol), it is found in the diet and has several important physiologic functions. A fundamental component of the cellular membrane, inositol is also necessary for correct functioning of the brain and nervous system, among other functions elsewhere in the body. Part of the reason inositol is important in proper brain function is because it serves as a precursor in the messenger system for some serotonin receptors. Inositol has been investigated as a treatment for several neurologically related disorders, and its role in bulimia continues to be uncovered. A group of bulimic patients were given 18 grams of inositol intramuscularly for six weeks.[13] Using symptomatic scoring tests, some of the people taking inositol improved by 50 percent in comparison to subjects taking placebo, and one subject who had not previously responded to pharmaceutical treatment (Fluoxetine) responded so favorably to the inositol treatment that they eventually achieved remission of bulimia after continuing inositol use. Side effects noted in this study were mild gastrointestinal upset, which was resolved by lowering the dose by 6 grams. In comparison to another clinical trial in which the efficacy of Fluoxetine in the treatment of bulimia was studied,[14] the results from the inositol study are comparable to the effectiveness of Fluoxetine in the treatment of bulimia.[15] This is an exciting example of the effectiveness and possible use of nutritional supplements in the treatment, prevention, and cure of disease. More research surrounding this nutrient is necessary in order to further define its role in bulimia and its effect on proper brain function. Regardless, it is interesting that as a major constituent of cells in the human body, adding this to the diet of persons with nuerochemical imbalances leads to the correction and balancing of those systems.

ZINC

Among other nutrients studied in bulimia, the role of zinc in this disease has been investigated in fair detail. The second most abundant trace element in the body (approximately 2 grams),[16] zinc is used as a catalyst in nearly 100 different enzyme systems in the body.[17] It serves as a cofactor in the synthesis of neuro-transmitters and plays a role in the regulation of gene expression and behavior and learning. Because of its important role in so many metabolic systems in the body, zinc deficiency may have several effects on the nature of bulimia. A defi-ciency of zinc was found in 40 percent of bulimic patients in one study and is speculated to enhance the chronic nature of altered eating behaviors in these patients.[18] Another study supplied bulimic patients with a large dose of zinc (120 milliliters of zinc sulfate for an average of 8.3 days) in order to determine its ef-fect on bulimia.[19] These patients experienced decreased indices on two separate scales designed to measure patients' self-perception (the Multidimensional Body-Self Relations Questionnaire and the Eating Disorder Inventory), meaning that the zinc supplementation was beneficial in reducing patients' self-reported feel-ings of disease symptoms. This same investigator reports that using a dose of 9.1 to 18.2 milligrams per day (supplied in a form of liquid zinc 40–80 milliliters) lead to improvements in both bulimic and anorexic symptoms. From the results of these studies, it appears that zinc may play a role in preventing the cycle of bulimia in various ways. More research of this nutrient is needed in the treat-ment and prevention of bulimia.

People with bulimia are often found to have several deficiencies of vitamins, minerals, and electrolytes in their bodies due to the purgative nature of the dis-ease. Constant binging followed by regurgitation continually depletes the body and leads to cumulative nutritional deficiencies. Although current research has not plied into these effects beyond regular physiologic illness due to deficiency, deprivation of nutrients may very well serve to continue the bulimic cycle, with more binging leading to increased deficiencies, never allowing the brain, where this disease originates, to gain a foothold in balancing the disease process. This phenomenon has been explained in the research, where investigators explored the relationship between vitamin status and clinical evaluation of both bulimic and anorexic patients.[20] These researches observed that vitamin deficiencies in patients with eating disorders lead to altered neuropsychological status and can be contributory to cognitive dysfunction. Not only are vitamins found in deficient amounts in bulimics, but minerals and electrolytes are notably decreased as well. Halting the bulimic cycle may be achievable when these essential nutrients are replaced in the patient. Another study investigating nutrient replacement in bulimia revealed that in comparison to stress management treatment, nutritional management causes a more rapid improvement in overall eating behavior, quicker decreases in binging frequency, and decreased binge eating overall, leading researchers to conclude that nutritional management should be the first line of therapy when treating the bulimic patient.[21]

Nutritional management for the bulimic (in an effort to prevent progression of the disease and to treat already depleted nutrient stores that lead to disaffective states of neurology that, in turn, lead to increased bulimic behavior) should include replacement of all vitamins and minerals in supplemental form, in addition, of course, to attempts at consuming and maintaining a healthy diet (including appropriate counseling). Electrolyte deficiencies, namely potassium, are another common result of fluid loss and dietary restriction. Hypokalemia (low blood levels of potassium) is a common occurrence in bulimics,[22] and deficiency of this electrolyte is life threatening, leading to cardiovascular complications (dysrrhythmia).

CONCLUSION

Research is just beginning to uncover the complexity of bulimia. We have much to learn regarding the role of nutrients in this disease. However, some research is beginning to show promise in the area of using nutritional replacement to attenuate some bulimic behavior. Placing more focus on this area (rather than treating bulimics as though they have a pharmacologic drug deficiency) may lead to improved physiologic and, in turn, neurologic functioning. Supplying bulimics with at least the earlier mentioned nutrients will undoubtedly assist them on their path to wellness, and even if such therapy leads to incremental improvement, this improvement may lead to just enough betterment to avert the chronic tendency of this disease.

Breaking the cycle of bulimia can take a very concerted effort on both the part of the patient and healthcare provider. In order to more easily achieve the goal at hand, supplementation with a good multivitamin and the nutrients mentioned above can ease the journey and allow for improved sense of "wellness" within the patient, allowing for heightened focus regarding the task at hand.

NUTRIENTS

- 5-HTP*
  150–300 milligrams per day

- L-tryptophan*
  1–1.5 grams per day
- Vitamin B-6
  45 milligrams three times per day
- Inositol*
  10–12 grams per day, divided doses
- Zinc
  15–20 milligrams per day

*Must be used under guidance of physician/provider if currently on medication.

Dementia

Dementia refers to the loss of cognitive or "thinking" neurologic function and is primarily attributable to changes in the brain resulting from disease or traumatic injury. Cognition is more properly defined as the process or act of thinking, perceiving, and learning; actions such as decision making, judgment, memory, spatial orientation, thinking, reasoning, and verbal communication are cognitive functions that are most often affected by dementia. Dementia can develop slowly over time or appear rather quickly. There are numerous causes of dementia (over 50 separate conditions are associated with dementia) that can either be reversible or irreversible. Irreversible forms of dementia include:

- Degenerative neurologic disorders: These include Alzheimer's disease (AD) (which accounts for 50–70 percent of all dementia cases), amyotrophic lateral sclerosis (Lou Gehrig's disease), Parkinson's disease, and other less-common degenerative diseases.
- Vascular disorders: Multi-infarct disease (the second most common cause of dementia) is a condition in which several small strokes occur throughout the brain leading to dementia and many other neurologic effects.
- Infectious disorders: AIDS dementia complex is a late form of HIV infection; Creutzfeldt-Jakob disease is a rapidly progressing fatal infection of the brain.
- Inherited disorders: These include Huntington's disease, which is a fatal hereditary disease that leads to the destruction of neurons and involves the emotional, intellectual, and movement centers of the brain.

Reversible forms of dementia include:

- Alcoholism: This can lead to thiamine (vitamin B-1) deficiency, causing Wernicke-Korsakoff syndrome.
- Infection: Infection by viruses, bacteria, and fungi that cause meningitis or encephalitis can temporarily lead to impaired cognition. Symptoms remit once the infectious process has been resolved.
- Chronic drug use/abuse: Pharmaceutical medications such as cough suppressants, barbiturates, benzodiazapenes, tricyclic antidepressants, monoamine oxidase inhibitors, anticholinergics, and digitalis can temporarily affect brain cognition.

Other causes of dementia include structural abnormalities, such as tumors, bleeding within the protective layers of the brain (chronic subdural hematoma), and increased pressure due to fluid retainment (hydrocephalus). Metabolic disorders including hypothyroidism (low functioning thyroid gland), hypoglycemia (low blood sugar), hypercalcemia (elevated blood calcium), and liver disease can all affect cognition and are generally reversible once the underlying causes are addressed.

INCIDENCE AND PREVALENCE

Dementia affects nearly 7 million people in the United States, and greater than 1 million adults in the United States are diagnosed each year with some form of dementia-causing brain disease.[1] Five percent to 8 percent of people over the age of 65 have some form of dementia, and in people over 65, the number doubles every five years over that age. Of people 85 years or older, 35.8 percent have moderate to severe memory impairment, and this population is the fastest growing sector of the American population.[2] Thirteen million to 16 million adults in the United States are currently affected with common brain disorders and diseases leading to dementia.[3] The prevalence of dementia has increased greatly over the last 20–30 years; this is possibly attributable to both increased diagnostic measures as well as increased longevity and its accompanying health factors.

RISK FACTORS

Several risk factors exist for dementia. Advanced age is often considered the greatest risk factor for dementia, and genetic inheritance (Alzheimer's or Huntington's diseases) accounts for a large portion as well. Whereas conventional medicine applies the cause of dementia to specific conditions of the brain, the focus of this chapter is to point out the origins of these conditions themselves. Medical problems such as tumors, cardiovascular disease, head injury, and other systemic diseases, although considered causes of dementia, are really only conditions that set the brain up for dementia. More specifically, deficiencies of the vitamins B-12, folic acid, and B-1 (thiamine) are definitively identified as risk factors that lead to the symptoms of dementia.

SYMPTOMS

A person affected by dementia will experience behavior and personality changes depending on the area(s) of the brain affected. Oftentimes, impairment of memory is the first sign of dementia, which can be manifested by forgetting one's own birth date or address or not recognizing familiar faces. As the dementia progresses, verbal communication, orientation in time and space, problem-solving judgment, and decision making may progressively decline. Sadly, personality is affected as well, wherein the person may make inappropriate remarks and have less emotional control.

NUTRITIONAL FACTORS

The role of nutritional factors in dementia has become popularized in the medical research. Investigative studies are discovering definitive links between nutritional deficits and dementia; vitamin deficiencies are clearly associated with some forms of dementia, and replacement of these factors leads to remission of dementia symptoms. Undoubtedly, nutrition plays a role in the aging process. Investigation into the role of nutrients and the aging process has indicated that subclinical deficiencies (lowered amounts of nutrients not quite high enough to cause physically apparent illness) of antioxidant vitamins like vitamins C, E, and beta-carotene, vitamin B-12, vitamin B-6, and folate may be evident long before dementia symptoms appear.[4] One of the best-established nutritional factors in dementia is folic acid. Folate, more specifically known as folic acid, refers to the various forms of this essential vitamin. Once absorbed by the body, folic acid is reduced to a form called tetrahydrofolate (THF). THF plays an integral role in the enzyme systems that deal with cellular metabolism. Folic acid is indirectly necessary for the final step in DNA synthesis and exerts a protective role on this vital genetic structure.[5] A deficiency of folic acid will lead to disturbances in the cellular division, leading to both early cell death (apoptosis) and hastened cell death.[6] It is clear from this information why a deficiency of this nutrient has an effect on the brain itself. Brain cells are notoriously fragile and are not replaceable.

The main role of folic acid in prevention of dementia lies within its ability to lower blood levels of the amino acid homocysteine. Homocysteine is a byproduct of incomplete methionine metabolism. Methionine is an essential amino acid (it is not produced in the body, therefore it is required in our diets). Elevated blood levels of homocysteine are considered a primary risk factor for atherosclerotic disease, and investigators are now looking at the link between hyperhomocysteinemia,* atherosclerosis, folate, and dementia. One such

*For hyperhomocysteinemia, vitamin B-12 in a dose of 500 mcg in combination with 0.5 to 5 mg folic acid and 16.5 mg pyridoxine has been used.

investigation looked at recent data that indicates people with low levels of folic acid and concordant elevated homocysteine levels have increased risk of Alzheimer's disease (of which dementia is primary symptom).[7] As a part of this same study, researchers determined that folic acid deficiency and homocysteinemia allowed for neuronal DNA to become more easily damaged by oxidation, setting them up for increased attack and resultant damage from amyloid beta-peptide, the protein form associated with altered neurological architecture (a primary anatomic finding in AD). This study in particular sheds some light on exactly how folic acid protects the brain from dementia. A large amount of research is being generated regarding homocysteine and its negative effects on cardiovascular health. Homocysteine, considered a primary risk factor for both atherosclerosis and stroke, is known to cause indirect and direct vascular damage that implicates elevated levels of homocysteine in vascular dementia and increased risk of multiple brain infarcts.[8] It is currently hypothesized that folate, homocysteine, cardiovascular disease, and dementia are interrelated, with folate deficiency being the initiating factor in this cascade of disease events leading to dementia. Homocysteine, as a direct link to dementia of both cognitive decline (age-related) and vascular dementia, can be controlled by other nutritional factors outside of folic acid (cobalamin [B-12] and pyridoxine [B-6]). Deficiencies of all three nutrients (folic acid, B-12, B-6) are common in elderly people, and a correlation exists between low levels of these nutrients and AD, a primary cause of dementia.[9]

B-6 AND B-12

B-6 (pyridoxine) is important in the brain because of its role in the synthesis and metabolism of neurotransmitters (GABA, serotonin, norepinephrine, and dopamine) and deficiencies can affect nerve transmission. Whereas vitamin B-12 is necessary to maintain neurologic health, a deficiency of this vitamin leads to neurologic damage via an inability to produce myelin nerve sheaths and, when progressive, leads to nerve degeneration (axon and nerve head).[10] Deficiency of this vitamin can also lead to functional deficiency of folate, as folate is not usable without B-12. Additionally, deficiency of B-12 can lead to memory loss, mood changes, and personality changes (key signs of dementia) without any overt clinical signs of the deficiency.[11] The nutritional cofactors pyridoxine and cobalamin play a role in the attenuation of homocysteine levels in addition to folic acid. For the most part, a large amount of the research on these vitamins and homocysteine attribute vascular damage to elevated homocysteine, rather that deficiencies of the vitamins. Although the point can be argued that low levels of B-6, B-12, and folate lead to high levels of homocysteine, which in turn damages the vasculature leading to dementia, other mechanisms of vitamin deficiency and dementia are being explored. A study investigating the application of B-12, B-6, and folate in people with mild cognitive impairment and elevated homocysteine levels determined that this treatment lead to improved functioning of the blood-brain barrier (a physiologic protective layer encasing the brain protecting it from unwanted/dangerous substances in the blood stream) and normalized homocysteine levels.[12] Additionally, none of the patients in this study progressed into dementia during the study period, and cognitive status appeared to stabilize. Studies such as this hint at the role of these vitamins in exerting a protective role against dementia for reasons possible other than their lowering effect on homocysteine. Another survey that examined the levels of B-12 in elderly people with varied levels of dementia demonstrated that lower B-12 levels were more common in older subjects and associated with significantly lower scores on mental status (Mini-Mental State Exam) and dementia scales (Blessed Dementia Scale).[13] These and other results lead researchers to conclude that low vitamin B-12 levels are associated with increased overall cognitive impairment in AD. Vitamin B-12 is known to be associated with other neuropsychiatric disorders and is probably more frequent in these conditions. An excellent example of the role of these vitamins in treating neuropsychiatric disorders including dementia is exemplified by the case of a patient with psychosis secondary to B-12 deficiency.[14] This patient exhibited no overt physical signs of the deficiency and experienced a complete remission of symptoms upon receiving a B-12 and folate replacement and remained stable for the next three months. Assessment of vitamin B-12, B-6, and folate should be determined in all patients at risk for or currently experiencing any form of dementia. This section only highlights a small portion of the positive literature surrounding the use of these vitamins in dementia states. Their efficacy in treatment further supports their role as preventive treatments in the development of dementia. Research clearly delineates their role in homocysteine metabolism and new investigations are discovering other ways in which these nutrients can prevent dementia.

MINERALS IN DEMENTIA

The role of minerals in dementia and brain function has been explored to some extent in the literature. Calcium, one of the major minerals in the body, plays a large role in nerve transmission as well as neurotransmitter and hormone release and storage. Research points to a deficiency of calcium as a contributing factor to dementia. Calcium is normally found in large amounts in the body (99 percent of which is located in the bones and teeth). Despite the high levels of calcium in these tissues, calcium is needed in so many areas of the body that compartmental deficiencies can be quite common (blood, extracellular fluid, muscle, and other tissues) and may or may not be accompanied by symptoms. A review paper theorized that chronically low levels of calcium might contribute to the development of plaques and neurofibrillary tangles (hallmarks of Alzheimer's disease) because of the role that calcium plays in the growth and development of microtubules in the brain.[15] (Microtubules, in a gross description, make up a basic part of brain microanatomy. Irregularities in microtubule formation may affect memory, learning, and development of plaques). This paper hypothesizes that because of this relationship between calcium and microtubules, adequate supplementation and availability of calcium may protect against cognitive decline. In a population study in an area of Japan with higher than average incidence of amyotrophic lateral sclerosis (ALS) and parkinsonism dementia (PD), the local environmental factors of low calcium and magnesium found in the soil and drinking water and their effect on the brain have been examined.[16] The results of this research have led the investigators to conclude that low dietary intake of calcium and magnesium over a long period of time may contribute to the formation of ALS and PD and consequent dementia.

Magnesium may play a role in the development of dementia in addition to calcium, and some relationships have been elucidated linking deficiency of magnesium and increased brain uptake of aluminum (aluminum may be considered a pathogenic factor in AD). As the most abundant positive ion in the body, magnesium takes part in over 300 cellular reactions,[17] and it is required for nervous and muscular electric potential generation as well as transmission of nervous impulses in the body.[18] Elderly people are at an increased risk for magnesium and other mineral deficiencies due to prescription drug use, inadequate intake of minerals, and less-than-optimal gastrointestinal function (absorption). Magnesium deficiency has recently been identified as a contributing factor in the aging process, and deficiency conditions are associated with AD and cardiovascular disorders in addition to other systemic illnesses.[19] Magnesium deficiency, as mentioned previously, may be solely due to inadequate intake and absorption. Other theories hold that intake of aluminum, a neurotoxic metal, may inhibit magnesium-dependent enzyme systems or that magnesium transport into the brain is altered, whereby aluminum transport is accelerated, leading to inadequate magnesium levels in the brain.[20] An additional study compared magnesium levels in various sections of the brains of control subjects versus those with AD-induced dementia.[21] Levels of magnesium were significantly decreased in the brain sections of the patients with AD compared to the control group. Aside from the roles mentioned here, magnesium is an important mineral for the cardiovascular system. Low intake of magnesium is associated with hypertension, atherosclerosis, and stroke.[22] This makes supplementation with magnesium even more important for anyone at risk for the previously mentioned diseases and especially for those at risk for dementia. Vascular dementia (a result of multiple ministrokes throughout the brain) has origins in hypertension, atherosclerosis, and, of course, stroke. Much more information is needed regarding the roles of both calcium and magnesium in the development of diseases that lead to dementia. The research gathered so far provides interesting insight to the problem; ensuring adequate intake of these minerals may very well supply a protective element against the development of dementia.

BOTANICAL MEDICINES

Ginkgo biloba

Several botanical medicines can be used in treating and preventing dementias. Perhaps the best-known (and researched) botanical medicine for dementia is *Ginkgo biloba*. The medicine from this plant is derived from the leaves and is used to treat many conditions, such as cerebral vascular insufficiency, memory loss, mood disturbances, cognitive disorders secondary to depression, and seasonal depression, associated with the vascular system in addition to vascular, mixed, and Alzheimer's dementia. The majority of research on ginkgo points to its efficacy in dementia. In fact, ginkgo is so effective at treating dementia, it is registered as the medication of choice in Europe for treatment of dementia.[23] Ginkgo's actions result in improved blood flow properties in the brain; protection against ischemia and hypoxia in the brain; improved nerve cell energy metabolism; protection against swelling and protection of myelin (the insulating layer surrounding nerve cells that allows for nerve transmission); antioxidant and free radical scavenging activity; and nonspecific effects on neurotransmitters and their receptors.[24] In an analysis of all studies performed on ginkgo and its effect on dementia, a review of the literature revealed that on an overall basis, improvement in cognition and function were associated with ginkgo, and no significant difference between ginkgo and placebo existed between study participants who experienced adverse effects. (There were no more negative side effects in those taking a placebo in comparison to those taking ginkgo.)[25] Ginkgo is a novel, safe medicine for treatment of dementia and has been shown to be as effective if not more so than standard antidementia medications currently employed, with comparably few side effects.[26]

Salvia miltiorrhiza

Salvia, also known as Dan Shen or red sage root, has been used historically in Chinese medicine for the treatment of dementia. *Salvia* has been shown by modern research to improve microcirculation, dilate blood vessels and improve circulation, and reduce blood clotting times.[27] *Salvia* was also employed traditionally for circulation problems such as angina and ischemic stoke; the root of the plant contains the medically active constituents. In experiments designed to test the ability of this plant medicine to prevent neurologic ischemia, extracts of the root were able to reduce the size of brain infarcts in animals by 30 percent and 37 percent using two standardized extracts (Tanshinones IIA [TsIIA] and IIB [TsIIB]).[28] Additionally, the size in reduction of the brain infarcts was accompanied by a comparable reduction in observed neurological deficit. Another animal study utilizing an extract of *Salvia* demonstrated a preventive action on age-induced learning deficit.[29] Such action may hint at possible uses for this herbal medicine in the treatment of age-related cognitive decline; however, further research is needed. Another study exploring the neuroprotective effects of *Salvia* demonstrated that an extract of the herb was 88.24 percent effective in treating cerebral infarction, possibly by reducing free radical damage in the brain.[30] Widely studied in China, *Salvia* is a botanical medicine that has potential protective and curative effects on dementia and may prove to be a significant treatment.

Huperzine A

Huperzine A is an alkaloid extract from the club moss *Huperzia serrata* and *lycopodium selago*. It works as a reversible inhibitor of acetylcholinesterase (AChE) and crosses the blood-brain barrier.[31] It can exert this activity for three to four hours and produces varying degrees of acetylcholine elevation in different brain locations, with maximal values of up to 125 percent.[32] In comparison to a prescription drug (tacrine) with a similar mechanism of action, huperzine A was found to be 64 times stronger and to have a longer duration of action.[33] In addition, huperzine A was shown to significantly improve memory in comparison to tacrine.[34] Huperzine A is used to treat AD and other causes of dementia, memory and learning impairment, and age-related cognitive decline and demonstrates protection against neurotoxic agents.[35] Huperzine is also used for improvement of cognitive function, behavioral function in AD, and myasthenia gravis due to its anticholinergic effects. Additionally, it may reduce cellular injury from strokes and epilepsy.[36] A study using huperzine A in AD patients showed improvement in memory, cognition, and behavioral function after only eight weeks of treatment.[37] In another study, huperzine A was able to significantly improve memory function in patients with multi-infarct and senile dementia after two to four weeks of treatment.[38] It is estimated that huperzine A has been used to treat over 100,000 people in China with AD and other forms of dementia. This botanical extract works similarly to prescription medications for dementia; however, it seems to be more effective with fewer side effects at this time. The benefits of using botanical medicines such as ginkgo, *Salvia*, and huperzine A are the wide-ranging protective effects in addition to their effects on dementia itself. By providing neuronal protection, the use of these medicines can serve to prevent the onset of disease and possibly restore function that would have otherwise been lost to the disease process. For other botanical medicines that are useful in dementia, refer to the chapter on Alzheimer's disease.

PHARMACEUTICALS AND DEMENTIA

One of the largest causative factors for dementia in the elderly (and all other ages as well) is the use of certain pharmaceuticals and the phenomenon of polypharmacy. The average number of pharmaceuticals that the average American was prescribed in the year 2000 was 10.4 (at an average cost of $45.27 each).[39] Prescriptions drugs are important cause of dementia. Seniors are already at an increased risk of pharmaceutical-induced dementia due to high levels of medication use, slower and less effective metabolism of drugs, and imbalances of neurotransmitters. A review article of the drugs with the highest potential for causing dementia in the elderly included medications such as benzodiazapenes, opiods, anticholinergics, and tricyclic antidepressants; other medication listed as having some effect on cognition include the older antihypertensive drugs reserpine and clonidine, as well as thiazide diuretics, calcium blockers, ACE inhibitors, and beta blockers.[40] However, this is not an all-inclusive list. Remember that individuals may be susceptible to dementia from any medication, and the effect of multiple drugs that do not cause dementia alone may lead to this symptom when combined. It is important to identify not only the more malevolent drugs when it comes to dementia, but also to investigate drug combinations in susceptible individuals as a possible cause of dementia. Close supervision of such prescriptions requires intensive management, and consideration of the nutritional side effects of these drugs (many pharmaceuticals are known to deplete stores of vitamins and minerals in the body) may lead to a more proactive management of dementia in these patients.

CONCLUSION

The treatment and prevention of dementia in its many forms is achievable using relatively simple vitamin replacement (folic acid, B-12, and B-6), the minerals calcium and magnesium, and several different botanical medicines. Combined use of these medicines can work to alleviate some symptoms of dementia, and if employed prior to the onset of disease symptoms, may very well offset or prevent disease advent and acceleration.

Cognitive decline and fluctuations can be brought on by many physiological circumstances and external environmental factors. Fostering optimal nutritional support is essential to achieve and maintain ultimate mental acuity and ability. There is also growing evidence that investing time into mental exercises and activities such as crossword puzzles, reading, and word finds can assist in maintaining "mental tone." Indeed, to a large degree the mind is also governed by the input-equals-output paradigm.

NUTRIENTS

- Folate
  5–10 milligrams per day
- B-6
  100 milligrams per day
- B-12
  500–1,000 micrograms per day
- Calcium
  300–400 milligrams per day

- Magnesium
  300–400 milligrams per day
- Antioxidant support
  A supplemental form of antioxidant nutrients should be consumed two
  times per day

BOTANICALS

- *Ginkgo biloba*
  300 milligrams twice per day
- *Salvia miltiorrhiza*
  Crude herb: 1–2 grams per day
- Huperzine A
  50–200 micrograms twice per day

Depression

The journey of life is painted with a vast array of emotions. Good, bad, and everything in between, it is a large part of the human condition that we all feel something, at all times. However, feelings of depression should not last for more than a few days to even weeks at a time at most, throughout the course of "normal" living. Approximately 19 million American adults suffer from clinical depression in a given year; this number is equivalent to nearly 9.5 percent of the adult population.[1] Almost twice as many women (12 percent) as men (6.6 percent) are affected by depressive disorders each year; these numbers are equivalent to 12.4 million women and 6.4 million men in the United States.[2] Depressive disorder (which includes major depressive disorder, dysthymic disorder, and bipolar disorder) accounts for three of the leading causes of disability in the United States and other developed nations (major depressive disorder ranks as number 1); many people who suffer from one mental disorder will suffer from additional disorders[3]; for example, many people with depression suffer from anxiety as well. The focus of this chapter is on major depressive disorder; treatment recommendations can be extended to dysthymia as well. Refer to separate chapters on bipolar and anxiety disorders for more information.

Major depressive disorder can develop at almost any age, but it occurs most commonly in a person's mid-20s; dysthymic disorder, however, often begins in childhood, adolescence, or early adulthood.[4] Depressive disorder is a mental illness that involves the mind as well as the body; it disrupts the way sufferers sleep and eat, as well as how they think of the world and themselves. It is not simply an extended "down" mood, the lack of mental or personal strength, or laziness. Untreated, people with depression can have symptoms for years on end. Defined according to the *Diagnostic and Statistical Manual of Mental Disorders*, fourth edition (*DSM-IV*),[5] depressive disorders can be defined in the following manner:

- *Major depression* has a combination of symptoms that occur with nearly every aspect of life (work, study, sleeping, eating, enjoyment) and can occur only once or several times throughout life.
- *Dysthymia* is a less severe form of depression that includes similar but milder symptoms that may be more chronic, preventing a person from ever feeling entirely "right." People with dysthymia can experience major depressive episodes as well.

SYMPTOMS

The American Psychiatric Association bases its diagnosis of depression on the following criteria:

- Loss of appetite and/or weight or overeating and weight gain
- Insomnia, early morning awakening, or oversleeping
- Physical inactivity or hyperactivity
- Loss of interest or pleasure in hobbies and activities that were once enjoyed, including sex
- Decreased energy or fatigue
- Feelings of guilt, worthlessness, or helplessness
- Difficulty concentrating, remembering, or making decisions
- Thoughts of death or suicide; even attempts at suicide

The presence of five of the cited symptoms is indicative of clinical depression, whereas the presence of four indicates probable depression. Symptoms must be present for at least one month to qualify as depression. Each person is different and experiences varying grades, severity, and types of symptoms that may even change over time. Other symptoms of depression may include: feelings of hopelessness or pessimism, persistent sadness, anxiousness or emptiness, and restlessness or irritability. Persistent physical symptoms that do not respond to standard treatment, such as headaches, digestive disorders, and chronic pain may also be present in depression.

CAUSES OF DEPRESSION

Depression has several origins. Some forms run in families, hinting at an inheritable (genetic) link; other forms can occur in people with no family history of depression. Regardless of form, however, both brain structure and function changes are associated with this disease. People with low self-esteem or who are overly pessimistic or easily overwhelmed by life stressors are prone to depressive illnesses—this may represent a possible personality susceptibility to depression. However, more often than not, various factors combine to cause a major depressive episode. Serious medical illnesses (heart disease, cancer, etc.), relationship stresses, a serious loss, financial problems, and even positive life changes may combine to cause a depressive episode. In addition, once a person has suffered from a major depressive episode, he or she may become more at risk from future episodes that may be triggered from lesser stresses. In short, combinations of psychological, environmental, and genetic factors can combine to bring about depression.

EVALUATION AND DIAGNOSIS

Determining if a person is suffering from depression involves a trained mental health professional taking a detailed history of symptom onset, duration, and severity; past or current treatments; and if they have ever occurred before. Other interview information regarding drug or alcohol use (pain, whether mental or physical, is often self-medicated), family history of depression, and suicidal thoughts should be obtained. Additionally, a mental status examination will be administered in order to determine the extent of depression from which the person may be suffering. Note: These steps and previously mentioned diagnostic criteria have been abbreviated in this text. Readers are directed to a more thorough workup of depression in the *DSM-IV*.

NUTRITIONAL FACTORS

Like every other mental illness, we all too often focus on the presenting symptoms of the disease. Treating symptoms in many cases can be highly beneficial for the patient. However, in order to delve deeper into medicine, we can look at body chemistry as the origin of dysfunctional neurologic function and depression; nutritional factors in depression have been researched in some detail and certain botanical medicines provide excellent treatment for depression and its origins.

Folic Acid

Folic acid's role in depression has been extensively investigated in the research. The information indicates that folate may play several roles in depression, as deficiency and low folate status have been linked in clinical studies to depression, persistent depressive symptoms, and poor antidepressant response. In a systematic review of research databases covering trials in which folate was used to augment treatment of depression, it was determined that folate has a potential role to supplement other treatments for depression; additionally it was determined that no adverse effects were encountered from the use of folate and other standard depression treatments.[6] The prevalence of folate deficiency in the United States may accompany certain numbers of people with depression; this establishes folate deficiency as an associated risk. A study investigating this link determined that people who met the criteria for either lifelong major depression or dysthymia had lower folate concentrations than healthy people without depression.[7] The sample group in this study was taken from different ethnicities ranging in ages from 15 to 39. From this study, the authors suggest that folate supplementation be administered to depressed people for a year following their episode. Because of the chronic nature of depression, and the associated future susceptibility, a lifetime supplement program seems to be more advisable (not to mention the other benefits of folate on homocysteine, etc.). Clinical observations and recent advances in the understanding of folate in brain metabolism have somewhat defined the role of folate and depression; folate deficiency commonly leads to neuropsychiatric symptoms of depression.[8] Additionally, low levels of folic acid have been demonstrated to result in poorer response to antidepressant medications, namely selective serotonin reuptake inhibitors.[9] Establishing an even greater tie to depression, serum and red blood cell levels of folate were found to be significantly lower in patients with major depressive disorder than healthy controls, and lower serum folate concentrations were associated with a greater severity of depression.[10] From just these few examples of studies tying folate to depression symptoms, it stands clear that folic acid should be one of the first supplements considered in the prevention and treatment of depression.

Pyridoxine

Pyridoxine (vitamin B-6) undergoes conversion in the body to two coenzymes, pyridoxal phosphate and pyridoxamine phosphate, and is subsequently used in numerous metabolic processes. One aspect of these reactions is the synthesis of brain neurotransmitters such as GABA, serotonin (a key neurotransmitter in depression), norepinephrine, and dopamine.[11] Pyridoxine is beneficial in lessening symptoms of depression in major depression as well as premenstrual syndrome.[12] The usefulness of pyridoxine in modulating central production of neurotransmitters is further evidence that deficiency, or inadequate supplies, may contribute to neurotransmitter dysregulation. High doses of pyridoxine may serve to ameliorate certain dysphoric mental states that are particularly associated with hopelessness or cynicism and to improve prognosis in this condition.[13] Pyridoxine more than likely exerts its beneficial effects on the brains of people with depression via its function as a cofactor for the enzyme 5-hydroxytryptophan decarboxylase, which serves in the production of serotonin (decreased levels of serotonin are one of the main physiologic causes of depression).[14] Although inadequate amounts of pyridoxine are implicated in depressive disorders, actual blood levels of this and other B vitamins associated with depression are not always found to be as low in patients exhibiting symptoms; blood vitamin levels do not reflect true brain vitamin function nor are they reflective of symptom severity in all cases.[15] Pyridoxine is another important vitamin with protective effects against depression in that it assists in the production of key neurotransmitters that may be deficient in this disease.

Vitamin C

Vitamin C, or ascorbic acid, is a nutrient that seems to always capture attention no matter what investigational study it undergoes. Part of the reason for this is that so many benefits are derived from vitamin C in such wide-ranging medical conditions. Although it is not new information, vitamin C does have benefits in depression and is also implicated as a precursor to the disease when deficient in the body. In a review paper studying the clinical effects of ascorbic acid deficiency in people, Hodges et al. noted that depression is one of the first symptoms of scurvy in humans who were experimentally subjected to deficient vitamin C diets.[16] Indeed, scurvy is relatively rare in modern life; however, diets low in vitamin C are not, especially with processed food diets on the rise. Further studies on vitamin C and scurvy revealed an interesting link between psychiatric patients and vitamin C levels. A study of psychiatric patients (some of whom had bipolar depression) revealed that many were in a state of low vitamin C saturation, or "subacute" scurvy.[17] This and another study involving a similar population of patients also demonstrated decreased vitamin C load, or borderline scurvy, without actually manifesting the symptoms of this disease.[18] Patients with depression and other psychiatric diseases may be in states of subacute scurvy; defining the actual point of insufficiency is difficult, especially today when RDAs are designed to supply the minimal amount of nutrients to prevent disease. Receiving just enough nutrients to prevent disease does not mean that a state of optimal health is achieved. In order to prevent illness and to be in a state of optimal health, sufficient amounts of nutrients are needed, above and beyond the amounts said to prevent disease only.

Cobalamin (B-12)

The role of vitamin B-12 in depression is similar to that of pyridoxine (B-6) and folate. Deficiency of B-12 may lead to symptoms of depression, among other neuropsychiatric symptoms.[19] In fact, deficiency of B-12 accompanies many depressive cases in which folate is low as well; deficiencies of both vitamins are common in major depression.[20] Although bodily stores of B-12 are higher (generally), a relative deficiency or inefficient utilization of this vitamin leads to a functional deficiency of folate[11] (folate depends on B-12 for its own metabolism). If this were the case, a person would have an especially difficult time manufacturing the neurotransmitters that are typically in short supply in depression (serotonin) because of the effect that folate has on serotonin production. Additionally, depression is a symptom of B-12 deficiency itself and may be manifested in addition to other neurologic symptoms when B-12 is deficient.[21] More specifically, B-12 is required in the synthesis of S-adenosylmethionine, which serves as a precursor to neurotransmitter production, as well as in the manufacture of proteins, DNA, and cellular phospholipids (components of cell membrane that regulate cellular metabolism).[22] A study of 700 older women designed to determine whether women with B-12 or folate deficiency were prone to depression revealed that those with a B-12 deficiency were more than two times likely to be severely depressed in comparison to nondeficient subjects.[23] Supplementation of B-12 along with folate is highly important to ensure that the effects of both vitamins are rendered effective. (Folate is more dependent on B-12 than vice versa.) Folate and B-12 are also necessary for the prevention of other neurologic diseases such as Alzheimer's disease and other dementias.

5-HTP

A precursor substance to the neurotransmitter serotonin is 5-Hydroxytryptophan (5-HTP). It is related to the amino acid L-tryptophan, which is converted in the body into 5-HTP, and it is able to cross into the brain and augment supplies of serotonin. Because of this, 5-HTP acts as an effective treatment for depression, as well as other conditions such as insomnia. Neurobiologists currently recognize insufficient activity of serotonin (including other neurotransmitters) as a key element in the pathogenesis of depression. One review article of the various precursor treatments for depression expressed that such therapies hold a therapuetic value in the treatment of depression and that more research is needed to confirm additional efficacy.[24] Another review article expressed the efficacy of 5-HTP as high in treating disorders like depression, in addition to binge eating and insomnia.[25] Employed as a nutritional food supplement, 5-HTP is a beneficial adjunctive treatment for patients with depression. Although the greatest task in medicine is identifying and removing the cause of disease (which in most cases of depression seems to be an inadequate activity/supply of serotonin), supplying this nutrient can act as a bridge to bolster the patient's neurochemistry while other nutritional treatments can be employed that may in principle restore brain neurotransmitter dysfunction. As the patient's symptoms decrease, tapering of supplemental 5-HTP will allow the patient to continue functioning normally, with fewer supplements.

BOTANICAL MEDICINE

Hypericum perforatum

One of the most investigated botanical medicines from a phytochemical aspect, St. John's Wort is a viable alternative to standard pharmacotherapy for depression. A literature review of the effects of St. John's Wort (Hypericum perfoliatum) reveals the efficacy of this herbal medicine in several biochemical pathways that play a central role in depression and its pathogenesis, including the monoamine oxidase (MAO), serotonin, gamma-amino butyric acid (GABA), and dopamine neurotransmitter systems.[26] Although no single constituent of the herb has been indicated in the plant's effectiveness in treating depressive disorders, the efficacy of St. John's Wort is similar to that of standard pharmaceutical therapeutics.[27] This being said, two main constituents of *Hypericum* are thought to play a major role in the plant's effect on depression. In addition to the originally identified active principle hypericin, other constituents such as hyperforin, adhyperforin, and other related compounds are thought to play an active role in the modulation of depression.[28] The extracts of this plant have been intensely studied for the last decade and are now considered a viable medicine in standard antidepressant therapy. A review of the mechanism of action(s) of *Hypericum*'s constituents include the abilities to bind to GABA receptors, down-regulate beta-adrenergic receptors, and up-regulate serotonin 5-HT(2) receptors; these effects lead to positive changes in neurotransmitter concentrations in areas of the brain that are implicated in depression.[29]

Hypericum displays a currently unparalleled broad profile in its effects on neurotransmitters. Because of this, *Hypericum* demonstrates effectiveness in a number of pharmacology models of antidepressant efficacy.[30] St. John's Wort is tolerated well by patients and has a very low incidence of adverse affects when taken properly. Despite this benefit, several drug interactions have been uncovered with *Hypericum* that are clinically significant. A recent double-blind, randomized, placebo-controlled trial involving 375 patients with depression taking 300 milligrams three times a day of standardized *Hypericum* extract produced a significantly greater reduction in Hamilton depression scale scores and was more effective in patients with higher depression symptom scores.[31] This study concluded that *Hypericum* extract was more effective than placebo in treating mild to moderate depression, and patients taking the extract had no more negative side effects than those people taking placebo. An effective medicine with few, if any, side effects, *Hypericum* can be employed as a frontline therapy in the treatment of depression. This herb represents an ideal treatment for depression, and nutritional causes are being pursued as well.

CONCLUSION

Depression is a disease that has various origins of varied nature. Treating the patient nutritionally provides a base for stabilizing brain neurotransmitter function and may lead to stabilization of symptoms when treatment is continuous. The role of vitamin factors in this disease is further backed by interesting research highlighting the various roles in which they are known to contribute. Nutritional neurotransmitter precursors such as 5-HTP provide a very specific source of fuel for the brain, supplying it with the building blocks it needs to function correctly. St. John's Wort provides a highly effective natural medicine that can augment depression treatment, with few side effects, and can serve in place of standard pharmaceuticals that are often poorly tolerated.

Depression has been well documented throughout human history; ancient civilizations varied their perspective as to both the etiology and the treatments. Among the various treatments were bloodletting, spiritual interventions, fasting, and even transfusions with the blood of animals that were perceived as being more potent. Indeed, the true cause of the depression needs to be addressed so that the root cause can be eliminated. A healthy mind, body, and spirit fostered via a good diet, mental hygiene, exercise, and pursuit of deepened spirituality can all help augment quality of life. It is always important to note that depression is a serious health concern and warrants close and careful management and that some patients, regardless of natural medicine interventions, may need additional assistance with pharmaceutical agents.

NUTRIENTS

- Folate
  1–2 milligrams per day
- B-6
  5–10 milligrams
- Vitamin C
  1,000–2,000 milligrams
- B-12
  500 micrograms per day
- 5-HTP
  150–300 milligrams per day

BOTANICALS

- *Hypericum perforatum*
  300 milligrams three times per day (standardized to 0.3 percent hypericin or 4 percent hyperforin)

Hormonal Mental Health

This chapter, unlike the others in this book, takes a different approach in looking at optimal brain function by focusing on the body's hormones and how they are affected by nutritional and botanical supplementation. Not an overt disease condition, hormone irregularities and their effects can highly impact one's health and mental state of being. Hormone irregularities are common throughout the human health spectrum, and there is much we can do to assist in returning patterns toward normal and to help the body to better utilize its hormones. This approach is important, as hormones exert powerful effects throughout the body, in both sexes.

The human body synthesizes approximately 20 different hormones, all of which are normally tightly regulated by a system of glands that produce them known as the endocrine system. Often overlooked in subclinical health conditions, the glands of the endocrine system secrete hormones that influence every cell, organ, and function in our bodies. Hormones are a specific set of chemical messengers that transfer information and instructions from one group of cells in our bodies to another. In addition to their many other functions, hormones influence our moods to a greater degree than many may think. The endocrine system's effects on the body are far reaching, and its control of body systems is comparable to that of the nervous system. Generally however, hormones operate more slowly, but have longer lasting effects in the body. Hormonal molecules are released and travel through the blood stream until they reach a specific cell that is programmed to be receptive to the hormone, allowing it to affect the cellular function. Hormones are produced in small amounts by tissues other than those of the endocrine system. The brain is one area, as well as the kidneys, liver, heart, lungs, and skin.

Hormone levels fluctuate on a variety of time schedules and are directly affected by stress, infection, and even shifts in electrolyte levels in the body. Additionally, hormones play a role in modulating our behavior, and when imbalanced, the endocrine system's effects are felt widely throughout the body. Both men and women are deeply affected by the levels of hormones in their bodies. Humans are deeply entrained to the ebb and flow of natural cycles both inside and outside of our bodies, and we are highly sensitive to our environment despite our perceived mastery of our surroundings. Women are especially affected, experiencing a monthly hormonal cycle that governs the menses, which allows for the continuation of a new life. New insights have also brought to light the hormonal cycles of men and the possibility of a "male menopause," known as andropause, which may affect them similarly to the way menopause affects women. Despite these findings, it is clear that women share a much greater burden from the ebb and flow of hormonal cycles and stand the greatest chances of being negatively affected by them.

Hormones play an important role in modulating our behavior, and the brain stands at the center of hormonal control, just as it does with the rest of our bodily processes. The brain controls the release of hormones through its connection with the nervous system. Located deep within the brain, an area known as the hypothalamus is able to "read" the state of affairs in the body and, in turn, is directly linked to the pituitary gland (often referred to as the "master gland"). The hypothalamus can either stimulate or suppress hormone secretions from the pituitary. The pituitary gland manufactures and secretes a set of hormones that directly control all of the other hormone glands in the body. The production and secretion of pituitary hormones can be influenced by factors such as emotions, physical states, and seasonal changes. To accomplish this, the hypothalamus relays information sensed by the brain (such as environmental temperature, light exposure patterns, and feelings) to the pituitary. One can think of the pituitary gland and hypothalamus as upper management of a corporation and the glands such as the ovaries, testes, adrenal glands, and thyroid as the employees. The pituitary and hypothalamus are continually monitoring work performance and adjusting their orders according to production. Much like master chefs, these glands "sample" the blood levels for various hormone levels and request shifts in the recipe accordingly.

The purpose of this illustration is to emphasize the importance of mental states (feelings, emotion, and external environmental clues) and the brain's influence on hormone secretion. A healthy mental state, which can be augmented by a proper intake of nutritional supportive factors, has an effect on the rest of the body via the endocrine system. Therefore, when treating a physical problem, it is important to explore the link between brain function and hormonal influences on the body. Similarly, the reverse is true; when the body is improperly nourished, hormonal levels may become improperly regulated as the body strives to control hormonal levels as precisely as it can. When in short supply, several nutritional factors may exert an effect on hormone levels, and therefore manifest physical and mental symptoms. Often times problems in the body arise from an inability to properly metabolize hormones and establish a beneficial level. Taking this a step higher, utilizing natural medicines in the form of herbs can produce excellent outcomes in the realm of hormonal balance as well.

PREMENSTRUAL SYNDROME AND PREMENSTRUAL DYSPHORIC DISORDER

Premenstrual syndrome (PMS) is perhaps the most commonly experienced symptom of hormonal irregularity. PMS is defined as a series of physical and emotional symptoms that occur in the second phase of the menstrual cycle. The most popular theory for the cause of PMS is an imbalance of hormones, namely deficiency of progesterone and excess levels of estrogen. Symptoms vary for each woman and may last typically from 4 to 10 days. The most common symptoms include acne, anger, anxiety, bloating, breast pain, uterine pain, depression, dizziness, fatigue, headaches, hostility, insomnia, irritability, mood swings, nausea, nervousness, and tension. The emotional symptoms of PMS are the most problematic and can have extensive effects on a woman's work and social and family life. Premenstrual Dysphoric Disorder (PMDD) is not a new condition and is in fact a more severe form of PMS. The symptoms are similar; however, they markedly impair a woman's ability to function in everyday situations at work and home and in social and relationship interactions. Research suggests that of the 80 percent of women that have PMS symptoms, 5–10 percent of them meet the diagnostic criteria for PMDD.[1] PMDD is included in the *Diagnostic and Statistical Manual IV (DSM-IV)*; whether this solidifies the condition as an "official" ailment is to be decided, but in simple terms it defines a need for better management of symptoms. Physical symptoms aside, the mental-emotional toll of PMS, if untreated, leads to significant disability on a monthly basis for millions of women. When PMS is treated in a fashion to alleviate the root cause (PMS is not an ibuprofen deficiency!), significant symptom resolution can be achieved.

Commonly occurring symptoms of premenstrual irritability, mood changes, anxiety, and appetite and sleep variation in women with PMS are experienced mostly during the premenstrual phase; however, it is thought that many other women having these symptoms may indeed suffer from mood and anxiety symptoms throughout the entire menstrual period. A study was designed in order to determine to what extent women who suffer from PMS and seek treatment for these symptoms have mood or anxiety disorders in addition to PMS. A survey of 206 women revealed that 39 percent met the criteria for mood or anxiety disorders, or both; it was determined that mood disorders were twice as common as anxiety disorders.[2] The significance of these findings reveals a possible link between PMS and other mental disorders. With the majority of PMS symptoms related to hormonal dysregulation, it is possible that this may lead to increased mental dysfunction if hormonal balance becomes so skewed in a segment of the population that the women may have additional mood and anxiety disorders in relation to PMS. Early diagnosis and treatment of mood and anxiety disorders (and with every other disease condition) provides the best chances at full recovery and lower chances of reoccurring.

NUTRIENTS IN PMS

Pyridoxine

Pyridoxine (vitamin B-6) was shown to be effective in relieving depression in women taking oral birth control in a number of studies in the 1970s.[3] In addition, these studies confirmed that women using birth control had an impaired B-6 status and that administration of 40 milligrams of B-6 restored normal levels and relieved clinical symptoms of oral birth control pill–induced B-6 deficiency.[4] In a review of several studies that investigated the efficacy of B-6 in treating PMS and PMS-related depression, it was determined that treatment with B-6 improved both PMS symptoms and PMS-related depression.[5] A separate studied examined the efficacy of B-6 in the treatment of PMS in comparison to three standard pharmaceuticals (alprazalom, fluoxetine, and propranolol).[6] The following results were obtained: Fluoxetine in 10 mg doses resulted in a mean reduction of 65.4 percent in symptoms, propanolol resulted in a 58.7 percent reduction, alprazalam resulted in a 55.6 percent reduction, pyridoxine resulted in a 45.3 percent reduction, and placebo resulted in a 39.4–46.1 percent reduction. Pyridoxine was used in a dose of 300 milligrams per day; this study demonstrates the efficacy of using one individual nutrient (with virtually no side effects at this dose) when compared to pharmaceuticals with wide-ranging side effects. In this example, pyridoxine appears to be a superior choice for PMS treatment, despite its lower percentage of symptom reduction, because it provides the greatest amount of benefit, with the least amount of side effects, at a fraction of the cost.

Magnesium

Magnesium, a wide-ranging mineral in the body, is another useful treatment for PMS symptoms. One of magnesium's greatest uses is in alleviating muscle cramping and tightness, as well as generalized musculoskeletal discomfort (Epsom salt baths, highly useful for treatment of sore muscles, contain mainly magnesium salts). The use of magnesium in PMS has also been studied extensively and is found to be clinically useful for this condition for several reasons. A study examined the effects of 200 milligrams per day of magnesium for the duration of two menstrual cycles for its effects on premenstrual fluid retention.[7] Each study participant kept a daily log of symptoms; no significant effect was noted during the first cycle; however, during the second cycle, a notable reduction in weight gain, swelling of extremities, breast tenderness, and abdominal bloating was noted by the participants. In addition to demonstrating the usefulness of magnesium for fluid-retention-related PMS symptoms, this study highlights a common theory that complete tissue saturation with magnesium can take several weeks to accomplish (and thus for the patient to benefit from the effects of supplementation). It should also be noted that this study utilized a small amount of magnesium; a dose comprable to approximately 300–500 milligrams is recommended for optimal results for PMS symptoms.[2] The beneficial effects of supplementation with magnesium on PMS symptoms may be due in part to magnesium's relative deficiency in women who experience PMS. A study measuring red blood cell levels of magnesium in women who experienced PMS in comparison to those that did not revealed a decreased level of both red blood cell and white blood cell magnesium content in the group of women with PMS.[8]

Most importantly, magnesium has an effect on the mental symptoms that can occur with PMS. Another trial focused on magnesium's effects on mood in PMS sufferers revealed positive results in this symptom category as well.[9] A group of women affected by PMS were supplemented with 360 milligrams of magnesium three times a day, from day 15 of the cycle to the onset of menses. Utilizing the Menstrual Distress Questionnaire, researches found that treatment with this dose of magnesium resulted in lower questionnaire scores, meaning that negative symptoms associated with mood were decreased in the women taking magnesium. Because of this finding, the researchers of this study concluded that magnesium supplementation could be an effective way to treat PMS-related mood changes. In another hallmark study, magnesium was administered in order to determine its effects on nervous sensitivity, which can accompany emotional instability as part of the mood changes that a woman may experience premenstrually. This study demonstrated a decrease in feelings of nervousness in 89 percent of the study subjects, and in addition, breast tenderness and weight gain were reduced in 96 percent and 95 percent of the subjects, respectively.[10]

A study combining the effects of both magnesium and pyridoxine was performed in order to elucidate the synergistic effects of both nutrients on PMS-related anxiety symptoms. A significant effect using 200 milligrams per day of magnesium in combination with 50 milligrams of vitamin B-6 was observed on anxiety-related PMS symptoms of nervous tension, mood swings, irritability, and anxiety.[11] This and the previously cited studies demonstrate clearly defined beneficial effects of both supplements; the aforementioned study that combined the use of magnesium and pyridoxine utilized relatively small doses of these nutrients, and further studies investigating higher doses of both nutrients may reveal even greater benefit for women with PMS-related mental symptoms. It is noteworthy that in order for magnesium to achieve proper optimal cellular effect, adequate B-6 must be present. Thus, supplementation with magnesium in some patients with a relative deficiency of B-6 will not yield adequate results unless B-6 is supplemented.

Other Nutrients

Vitamin E is a fat-soluble vitamin that has demonstrated usefulness in PMS. Although not directly related to mental states, vitamin E has been shown to significantly decrease PMS-related breast symptoms of pain and soreness (doses ranged from 150 to 600 International Units per day).[12] When studied in relation to other PMS-related mental emotional symptoms, the use of 400 International Units of vitamin E per day was able to produce a 38 percent reduction in anxiety and a 27 percent reduction in depression after three months.[13] In addition, the test group taking vitamin E reported an increase in energy levels, fewer simple carbohydrate (sweets) cravings, and fewer headaches.

One suspected contributor to PMS symptoms, in addition to excess estrogen, is an excess of another hormone known as prolactin. Prolactin, in a simplistic description, prepares the breast tissue to begin producing breast milk in anticipation of pregnancy. A surge in prolactin may occur in some women with PMS, which may be partially responsible for some of the breast swelling and tenderness that accompanies PMS; researchers have noted that many symptoms of PMS are similar to those caused by an injection of prolactin and theorize that some women may be excessively sensitive to prolactin. Additionally, it is known that a derivative of essential fatty acids (prostaglandin E1) can inhibit some of the effects of prolactin in the body and that an absence or deficiency of prostaglandin E1 will allow for exaggerated prolactin effects. Because of this, several studies were performed in order to determine the effects of treating women's PMS symptoms with gamma-linolenic acid, an essential fatty acid precursor of prostaglandin E1. In addition, evening primrose oil (also an essential fatty acid precursor of prostaglandin E1) was shown to be highly effective in treating depression and irritability, as well as breast pain and tenderness and fluid retention associated with PMS.[14] A later study was able to reproduce these findings using gamma-linolenic acid in women with what was described as incapacitating PMS.[15] This treatment produced a reduction in PMS-associated depression as well as other general PMS symptoms. In order to assist the conversion of essential fatty acids into prostaglandin E1, it is recommended that adequate amounts of magnesium, B-6, and zinc be included in the person's diet, as the benefits of these nutrients on PMS symptoms may be partially derived from their effects on essential fatty acid metabolism.

Zinc levels may be associated with PMS symptoms as well. A study designed to determine whether changes in zinc and copper levels are associated with PMS symptoms revealed that zinc levels remained stable throughout the month in control subjects (women without PMS) but in the PMS patients, zinc levels were significantly lower during the luteal phase (the second half of the menstrual cycle, in which PMS symptoms occur) in comparison to the follicular phase (the first half of the menstrual cycle).[16] Additionally, zinc levels were lower in PMS patients than in the control subjects during the luteal phase. Another interesting aspect of this study was the relationship between copper and zinc levels during different menstrual phases. Copper levels were found to be higher during the luteal (PMS symptoms) phase in PMS patients when compared to the control subjects; this is noteworthy because copper competes with zinc for absorption in the body and therefore the ratio of zinc to copper is a direct measurement of zinc levels. These findings indicate that women with PMS experience a zinc deficiency during the symptomatic phase of the menstrual cycle due to the elevated levels of copper. These findings tie into the earlier section on optimal essential fatty acid metabolism, indicating further a need for micronutrients such as zinc in women with PMS. Additional studies have confirmed lower zinc-to-copper ratios in women with PMS, especially in the symptomatic phase of the menstrual cycle.[17]

HERBAL SUPPORT FOR HORMONAL MENTAL FUNCTION

Black Cohosh (*Cimicifuga racemosa*)

Black cohosh is known to have mild estrogenic effects and has been shown to be beneficial in the treatment of PMS-related depression, anxiety, tension, and mood swings.[18] Black cohosh is typically prescribed in a standardized form known as Remifemin; the majority of clinical studies on the effectiveness of black cohosh have used a standardized formulation that contains 1 milligram triterpene glycosides, calculated as 27-deoxyacetin. Black cohosh can alleviate hot flashes associated with the perimenopause state.[19] These effects serve to help regulate hormone levels that have gone awry, leading to less mental emotional symptoms.

Chasteberry (*Vitex agnus-castus*)

This herb has been used for menstrual irregularities (caused by hormonal dysregulation) as well as PMS and menopausal symptoms. The efficacy of this herb in these conditions may be partially explained by it ability to suppress prolactin hormone release, which may serve to normalize excessive hormonal symptoms during the luteal (symptomatic phase) of the menstrual cycle.[20] Other studies have indicated that chasteberry may have both estrogenic and progesteronic activity, which when supplemented may serve to regulate hormonal levels.[21]

Licorice (*Glycyrrhiza glabra*)

Licorice has a variety of uses in human health, and hormonal regulation is a primary indication for its use. In the treatment of PMS-related hormonal dysregulation, licorice has been shown to lower estrogen levels and at the same time increases levels of progesterone (PMS is thought to be caused by elevated estrogen with lower levels of progesterone).[22] Licorice can elevate progesterone levels by inhibiting an enzyme that is responsible for dismantling it in the body, and at the same time licorice can increase water retention via its effects on another bodily hormone, aldosterone. Aldosterone is responsible for assisting the body in retaining salt, which in turn allows the body to store more water. Therefore, licorice should be used cautiously in PMS with water retention as a major symptom.[23]

All of these herbal medicines are effective at relieving PMS-related mental emotional symptoms through their effects on hormone levels that become dysregulated. Supplementation can serve to adjust these hormone levels such that patients do not as easily notice the extensive effects of hormonal imbalance.

Hormonal mental health can be achieved by using nutritional and herbal supplements that act to assist the body in regulating its hormone levels. The brief research reviewed in this chapter provides a clue to how one can control previously unregulated hormones. When in a state of disarray, hormones can begin to affect mental processes that may result in serious consequences in regard to a person's professional and social functioning. The case of women's monthly hormone cycles was only partially illustrated herein; with the approximate 20 different hormones in the body, there are many other conditions of hormone dysregulation that have different effects on the mental state that were not touched upon in this chapter. The previous research demonstrates the relatively simple, yet highly effective modes for which nutritional factors can be employed to alter hormonal dysfunction, leading to fewer mental symptoms.

MALE HORMONES AND BEYOND FOR BOTH SEXES

Both men and women have a composite of estrogen, progesterone, and androgens such as testosterone. Men also cycle; testosterone levels are typically highest in the morning and decrease throughout the day. More significantly, overall testosterone levels decrease beginning in the fourth decade; it is noted that low testosterone yields a male menopause and, likewise, shifts in metabolism of the testosterone lead to significant health issues such as hot flashes, decreased erections, libido, and stamina. If zinc levels are low in both men and women, testosterone metabolism does not occur properly, causing acne, mood changes, prostate changes, and, in the case of men particularly, a circumstance called gynecomastia, which is the development of enlarged breasts due to insufficient levels of testosterone that normally counters the effects of estrogen in men.

Adrenal gland function affects both male and female hormonal health. Adrenal health not only affects hormones such as cortisol and related stress response hormones (epinephrine and norepinephrine), it also buffers steroidal hormone blood levels. Indeed DHEA and other precursor hormones produced by the adrenals are essential for the entire cascade of steroidal hormone production that all start from the humble beginnings of cholesterol as the principal building block. Adrenal function can be supported nutritionally with the following nutrients.

Vitamin C

The adrenal glands concentrate more vitamin C in them than any other part of the body. Because of this, large amounts of research have delved into the function of vitamin C and the adrenal glands. Vitamin C has numerous beneficial affects in this multifaceted organ. Controlling the release of several different hormones, vitamin C serves to support the tissue of the adrenal glands by both protecting and enhancing the responsiveness of this tissue.[24] This is important as a specific group of hormones, the catecholamines, are released from the adrenals to mediate the body's stress response. As mental and physiologic stress increases, more of these hormones are released, which can assist us in dealing with our stressors. When constantly exposed to stress, as much of us are, it is important to provide the adrenal glands with the nutrients it needs to continue manufacturing these supportive hormones. Vitamin C is essential for the production of hormones in the adrenals, as well as the conversion of these precursor hormones into their active forms. A study of animals that did not have the ability to utilize vitamin C in their adrenal glands showed that they were unable to produce adequate amounts of catecholamines and soon thereafter died from inadequate adrenal function.[25]

Phosphatidylserine

Known as a phospholipid, phosphatidylserine is manufactured in the human body in a complex series of reactions. Despite this, the body obtains most of it through the diet. This molecule has several functions, some of which include proper brain cell membrane function, cell-to-cell signaling in the nervous system, and secretory vessicle release (hormones are sent into the blood stream in " waterproof" vesicles for transport to other parts of the body).[26] Therapeutic use of phosphatidylserine increases catecholamine release in diseased animals.[27] Phosphatidylserine can assist in supporting adrenal gland function by blunting the response of the gland to exercise-induced stress.[20] This study demonstrated that phosphatidylserine attenuated the release of adrenocorticotropin by the brain (a hormone that stimulates the adrenal gland) and cortisol (the main "stress" hormone made by the adrenal glands).

Cordyceps Sinensis

A fungus harvested in mountainous regions of China, Cordyceps is said to be an adaptogenic agent. An adaptogen is an agent that assists a person in counteracting adverse physical, chemical, or biological stressors by generating nonspecific resistance. More simplified, adaptogens bolster our body's defenses against stress, helping us to stand up to it. Cordyceps was used to measure the physiologic stress response in animals in one study, utilizing the weight of the adrenal gland as a guage.[29] It was found that the adrenal glands of the animals given the Cordyceps and exposed to stress were not as large as those that were not supplemented and exposed to stress. (The adrenal glands grow in response to stress in order to compensate for increased demand on this gland.) Cordyceps can be used to assist the body in dealing with stress, and the hormonal consequences of this, by supporting the function of the adrenal gland.

CONCLUSION

We are a composite of the total sum of our overall health quotient. Unless each segment of our body is biochemically balanced, the net result is an imbalance. Much like a bank account is managed to maintain a proper balance—debits and credits must be adjusted to achieve one's financial goals—our health accounts must balance as well. Indeed the balance to be carried in one's health account is not a net zero, for that would be merely survival on the brink; rather, we must each have a significant positive credit to maintain a disease-free state and to avoid the circumstances of becoming overdrawn that may lead to chronic disease or worse. There is an important differentiation to be made between biological and chronological age. Chronological age is simply how old we are relative to our date of birth. Yet, biological age is the sum of genetics, diet, and lifestyle and can differ in those of similar chronological age. Indeed, genetics may load the gun, but diet and lifestyle pull the trigger. Investing in one's hormonal health yields big dividends and is well worth the interest.

NUTRIENTS

- Pyridoxine
  50 milligrams per day, maintenance
  300 milligrams per day during second half of menstrual cycle, in divided doses
- Magnesium
  300–400 milligrams per day
- Vitamin E
  400–800 International Units per day
- Essential Fatty Acids
  2,000–3,000 milligrams per day
- Zinc
  30–40 milligrams per day
- Vitamin C
  1,000–2,000 milligrams per day, divided doses
- Phosphatidylserine
  100 milligrams three times a day

BOTANICALS

- Black cohosh (*Cimicifuga racemosa*)
  40–80 milligrams, standardized to 4–8 milligrams triterpene glycosides per day
- Chasteberry (*Vitex agnus-castus*)
  Crude herb: 20–240 milligrams per day up to 1,800 milligrams per day in two to three divided doses

Fluid extract: 40 drops daily
Tincture (1:5–1:2): 1 milliliter three times daily
- Licorice (*Glycyrrhiza glabra*)*
Crude herb (powdered root): 2,000–4,000 milligrams per day, divided doses
Tincture: 2–4 milliliters two times per day
- Cordyceps sinensis
2,000 milligrams per day

*May increase blood pressure, monitoring is essential.

Insomnia

The average adult sleeps approximately 7.5 to 8 hours each night.[1] Researchers are still determining the true function of sleep; however, much evidence has shown that a lack of sleep has serious consequences including medical and mental health problems, as well as memory deficits, accidents, and impaired occupation and social functioning.[2] Simply put, rest is the source of "*restoration*" for the mind and body. Without it, the normal healing and supportive pathways of the body are not sustainable.

Although not technically a disease condition, insomnia is actually a symptom of deeper neurologic dysfunction. Insomnia can include the perception or complaint of poor quality or inadequate sleep due to difficulty in falling asleep, frequent waking during the night with difficulty falling back asleep, waking up too early in the morning, and having unrefreshing sleep. Not defined by the number of hours of sleep that one receives or how long it takes to fall asleep, insomnia can vary from person to person because sleep needs are highly individualized. The prevalence of insomnia is thought to be 32 million people, which figures to approximately 1 out of 8 people or 11.76 percent of the population having insomnia at any one time.

Insomnia is classified into three main groups:

- Transient: This is short lived, lasting from days to weeks.
- Intermittent: This entails clusters of transient insomnia that occur periodically.
- Chronic: This insomnia occurs nearly every night, lasting for a month or longer.

More specifically, insomnia is thought of as either primary, in which sleeplessness is not attributable to a medical, psychiatric, or environmental cause (a more expanded definition can be found in the *Diagnostic and Statistical Manual of Mental Disorders*, Fourth Edition (*DSM-IV*), or secondary, which is caused by a physical condition or psychological problem such as depression. Secondary insomnia is thought to be much more common than the primary form.[3]

The characteristics of primary insomnia are:

- A predominant complaint of difficulty initiating or maintaining sleep for a least one month
- Sleep disturbance that causes clinically significant distress or impairment in social, occupational, or other important areas of functioning
- Sleep disturbance that does not occur exclusively during the course of narcolepsy, breathing-related sleep disorder, circadian rhythm sleep disorder, or a parasomnia
- Sleep disturbance that does not occur exclusively in the course of another mental disorder (major depressive disorder, generalized anxiety disorder, a delirium)
- Sleep disturbance that is not due to direct physiological effects of a substance

A common complaint with fairly significant medical and psychologic complications, insomnia is often a symptom of an underlying medical, psychiatric, or environmental condition. More specifically, anxiety and depression are thought to be among some of the most common causes of insomnia; however, neurologic disorders like restless leg syndrome and limb movement disorder can contribute to insomnia as well. Proper management of secondary insomnia is entirely dependent on accurate diagnosis and appropriate treatment of the underlying condition whereas primary insomnia can usually be directly treated.

Insomnia tends to occur more often in those of advanced age (it is more frequent in those over 60), females, and those with a history of depression. Generally, the most common predisposing factors for primary insomnia are stress, environmental noise, changes in surrounding environment, jet lag, and medication side effects. Secondary, or chronic, insomnia is generally more complex in nature and results from underlying mental or physical disorders. These include depression (one of the most common causes of insomnia), arthritis, heart disease, asthma, hyperthyroidism, and many other diseases. Chronic insomnia can be due to behavioral factors as well, such as overuse of alcohol, caffeine, or other substances and interruptions in sleep-wake cycles from shift work or extended nighttime activities.

Behaviorally, insomnia seems to be perpetuated by the following behaviors; sometimes curtailing these activities can make a large difference.

- Drinking alcohol before bedtime
- Smoking cigarettes before bedtime
- Excessive napping in the afternoon or evening

- Irregular or continually disrupted sleep-wake schedules
- Expecting to have difficulty sleeping and worrying about it
- Ingesting excessive amounts of caffeine

Insomnia is diagnosed through a medical and sleep history intake. Usually, the patient or the patient's bed partner completes a diary regarding the quality and quantity of sleep. In addition, specialized sleep studies may be needed to diagnose other sleep-related disorders such as sleep apnea (the cessation of breathing while sleeping) or narcolepsy (excessive daytime sleepiness, lack of REM sleep, and transient sleep like states during the daytime).

Initial treatment of insomnia involves identifying the cause, whether physical or mental. Depending on this diagnosis, additional medical intervention will be necessary to alleviate the underlying disorder. Medical problems typically cause insomnia due to physical discomfort, which may or may not be relieved, depending on the nature of the problem; surgical pain is amenable to medications that blunt the brain's recognition of pain, whereas insomnia due to asthma may be curtailed by removing nocturnal symptoms. Although not the focus of this chapter, the resolution of insomnia by treating the underlying disorder stands to reason as the most efficacious approach. The highlights in this chapter can be utilized to resolve insomnia that originates from any number of causes, whether primary or secondary. These approaches are more favorable than the use of medication designed to bring about sleep; medications are addictive, have a rebound effect, and are typically only prescribed in small doses for short periods of time for the aforementioned reasons—they are not curative. Treating insomnia with another popular standby, alcohol, is strongly discouraged. Alcohol is commonly thought by the general public to help with sleeping. However, alcohol consumption can diminish the quality of sleep by disrupting the sequence and duration of the various sleep states, altering total sleep time and sleep latency (time to fall asleep). Consumed near bedtime, alcohol may decrease the time it takes for one to fall asleep. However, when consumed within an hour of sleep, it appears to cause disruptions in the second half of the sleep period.[4] Sleep may be more fitful, charachterized by frequent awakening from dreams and difficulty falling back asleep. As one continues to rely on alcohol at bedtime, the sleep-inducing effects may decrease while sleep-disrupting effects increase.[5] Seniors are more at risk from these effects, as alcohol is not metabolized as quickly in them compared to younger people, leading to higher blood/brain alcohol levels from the same amount consumed.

The effects of alcohol on sleep (wakefulness during the second half of sleep) can be induced by consuming a moderate dose of alcohol as much as six hours prior to bedtime.[1] At this point, all alcohol has been eliminated from the body, which suggests a long-term change in bodily sleep regulation and mechanisms. Alcohol consumption in pregnant women has even been shown to induce sleep disruptions in the newborn baby.[6] Measurements of brain activity showed that the infants of mothers who consumed at least one drink per day during the first trimester of pregnancy had sleep disruptions and increased arousal compared to the infants of mothers that abstained from alcohol. Even more, infants exposed to alcohol in breast milk fell asleep sooner but slept less than those infants not exposed to alcohol.[7] Avoidance of alcohol for insomnia is strongly recommended; it only serves to increase the problems of sleep difficulty and, over the long-term, may lead to abuse and dependency.

NUTRITIONAL CONSIDERATIONS

Vitamin B-12

Cobalamin, otherwise known as vitamin B-12, plays a role in insomnia development and control. B-12 plays a role in numerous neurologic conditions and appears throughout this book; it is not surprising that B-12 is also involved in insomnia as well. In a study to determine the effect of supplementing methylcobalamin (a coenzyme form of B-12) on sleep-wake rhythm disorders, researchers found a large dose of B-12, significantly improved sleep-wake cycle measures as well as clinical symptoms.[8] Although noted as inconsistent, both groups (high-dose and low-dose B-12) exhibited improvement in their sleeping patterns; B-12 did provide improvements at both a high and low dosage in this particular study. An interesting extension of this study might include examining patients' B-12 status (i.e., blood levels) and folate levels, as these two vitamins are intimately involved in metabolism.

In a more specific study, B-12 supplementation was used in two separate patients with chronic sleep-wake rhythm disorders.[9] The first patient, a 15-year-old blind girl, had been entrained to a free-running sleep-wake rhythm of 25 hours. (This is a common period of time that humans, when deprived of external light cues to time, will shift their bodily rhythms toward; this creates difficulty in establishing set patterns such as falling asleep and waking.) She was supplemented with 1.5 milligrams B-12 three times a day and soon thereafter shifted to a 24-hour rhythm that was maintained as long as she continued the supplement regimen. However, at two months post-discontinuation of the B-12, her previous 25-hour pattern reemerged. Interestingly, her serum levels of the vitamin were within the normal range before and after the treatment. The second patient in this study was a 55-year-old man who experienced delayed sleep for much of his life. When supplemented with 1.5 milligrams B-12 one time per day, his sleep pattern was improved, and this effect lasted for the six months of follow-up that the patient underwent. In a combination study employing B-12 along with light therapy (exposing patients to light at preset times) and time therapy (entraining time patterns), 106 patients with various forms of insomnia that included sleep-wake rhythm disorders, delayed sleep phase syndrome, irregular sleep-wake pattern, and prolonged sleep pattern experienced improvements of 32 percent, 42 percent, 45 percent, and 67 percent, respectively.[10] These subjects also experienced improvements in subjective feelings of lack of adequate sleep, unpleasant feelings at waking, and daytime sleepiness. The use of vitamin B-12 as an adjunctive factor in treating insomnia appears to have some merit from these limited studies. Ensuring that a person has adequate B-12 in the diet and via supplementation may serve to alleviate a large portion of their insomnia, and this approach seems to have efficacy in several different forms of insomnia and sleep disorders.

Folate

Folate (folic acid) is also intimately related to proper neurologic function plays several roles in the development and resolution of numerous neurologic disorders, and appears throughout this book. Its roles in amino acid metabolism, nucleic acid synthesis (DNA and RNA), and catecholamine neurotransmitters are considered essential. Among the neurologic disorders implicated in folate deficiency, insomnia is mentioned in the literature.[11] The role of folate has been studied in the context of alleviating restless leg syndrome, which can be a primary cause of insomnia. Restless leg syndrome is characterized as a neurosensory disorder that begins in the evening and prevents the person from falling asleep due to the continuous need to move the legs. In a study of pregnant women with restless leg syndrome, a folate deficiency was associated with the occurrence of the syndrome, significantly delayed sleep onset, and depressed mood.[12] This association was excluded from other factors such as B-12 and iron deficiency in these women, and because of these findings, investigators recommend a reevaluation of suggested folate levels during pregnancy in order to alleviate restless legs and subsequent insomnia. It is known that in psychiatric patients, symptoms are more severe and increasingly frequent in those with suboptimal folate levels in comparison to those patients with normal levels. Folate supplementation has been demonstrated to have a therapuetic effect in psychiatric symptoms, insomnia being a prime symptom.[13] Although limited in research, the application of folic acid supplementation in insomnia, especially that related to a psychiatric disorder, may serve to decrease symptoms. The interworkings of folate and the nervous system continue to be elucidated, and primary research hints at the usefulness of this supplement in conditions like insomnia.

Magnesium

Magnesium is the most plentiful positively charged electrolyte in the body. It is used in over than 300 different cellular reactions required for movement of ions across cellular membranes,[14] and it is a crucial part of maintaining nerve and muscle electrical potentials as well as in the transmission of nervous impulses.[15] Because of its usefulness in the nervous system, the role of magnesium in insomnia has been intensely studied throughout the literature. Recognized as affecting sleep and sleep-related nueroendocrine functions as well as altering EEG (electroencephalogram) sleep patterns, magnesium was studied to determine its usefulness in the treatment of insomnia in the elderly.[16] The authors of this study noted that aging results in decreased sleep indices, namely, slow wave sleep and delta and sigma wavelength power, and that these three measures of sleep quality were improved by magnesium supplementation. Additionally, the authors suggest that magnesium, in this circumstance, may affect the glutamaterigic and GABAnergic neurotransmitter systems and that treatment with magnesium may reverse age-associated sleep changes. Magnesium deficiency and depletion is thought to disrupt normal biological rhythms, including sleep. Low magnesium correlates with both hypofunction and hyperfunction of the biologic clock; hyperfunction of the biologic clock in association with magnesium depletion is associated with nervous hypoexcitability, resulting in depression, nocturnal headaches, and excessive sleepiness, whereas hypofunction of the biologic clock associated with magnesium depletion is associated with nervous hyperexcitability, and may cause delayed sleep onset, age-related insomnia, jet lag, anxiety, and migraines.[17] Researchers speculate that the role of the biologic clock and magnesium levels are linked in such a way that a balance of magnesium is necessary for the efficiency of the pineal gland and suprachiasmatic nuclei.[18] Furthermore, they hypothesize that magnesium may have effects such as stimulation of inhibitory neurotransmitters such as GABA and taurine and may antagonize "neuroactive" gases such as carbon monoxide and nitric oxide. Magnesium plays an intricate role in the regulation of the biologic clock; much more research into this area is needed to further elucidate its role. Regardless, current research demonstrates a causative effect of low magnesium status and insomnia.

Tryptophan, 5-HTP, Melatonin, and Serotonin

Tryptophan is an essential amino acid not produced in the human body and is therefore required in the diet. A precursor of the neurotransmitter serotonin, tryptophan has a sedative effect.[19] A highly useful dietary supplement, tryptophan was stigmatized in 1989 when one particular manufacturer's batch of tryptophan was associated with a disabling and fatal condition known as eosinophilia-myalgia syndrome (EMS). Despite the evidence that this outbreak of EMS was largely thought to be a result of contamination in the manufacturing process,[20] the FDA removed over-the-counter tryptophan supplements from the market in 1990. Tryptophan is available by prescription, however, from a compounding pharmacy.

Tryptophan is useful in the treatment of insomnia, as well as seasonal affective disorder, a condition charachterized by seasonally related insomnia and either oversleeping or insomnia.[21] The most frequently used dose of tryptophan is 1 gram, and this has been shown to increase subjective feelings of sleepiness and decreased waking time.[22] Tryptophan is thought to induce sleep through its ability to increase serotonin levels in the brain (tryptophan is a precursor molecule to serotonin). Serotonin plays numerous roles in the brain, primarily modulation of the circadian rhythm and sleep and wake cycles. Depending on location in the brain, serotonin and serotonergic effects include sleep, wakefulness, and behavioral states.

5-hydroxytryptophan (5-HTP) is an intermediary precursor to serotonin and is derived from tryptophan. Available as a supplement, 5-HTP crosses the blood-brain barrier and thereby increases serotonin synthesis. One study demonstrated this effect when a dose of 100 milligrams was shown to increase slow-wave sleep.[23] 5-HTP enters the brain easily and effectively augments serotonin levels; this has been shown to be of clinical benefit in insomnia as well as conditions such as depression, fibromyalgia, and binge eating.[24] Because of these effects, 5-HTP may be an effective agent for reducing insomnia symptoms resulting from serotonin dysfunction.

Melatonin is a hormone that is produced from serotonin. Melatonin seems to affect the neurotransmitter GABA by assisting its binding to its receptors and by decreasing neurotransmissions by directly affecting neurons in the brain.[25] Primarily, melatonin appears to regulate the circadian rhythm and sleep patterns, as well as endocrine secretions. Melatonin levels are influenced by day and night cycles; light will inhibit melatonin production and darkness will stimulate its secretion.[26] This may partially explain increased somnolence in wintertime, especially in northern climates. Production of melatonin decreases in the elderly, and serum levels are decreased in people with insomnia and depressed moods.[27]

Low-dose supplementation of melatonin, enough to achieve normal nighttime levels (in those with low melatonin levels), will promote sleep onset and maintenance without altering neurologic sleep indices (sleep architecture).[28] Additionally, melatonin can advance or delay circadian rhythms (when given in the evening or in the morning, respectively). Melatonin has been shown to benefit insomnia as a result of numerous factors and conditions. For instance, melatonin supplementation is effective for relieving insomnia that results from jet lag,[29] in the elderly,[30] in children with mental retardation,[31] and in those with Asperger's syndrome,[32] as well as in children with chronic sleep-onset insomnia.[33] Melatonin has been shown in the research to be beneficial in insomnia from a variety of additional causes; these are only a few of the most recalcitrant causes of insomnia in which melatonin has been shown to be of benefit.

BOTANICAL MEDICINES

Passiflora incarnata (Passionflower)

Passionflower contains several active constituents, including the flavonoid compounds and harman alkaloids.[34] Passionflower acts as a sedative and hypnotic and anxiolytic agent and also has antispasmodic and pain relieving effects.[35] Some research shows that a constituent of passionflower, apigenin, is capable of binding to benzodiazapenes receptors in the brain, thereby acting as an anxiolytic.[36] Other research points to the ability of passionflower to reduce restlessness and aggressiveness while raising the pain threshold.[37] Passionflower extracts are widely used as a sedative agent in complementary sleep-aid products. Several pharmacologic investigations have demonstrated the sedative effects of passionflower as well as an anxiolytic effect, underlying its role as an important agent in restlessness, irritability, and insomnia as a result of anxiety.[38]

Valeriana Officinalis

Valerian root is commonly used for sleeping disorders due to its known sedative-hypnotic and anxiolytic effects.[39] The active constituents of valerian include the valepotriates, volatile oils, and monoterpene and sesquiterpene constituents.[40] Despite the identification of several possibly active constituents in valerian, the effectiveness of the herb is probably more accurately attributable to more that one compound (as is the case for most herbal medicines). Valerian is effective when used to alleviate insomnia by reducing sleep onset time and by improving reported sleep quality.[41] In addition, valerian is effective at improving sleep quality in people undergoing withdrawal from benzodiazapenes (for treatment of insomnia).[42] Valerian is most effective for insomnia when taken over a period of several days to weeks rather than a one-time-only dose; however, this approach can be effective at increasing sleep as well.[43] The effectiveness of valerian in treating insomnia is more than likely attributable to both its anxiolytic effects (thereby reducing anxiety) and its sedative-hypnotic effects on the brain.

Matricaria recutita (Chamomile)

Known as a mildly sedative herb, chamomile is useful in inducing sleep in a gentle manner, with no morning side effects. Categorized as a sedative in the medical literature,[44] chamomile is beneficial for reducing nervous activity in the evenings, allowing a person to fall asleep with greater ease. Chamomile's effects appear to be carried out on the central nervous system and may reduce aggressive behavior, thereby curtailing anxious energy.[45] The sedative activity of chamomile has been proven in a number of studies, making chamomile a good choice for those suffering from insomnia that delays sleep onset.[46]

Combination Homeopathics

There are a few combination homeopathic medicines that can be used for the treatment of insomnia. Containing homeopathic doses of passionflower, oats (a mildly calming herb), chamomile, and homeopathic salts, these combinations are found to be useful by some people. In the treatment of insomnia, using homeopathic medicines provides a nontoxic form of treatment with no side effects. These medicines are effective in roughly 33 percent of the people who use them and are very inexpensive.

SLEEP HYGEINE

The importance of sleep hygiene, or maintaining a healthy sleeping environment, can be vital to correcting patterns of insomnia. Many people, when going about their routines of going to bed, follow certain patterns each night. The development of a healthy pattern is essential in allowing the body and mind to adjust to a different physiologic phase. Just as an athlete goes about a ritual of warming up, stretching, and mental preparation before an event, a person should have similar processes in preparation for sleep. As part of this process, one should:

- Avoid television just before or in bed (especially the nightly news, which always contains stories of mayhem)
- Avoid eating late at night
- Organize the day ahead on paper, and preview the next day, so that you can rest knowing you are prepared
- Keep a clean, soothing bedroom. Work clutter and other unnecessary items only keep your mind running when it should be winding down

CONCLUSION

Insomnia is both a symptom and a condition. Depending on the nature of its origins, insomnia can be treated as a symptom of another disease process or as a primary symptom. Ideally, treatment of insomnia will involve addressing the initial cause (of which a majority of insomnia is attributable) before direct modulation of sleep patterns is carried out. Conversely, assisting the person in overcoming insomnia and obtaining sleep is highly important in the treatment of almost every disease processes. Utilizing natural therapies rather than standard pharmaceutical medications (which are costly and can be addictive) to treat insomnia can be achieved with a variety of nutritional and herbal applications.

NUTRIENTS

- B-12
  500 micrograms daily
- Folate
  400–800 micrograms daily
- Magnesium
  300–400 milligrams, ½ hour before bed
- 5-HTP
  150–200 milligrams in the evening
- Tryptophan
  1–3 grams in the evening; start with the lowest dose and work up to 3 grams, if necessary

- Melatonin
  0.3–5 milligrams in the evening; start with the lowest dose and work upward

BOTANICALS

- Passionflower
  Crude herb: 0.25–2 grams, three times daily; or one cup of tea three times daily, with the last dose half an hour before bedtime
  Liquid extract (1:1 extract): 0.5 to 1.0 milliliter three times daily
  Tincture: 0.5–2 milliliters three times daily
- Valerian
  400–900 milligrams valerian extract up to two hours before bedtime
- Chamomile
  Crude herb: 0.25–2 grams, three times daily; or one cup of tea three times daily, with the last dose half an hour before bedtime
  Tincture: 2 milliliters half an hour before bedtime

Learning Disability

Learning disability (LD) is a neurological disorder that may arise as a result of numerous reasons, ultimately affecting the ability of the brain to receive, process, store, and respond to information it receives. Disability refers to the unexplained difficulty a person with normal intelligence has in obtaining basic academic knowledge and skills. Not a solitary disorder, LD comprises numerous disorders that can affect the person in a variety of learning areas. Limitations in learning can appear as difficulty in listening, speaking, reading, writing, coordination, self-control, or attention. These, of course, can impede the ability to master reading, writing, arithmetic, and other academic or social material. LD can occur throughout life and affect numerous aspects, especially if the person has more than one LD. However, if a person has only one LD, it may have little effect on the rest of the person's life. Some features of learning disabilities include:

- Difficulties may emerge differently in different people.
- Difficulties may emerge in a variety of ways throughout development.
- The person may have socioemotional skills and behavior difficulties.
- There may be a distinct gap between expected and actual achievement level.

Learning disabilities affect nearly 2.9 million schoolchildren in the United States, and a portion of them receive some type of special education. This number comprises nearly 5 percent of children in public schools; this does not account for those in private and religious schools or homeschooled children.[1] Thus the actual number of affected individuals is likely to be meaningfully higher, as supported by clinical observations. LDs do not affect racial and ethnic groups equally; only 1 percent of white children compared to 2.6 percent of black children received special education services in 2001. This disparity has been attributed to economic background rather than ethnicity. Furthermore, LD is not caused by socioeconomic status, but exposure to known toxins such as tobacco, lead, and alcohol during early phases of development are more prevalent in low socioeconomic areas.

Learning disabilities have several causes, none of which are specific. As previously mentioned, environmental factors such as exposure to known neurologic toxins, nutritional deprivation, and injuries may all contribute. Additionally, LD may be the result of illness or injury before or during birth, drug and alcohol use during pregnancy, low birth weight, lack of adequate oxygen, and labor difficulties. Additionally, LDs can run in the family, hinting at a hereditary pattern. Most often, however, no specific cause or incident can be attributed to developing a learning disability.

TYPES OF LD

The exact diagnostic criteria for LD is listed in the *Diagnostic and Statistical Manual of Mental Disorders IV* (*DSM-IV*). Generally however, LDs can be divided into three broad categories of:

- Academic skills disorders
- Developmental speech and language disorders
- "Other" disorders that include coordination and learning disabilities not covered in the previous terms

Each category can be broken down into several more specific disorders. The most common disorders include dyslexia, characterized by difficulty in processing language, leading to problems in reading, writing, and spelling; dyscalculia, characterized by difficulty with math skills, leading to problems in computation, math facts, and concepts of time and money; dysgraphia, characterized by difficulty in written expression, leading to problems in handwriting, spelling, and composition; and dyspraxia, characterized by difficulty with fine motor skills, leading to problems with coordination and fine manual dexterity. Other common subgroupings include auditory and visual processing disorders that are marked by problems in processing auditory and visual information.

DIAGNOSIS

Not every learning problem is considered a learning disability. Many children are slower in developing certain skills and natural differences in development rates may appear to be learning disorders but are only maturation delays. A learning disability can only be diagnosed by meeting certain diagnostic criteria. Observations by parents, teachers, and anyone else who regularly interacts with the person will be taken into account when considering a diagnosis. If a pattern emerges, a learning specialist can then evaluate the person. Nearly a third of the people with learning disabilities also have attention deficit hyperactivity disorder (ADHD), which serves to confound the condition even more.

Not a disease process, learning disabilities are not necessarily curable and do not go away. Typically, LDs are treated with a combination of special education, coping skills, and medication protocols. If vigilantly adhered to, such programs can help those with learning disabilities achieve "normal" goals similar to others in their age and education group. Keeping in mind that learning disabilities and how they affect each individual is highly varied, different approaches and techniques work differently in each person.

The object of this chapter, similar to those prior to it, is to highlight possible nutritional deficiencies that may predispose a person to a learning disorder and to explore other natural medications that may alleviate the onset or symptoms of learning disabilities.

NUTRITION

Seemingly commonsensical, the idea that optimal nutritional status has an effect on learning capability appears to be commonly overlooked in modern society. Children are more often than not fed nutritionally bankrupt foods not only for breakfast, but also throughout the day. Many meals comprise food items that have been processed and laden with sugars but are passed off as "nutritious" because of a certain fiber content or amount of fortification with B-vitamins. The importance of breakfast on school performance and learning has been studied and appears throughout the literature. A large study involving nearly 6,500 Korean schoolchildren revealed the importance of breakfast and lunch as being related to academic performance; a positive association between height and physical fitness to academic performance was noted as well.[2] Academic performance was strongly associated with dietary behaviors, namely, with meal regularity even after controlling for parent's level of education.

Another study investigating the effects of a universal, free school breakfast program on academic performance revealed interesting results as well.[3] Students who had total energy intake below 50 percent of the recommended daily allowance (RDA) and/or intake below 50 percent of the RDA of two or more micronutrients were considered to be at nutritional risk. Prior to the beginning of the breakfast program, 33 percent of the students were classified as being at nutritional risk and had significantly worse attendance, punctuality, grades, and behavior problems and were less likely to consume breakfast at school than the children not considered at nutritional risk. Six months after the initiation of the breakfast program, the nutritional risk students exhibited greater improvements in attendance, math grades, behavior, and decreased hunger than children who did not decrease their nutritional risk. This study demonstrates the importance of nutrient intake and its effect of academic and psychosocial functioning.

The importance of breakfast nutrition on cognitive performance by school-children appears throughout the literature with additional positive effects on attendance, punctuality, and behavior. If eating breakfast can produce positive results in these areas, it is not surprising that adequate morning nutrition will lead to general educational improvements. Needless to say, better attendance, behavior, and cognitive performance all contribute to better school performance. Although these studies do not assess the effects of breakfast nutrition on learning disabilities, it stands to reason that the aforementioned benefits will be of use to the child with learning difficulties as well.

IRON

Several individual nutrients have been implicated in learning disorders; whether associated with or directly related to, these nutrient studies provide us with interesting clues in the treatment and nutritional etiology of learning disabilities.

The association between iron deficiency and learning disorders has been studied for some time now. In one study, the relationship between learning disability and iron deficiency was studied in preschool-aged children.[4] The prevalence of iron deficiency and learning disability and the different areas of mental development were assessed in 136 children ages four to five. Nutritional status, iron storage status, and psychomotor, socioeconomic, and cultural posts were taken into account, and a positive correlation between iron deficiency greater than 22.8 percent and disability in the area of speech analysis and synthesis was noted.

Another study investigated the effect of iron supplementation on school performance measurements in iron-deficient anemic children and nonanemic children.[5] The two groups of children were divided into placebo and iron-supplemented groups; notable increases in mean hemoglobin and in hematocrit and transferrin saturation were noted in the anemic children, and the iron status of these children was associated with significant positive changes in school achievement as measured by improved test scores. (The iron-treated students demonstrated slightly higher test scores than the untreated group.)

A review article focusing on the role of iron and learning potential in childhood covered several interesting aspects of this relationship, namely that iron deficiency will adversely affect behavior by impairing cognitive function, producing noncognitive disturbances, and limiting activity and work capacity.[6] In regard to cognitive function, there is evidence that mental and motor development is lower among infants with iron-deficiency anemia, and there seems to be an alteration in processes involving attentional focus in older children and adults with iron deficiency. Noncognitive effects of iron deficiency in infants revealed a short attention span, failure to respond to test stimuli, and unhappiness. This research reinforces the need to ensure proper nutrient intake starting with the youngest children, as iron deficiency can begin to affect the neurodevelopmental process in infancy.

Youdim and colleagues elucidated speculation into just how iron deficiency affects learning in an animal model.[7] A noticeable characteristic of iron deficiency is a specific decrease in central dopamine neurotransmission that results from a decline in the number of dopamine D2 receptors in certain areas of the brain (caudate nucleus, nucleus accumbens, pituitary, and possibly the frontal cortex). When diminished, dopamine neurotransmission will serve to negatively modify dopamine-dependent behaviors, most notably a reduction in learning processes. The authors speculate that iron plays a vital role in maintaining healthy function of dopamine neurons, which are intimately involved in cognitive processes.

OTHER NUTRIENTS

Magnesium

The mineral magnesium has been implicated as a causative factor in symptoms that are inconsistent with learning, such as anxious restlessness, fidgeting behavior, psychomotor instability, and learning difficulties, all of which were noted in children with normal IQ levels.[8] Magnesium is a potent mineral with numerous physiologic functions; its role in learning disabilities requires more intense investigation.

Zinc

Zinc is a cofactor in the synthesis of neurotransmitters and is indirectly involved in dopamine metabolism (low levels of dopamine are associated with ADHD and supplementation of dopamine has alleviated the symptoms of this learning disability),[9] and several studies reveal that zinc is deficient in people with ADHD.[10] ADHD is considered to be an "other" form of learning disability and occurs in up to one-third of the people who have other learning disabilities. Two separate animal studies demonstrated the initiation of learning disabilities in both young and adult animals when deprived of zinc in their diets for a period of time.[11]

Vitamin C

In an older study, a large group of students ranging from kindergarten to college age were divided into two groups based upon plasma ascorbic acid (AA) levels.[12] The average IQ for the higher AA group was approximately 4.51 points higher than in the lower AA group. The two groups were then divided and were given supplemental orange juice for a period of six months. The average IQ for the higher AA group rose only 0.02 points, whereas that of the lower AA group rose by an average of 3.54 points. This study was continued into a second year, and IQ was raised by an average of 3.6 points when plasma AA levels were increased by 50 percent.

Iodine

Iodine is an essential element in human health. Obtained through a variety of foods, iodine is one on the most highly absorbed elements in the human body. Essential for proper function of the thyroid gland, gross deficiency of iodine has devastating effects on growth and development; deficiency is associated with mental retardation and cretinism in extreme cases.[13] Because of these effects, hypothyroidism (which can result from low iodine intake) is screened for at birth in most developed countries. The richest sources of iodine come from marine animals, but it is found elsewhere in other foods. However, iodine is added to many foods to ensure that the population receives enough of this important mineral; certain geographic areas produce what is known as endemic goiter, or a condition in which iodine rarity leads to a goiter condition of the thyroid gland.

Despite being added to table salt, there is some speculation that this may not be enough, and dietary patterns that focus on low-iodine content may have an effect on the learning and cognitive development of children. A study examining the long-term effects of subclinical iodine deficiency on learning and motivation in male children was undertaken to demonstrate the importance of iodine in these processes.[14] The children were divided into a severely deficient iodine group and a mildly iodine-deficient group. After undergoing a battery of tests designed to measure learning and motivation abilities, the results demonstrate that the severely deficient children were slower learners and scored significantly lower on the achievement motivation scale in comparison to the mildly deficient children. The researchers in this study suggest that subclinical iodine deficiency causes impaired neural development and poor sociopsychologic stimulation, which results in learning disability and decreased learning achievement motivation in these children. In another study carried out in a region of endemic goiter in Sicily, visual perceptual integrative motor ability (a measurement of reading and speaking comprehension) was measured in over 700 clinically normal 6- to 12-year-old children (with normal thyroid function) who live in iodine-deficient endemic goiter areas.[15] Neurologic testing revealed that nearly 14 percent of these children were found to have some type of neurologic deficiency (as compared to only 3 percent of children living in a control area adjacent to the sea-iodine is plentiful in marine-based foods). Additionally, 19 percent of children exhibited signs of neuromuscular and neurosensorial abnormalities as measured by other neurologic tests. The results of this study suggest the presence of an endemic cognitive deficiency; this was speculated to be due to the low iodine availability in the area study.

These studies suggest that suboptimal levels of the above nutrients may have an effect on the learning capabilities of children, especially in the developmental years. These studies are also interesting in that the nutrients examined are relatively common in healthy diets, suggesting that either food contain inadequate amounts of these nutrients or that optimal amounts need to be reconsidered. This brings home the importance of supplying children (and adults) with the very best nutrition possible, even more so in those with a family history or predisposition to learning disorders.

METAL TOXICITY

The accumulation of metals in the neurologic system is a fairly well-recognized cause of neurological impairment in children. Children affected by metal toxicity are even more severely affected than those with organic forms of learning disorders. Society has done much to lower this risk; lead has been removed from household paints and automotive fuels; however, children exposed to lead paints in older, unkempt homes remain at risk. Other environmental metals that pose a neurologic threat include selenium, cadmium, and aluminum. Hair samples were taken from groups of children with learning disabilities and another group without learning disabilities and compared for metal content.[16] The group of children with learning disabilities was found to have elevated levels of lead and cadmium in comparison to the non–learning disability group.

Lead exposure is known to cause learning impairments and behavioral problems.[17] Lead is thought to affect neurotransmitter receptor sites in the brain and the availability of the neurotransmitter dopamine. Lead exposure leads to learning disability and other problems, not only in children. A review of the effects of chronic low-grade lead exposure (which is common in the general population and is thought to still affect 10–50 percent of American children [over 3–4 million]) hypothesized that long-term effects include difficulty in mentation (thinking processes), behavioral difficulties, and the development of hypertension.[18] The prevalence of metals in the environment (as a result of industrial pollution) is fairly widespread and will undoubtedly have an effect on neurologic development as long as it is present. However, because of the multiple causative factors in learning disabilities, it is difficult to pinpoint a solitary factor in their development, especially when they are the result of environmental factors.

ESSENTIAL FATTY ACIDS

The development of the brain is a highly interactive process, and events that disrupt this development early on can have significant, long-lasting effects on later development. Neuronal development follows a network of signaling pathways, and the ability of the brain cell to accurately relay signals is dependent on the complex interactions of the cell membrane. The brain is composed of nearly 60 percent lipids; the majority of these fatty acids are arachidonic and docosahexaenoic acid and are known to be vital for the growth, function, and integrity of the brain structure. Polyunsaturated fatty acids, most specifically arachidonic acid and docosahexaenoic acid (DHA), are accumulated in large amounts in early brain development, which reflects dietary intake of these nutrients. (Both fatty acids are found in human milk.) These fatty acids are incorporated into the cell membrane, and their relative content can influence signaling pathways and efficiency. Researchers have shown that fatty acid imbalances and deficiencies have an adverse effect on brain development, including the ability to respond to environmental stimulation (i.e., teaching and other learning processes).[19] Additionally, this research indicates that omega-3 fatty acids deficiency can influence neurotransmitters such as the dopamine system, which negatively affects specific learning that takes place in the prefrontal lobe of the brain. This and other studies of human infants suggest that dietary deficiency of DHA may play a role in cognitive development and in neurodevelopmental disorders that may, in turn, play a role in the development of learning disorders.

Animal studies demonstrate that when essential fatty acids such as AA and DHA are supplied in insufficient amounts, neurologic development is inhibited, and this effect is permanent.[20] Risk of neurodevelopmental disorders are highest in the lowest birth-weight babies, and these babies tend to have deficits of AA and DHA, which contribute to long-term developmental deficits.[21] Another study investigated the effects of withholding omega-3 essential fatty acids from the diets of test animals. The researchers noted a decline in cognitive performance as brain content of DHA decreased.[22] The importance of AA and DHA in brain development is evidenced by the permanent effects noted when these fats are deficient in the diet of developing brains. Supplementation at an early age, beginning immediately following breast milk weaning, should be employed to avert any long-term neurologic defects.

OTHER FACTORS

Other environmental factors can affect learning and development as well. There is some evidence that caffeine ingestion may impair the brain's ability to form memory, which is a large part of learning and development. In one study, caffeine impaired the memory retention scores in test subjects when administered 30 minutes before a learning situation occurred.[23] This study demonstrates the ability of caffeine to affect learning by challenging the process of memory making. Other factors, such as television and video games, definitely have a negative effect on learning, solely because of time spent away from productive study habits. These influences have been shown to also affect behavior in ways that are not conducive to learning. Children with learning disorders were exposed to either aggressive or control cartoons in one study.[24] After assessing five different categories of social behavior following the cartoon viewing, it was noted that the children most affected by their leaning disorders were more physically aggressive after viewing the aggressive cartoons. Studies such as this indicate that what children view on television may impair their ability to learn.

CONCLUSION

Learning disability, although not a disease, can affect people throughout their lifetimes and comes with significant effects on quality of life. Affecting people in a variety of ways, learning disabilities can occur singly or in combination. Causes for learning disabilities include hereditary and environmental and nutritional factors. Paying particular attention to nutrition, especially in our youngest children, may serve to blunt the effects that other contributing factors may contribute to the development of learning disability and may even prevent some disabilities. Research has provided several interesting insights into nutritional deficiencies and their effects on neurologic development. Clinically, we routinely observe significant improvements with simple dietary and supplemental interventions. Indeed, much like a car requires the "right" grade of fuel for peak performance, so does the human body. Just as each car is designed for certain "octane," individuals need varying levels of nutrients. Thus, whether due either to genetic or environmental factors, additional nutrient needs may differentiate those that manifest with LD and those that do not. This clinical observation is by no means intended to oversimplify the complexity of the LD, but without a strong nutritional intervention, work with LD can often be unnecessarily more challenging than needed. Children, particularly, have a tremendous ability to adapt and neurologically are very able to make significant strides when the condition is addressed at the root cause.

NUTRIENTS

- Multivitamin/Mineral
  Two tablets twice daily with food (or as directed)
  Containing nutrients meeting at least the suggested RDA for each
- Iron
  Children should be assessed for iron deficiency prior to supplementing with this nutrient
  RDA doses for iron: (iron is leading cause of childhood poisening)
  Older infants and children:
    7 to 12 months, 11 milligrams per day
    1 to 3 years, 7milligrams per day
    4 to 8 years, 10 milligrams per day
    9 to 13 years, 8 milligrams per day
    Boys 14 to 18 years, 11 milligrams per day
    Girls 14 to 18 years, 15 milligrams per day
  Adults:
    Men aged 19 and older and women aged 51 and older, 8 milligrams
      per day (best to get test prior to supplementing)
    Women aged 19 to 50 years, 18 milligrams per day
- Magnesium
  5 milligrams per kilogram of weight, or roughly 100–200 milligrams per day
- Zinc
  10 milligrams per day

- Vitamin C
  250–500 milligrams per day
- Iodine
  150 micrograms per day
- Essential Fatty Acids
  1–2 grams per day in the form of DHA starting just after weaning

Mental Fatigue

Mental fatigue is a condition that virtually everyone has experienced at some time in his or her life. For many others, however, peak performance in life is attenuated by constant mental fatigue resulting from several factors. Among the obvious are overwork, and "burning the candle at both ends," a scenario that many of us in the modern working world experience. For many, life is a series of fast-paced events and situations that demand absolute attention; personal, family, and work priorities all demand 100 percent of our focused energy. For the majority of Americans, mental fatigue is a fact of life. Our dependence on mental labor today has strong effects on the neuroendocrine and immune systems; it is no wonder people are in the midst of psychological and emotional dysfunctions that result in depression, anxiety, and fatigue.

Mental fatigue affects people in different ways for differing periods of time. Primarily the result of brain overactivity, mental fatigue is really an exhaustion of the neurologic system, which is very similar to exhaustion of the physical body from physical labor. Mental fatigue is caused by continuous mental effort and attention on a particular task or related tasks or from high levels of stress or emotional states. Really, any excessive mental process can result in this disorder. The most common manifestation of mental fatigue occurs near the end of the working day (which can extend late into the evening). Fatigue appears as duties seem more complicated and impedes thought processes, making concentration low and raising the occurrence of mistakes.

Mental fatigue at first seems easily taken care of by just resting or switching one's concentration. Unfortunately, the events that lead one to become mentally fatigued are usually lifestyle based (job and home life) and are not easily left alone for any extended period of time. The brain, being the incredible creation that it is, is highly able to respond to slight changes in the way we take care (or for that matter, do not take care) of ourselves. Supporting this organ nutritionally will provide the nutrients that contribute to mental energy processes and will also replace those nutrients that are consumed in the process of mental activity.

The definition of mental fatigue is the subjective feeling of fatigue, combined with negative effects on performance due to time spent on cognitively demanding tasks.[1] Additionally, these feelings of fatigue and performance changes can occur independently from influences such as the time of day, learning capabilities, or physical effort. (This may explain why those with mental fatigue can feel exhausted even after a solid night of sleep; the process is chronic and not easily ameliorated.) Researchers in this area note that among the most important changes in performance in mental fatigue is a deterioration of the organization of behavior; behavior appears to lose cohesion when people become mentally fatigued.[2] The following characteristics are noted as defining factors of mental fatigue:

- Subjective feeling of fatigue
- Negative change in performance due to time spent in cognitively demanding tasks
- Independence from time of day, learning, or investment of physical effort

Neurologic processes that are thought to be affected by mental fatigue include[3]:

- Inhibition of interfering stimuli
- Inhibition of prepotent responses (irrelevant information that "pops" into one's mind)
- Working memory processes that enable retrieval of information
- Working memory processes concerning preparation of responses

DIET AND FATIGUE

Mental energy, based on similar physiologic mechanisms as is physical energy (muscular), would seem to be responsive to similar nutritional guidelines that are followed for physical fatigue. Therefore, similar dietary recommendations for peak physical energy also should be adhered to in persons with mental fatigue. True, neurochemistry is starkly different from muscular and metabolic physiology, but both systems derive energy from the same general sources: carbohydrates, proteins, fats, and the vitamins and minerals they contain. One of the fist places a person with mental fatigue should look (other than the overindulgence in activities that led to the fatigue) is at their nutritional status (i.e., dietary intake). The topic of mental fatigue is one that demands an evaluation of overall macronutrient intake and its effect on this condition. Not defined as a standard disease, mental fatigue is definitely a symptom of overwork and undernutrition and may someday be considered an associated risk factor for true mental disease.

Regaled in the media as of late as a highly undesirable food component, carbohydrates are necessary for human (and for that matter, animal) metabolism. Overindulgence in simple carbohydrates and resultant insulin resistance is without a doubt one of the main reasons for much of the diabetes, obesity, hypertension, and cardiovascular disease seen in modernized countries today.[4] However, carbohydrates are a primary and necessary fuel source that must be consumed for proper energy metabolism. An interesting study compared the effects of various macronutrient balanced lunchtime meals on perceived fatigue in people consuming them.[5] Specifically, healthy subjects consumed lunchtime meals (after fasting overnight and then consuming a normal breakfast) consisting of either a high-carbohydrate, low-protein meal, a similar meal containing equal amounts of both carbohydrates and protein, or a high-protein, low-carbohydrate meal, or they continued to fast. All meals consisted of the same amount of calories and had equal fat contents. The only meal to cause a significant, immediate increase in fatigue was the high-carbohydrate lunch; this was not attributed to reactive hypoglycemia as patient blood glucose levels remained elevated. Investigators were able to partially explain the postcarbohydrate fatigue as being relative to elevations in plasma tryptophan levels; however, the fatigue ceased even though tryptophan levels remained high within the time frame of the study.

In another related study, subjects consumed breakfast meals consisting of low-fat, high-carbohydrate content; medium-fat, medium-carbohydrate content; and high-fat, low-carbohydrate content, or they had no meal.[6] These people were then tested on a number of tasks designed to measure cognitive performance and mood following the breakfast meal. Although no differences in cognition were noted, significant changes in mood were noted, specifically demonstrating that macronutrient content of foods can affect mood states following consumption. The significance of these findings is that food intake can alter mood, and there is no doubt that mood state can affect one's performance at work and in other areas of life.

Providing a low-glycemic diet may be helpful in offsetting any food-induced cognitive deficits following the food intake. Foods high in sugars such as simple carbohydrates (cakes, cookies, soda, etc.) create the well-known phenomenon of reactive hypoglycemia in which, following consumption of such foods and the resultant insulin response, blood sugars are left lower than their previous levels.[7] This is undoubtedly detrimental to mental function, as glucose is the brain's main fuel supply; many people are familiar with the late-afternoon hypoglycemic "crash" in which they become hungry and irritable and have decreased performance.

An interesting study investigated the cognitive effects of different macronutrients (fat, protein, and carbohydrates).[8] In this study, fat ingestion lead to the best postprandial (after eating) cognitive performance, whereas carbohydrates and protein consumption resulted in lower overall cognitive performance. However, different cognitive functions were affected by each macronutrient; carbohydrate ingestion caused better short-term memory and task accuracy, whereas protein ingestion led to better attention and task efficiency. Such findings support the idea that both stable and best cognitive performance is related to balanced glucose metabolism and metabolic states.

Another analysis of breakfast meals was performed and highlighted in a review article that compared the findings of three separate studies investigating the importance of adequate blood glucose in improving memory function in people who ate breakfast.[9] The findings from this review revealed that eating breakfast influenced cognition through several mechanisms, one of which was increased blood glucose. Eating breakfast (and maintaining adequate blood glucose levels) resulted in improved memory function, whereas fasting was found to adversely affect recall; this performance decline was reversible by consuming a glucose-rich food. Luckily, failure to eat breakfast did not affect performance on intelligence tests.

There is much research regarding the role of folate in mental health; the role that folate plays in the synthesis of neurotransmitters can be applied to its use in mental fatigue as well. Neurotransmitters are essentially the language of the brain, and theoretically, very little neurologic work could happen in their absence. Previous chapters have highlighted the role of folate in brain metabolism and their improvement when deficiencies are corrected. The role of folates in neurotransmitter synthesis and function, as well as their role in neuronal structure, stresses the importance of this vitamin and its forms in proper neurologic function and that deficits are associated with mental health problems. Among the other functions of folate, it contributes to the formation of glutamate, and excitatory neurotransmitter, just to name a few.[10]

BOTANICAL MEDICINES

There are several herbs with so-called nootropic effects, meaning they have an affinity for improving brain function. Although the role of proper nutrition in mental health and prevention of mental fatigue cannot be disputed, the addition of botanical medicines that further assist the brain on a metabolically enhanced level are important to consider. The botanical medicines mentioned herein do not act as stimulants; several stimulants (caffeine, ephedra) have been intensely studied and show a definite increase in cognitive function. However, the metabolic premise of these and other neurologic stimulants can be likened to robbing Peter to pay Paul. Rather, stimulants only increase energy at the expense of the brain's nutrient supply; pushing on the accelerator makes the car go faster, but it also uses the fuel more rapidly and accelerates wear and tear on the vehicle. Botanical medicines that are used to avert mental fatigue do so primarily by supporting cognitive function through their effects on neurologic metabolism.

Rhodiola rosea

A native plant to the Arctic regions of Siberia, Scandinavia, Lapland, and Alaska, *Rhodiola* has a long history of medicinal use dating back to the first century A.D.[11] This herb has been used to increase energy and stamina as well as mental capacity; it is classified as an adaptogen, or substance that assists the body in resisting physical, chemical, and environmental stressors. Recent research has investigated the efficacy of this plant as applied to modern-day life stresses with interesting results. One study investigated the antifatigue effects of *Rhodiola* on mental work capacity in a situation of background fatigue and stress (military cadets).[12] The study results demonstrated a significant antifatigue effect in the cadets taking the herb, and this effect was statistically significant in comparison to the placebo group. Another study more applicable to mental fatigue investigated the effect of a standardized extract of *Rhodiola* on fatigue during night shifts among healthy young physicians.[13] Mental performance in this study was measured using tests designed to monitor mental fatigue involving perceptive and cognitive cerebral functions such as associative thinking, short-term memory, calculation, concentration ability, and audiovisual perception. Results demonstrated statistically significant improvements in mental performance as measured using the mentioned objective points; no side effects were reported in subjects using the herb.

Studies such as these demonstrate the fascinating effects of this plant on stress-related mental function; this is applicable, of course, to many people's everyday lives that are full of stressful events, with little reprise. Another study used *Rhodiola* in students during an acute stressful period of test taking that occurred over a period of several weeks.[14] *Rhodiola* was used to attenuate the effects of stress as measured by mental fatigue, neuromotor tests, and physical fitness, before and after supplementation, over a 20-day period. Self-assessment of general well-being improved following the study period, and significant improvements were noted in the areas of physical fitness, mental fatigue, and neuromotor test categories as well. *Rhodiola* is an interesting adaptogenic botanical medicine with definite uses in those that suffer from mental fatigue. A large amount of research was performed on this herb in the late 1960s and 1970s, primarily in Russia, with interesting results in fitness and mental work performance. Researchers are again investigating the promising effects of this herb; it has properties that make it an ideal supportive aid for mental fatigue.

Ginseng

Ginseng is derived from three main varieties of this herb (Panax, Siberian, American). Another traditionally used botanical with thousands of years of use, the ginsengs are also considered adaptogenic botanicals. The term "adaptogen" covers a huge area of physiologic responses and is elicited differently with individual herb species. Past research on ginseng reveals physiologic effects that may benefit cognitive performance and mood; animal studies indicate modulation of stress, fatigue, and learning capacities, and single doses administered in human subjects have been shown to improve memory.[15] Components of ginseng, known as ginsenosides (which are derived from all three species of ginseng), have numerous pharmacologic actions on the brain and nervous system (in addition to other areas of the body). A study using a ginseng component was shown to enhance the growth of neurons and protect them from damage induced by a commonly used experimental neurotoxin (MPTP).[16] Results from this study suggest that the neuroprotective and neurotrophic (nerve-growing) effects of ginseng may account for the enhancement of cognitive function that is experienced in people using ginseng as a supportive agent. Another effect of ginseng that may contribute to the herb's benefit on brain function is the ability of one ginsenoside to facilitate the release of a neurotransmitter (acetylcholine) from an area of the brain known as the hippocampus.[17] Researchers noted that this increased release of acetylcholine might be associated with the ability of ginseng to prevent memory loss by modulating the metabolism of this neurotransmitter.

Ginkgo biloba

Ginkgo biloba is best known for its preventive effects on the brain in various forms of dementia (please see the chapter on Alzheimer's disease for more information). Not surprising, this herb also has neurologic benefits prior to the onset of age-related decline; it is a challenge to recall that many herbs, containing several active constituents, have various effects on same-organ systems, as well as other bodily systems. Ginkgo is beneficial in conditions of mental fatigue perhaps in part due to its ability to increase blood flow and oxygenation to the brain, among other functions. Its combination with ginseng demonstrates additional neurologic benefit that has been highlighted in several studies.

Ginkgo extract, in addition to being effective in preventing Alzheimer's disease, vascular dementia, and age-related cognitive decline, also has potent antioxidant activity and directly affects the cholinergic neurotransmitter system; recent research demonstrates that ginkgo acts as a nootropic agent that works to improve brain function. A randomized, double-blind, placebo-controlled study utilizing ginkgo extract for 30 days demonstrated significant improvements in working memory, rapidity of information processing, and mental processing.[18] These results are suggestive of the ability of ginkgo extract to improve brain functions that are associated with both mental fatigue and measurements of intelligence.

Research involving combinations of both ginkgo and ginseng have provided fascinating results regarding mental performance. Although not surprising, combinations of these two powerful brain-specific botanical medicines provide further benefits for combating the fatigue of mental exertion. Utilizing a combination of the two herbs, one study attempted to define calculation skill improvements following serial doses of the two herbs.[19] Study subjects experienced significant and sustained increased ability to calculate (Serial Sevens) following dosing of the herb combination at one, two, four, five, and six hours following administration. Another study revealed that after receiving a combination of the two herbs, those receiving the active compound experienced a dose-dependent improvement in performance in the "quality of memory" test factor in cognitive performance.[20] This effect was specifically more prominent at longer term memory function. These results are quite profound in that a near-immediate effect on specific brain functions were realized following administration, and it lasted for some time thereafter. Keeping in mind that the effects measured in these particular studies represent only a miniscule fraction of cognitive function, it is exciting to see such outcomes; extrapolation of these results in relation to mental fatigue seems quite promising as this study demonstrates the utility of these herbs as an immediate remedy. Ginkgo and ginseng are both safe botanical medicines with very specific effects on cognitive function. These effects can be interpreted as improvements in cognitive function that makes them superior choices in combating mental fatigue. These herbs seem to have several effects on the brain. Whether increasing cognitive function in the healthy or ameliorating the effects of dementia, they present an as of yet unparalleled nutritional treatment that is not matched by any other compound.

OTHER CONSIDERATIONS

In addition to avoiding low blood sugar symptoms by consuming regular, balanced meals, certain nutrients may help to assist the body in maintaining its blood sugar. Chromium is an essential trace element that the body uses to utilize blood glucose. Part of a complex of molecules known as glucose tolerance factor, chromium is thought to be the active part of the complex. Chromium is thought to enhance the activity of insulin, a bodily hormone that is responsible for transporting glucose into the cells. Chromium increases the number of insulin receptors, or doorways through which insulin and glucose enter cells, as well as receptor affinity to glucose.[21] Without chromium, insulin does not bind as well to cells, and the number of insulin receptors decrease. Chromium also serves to assist with the metabolism of glucose itself, as well as its transformation into fatty acids and cholesterol.[22] What all of this means is that taken supplementally, chromium helps the body utilize foods (primarily carbohydrates) more efficiently, thereby preventing hypoglycemia (decreased blood sugar) that contributes to decreased mental focus and attention.

CONCLUSION

Mental fatigue is primarily the result of overburdening the central nervous system. However, with modern life and its constant demands, people require additional support of their cognitive functions in order to cope with daily stressors and to avert future mental dysfunction. Appropriate support of the brain begins with an adequate nutritional plan; research demonstrates the importance of balanced, regular meals as a first step in achieving this goal. As always, healthy nutrition should be reinforced with a multivitamin and mineral supplement, as a supportive element. In addition to nutrition, the botanical medicines *Rhodiola rosea, Ginkgo biloba,* and ginseng species provide adaptogenic as well as specific neurologic function support for combating mental fatigue. The person suffering from fatigue can effectively employ combinations of these botanical medicines as a preventive strategy against mental fatigue and decline.

The key to helping treat mental fatigue is to eliminate deficit spending. Or put another way, if a car burns a higher rate of gasoline than is put in the tank, it will run on vapors until it ultimately runs out of fuel. The human body is very comparable. Indeed, proper fueling of the body is critical, yet, even with a full tank of fuel, a body that has become deconditioned from overuse, excess stress, insufficient rest, or underlying other health issues will increase the likelihood of potential catastrophic failure of the neurological functioning resulting in diminished mental alertness and foundational energy. On the positive note, the body is remarkably recuperative, and with the slightest inclination, significant strides can be made to regain lost ground. The take-home message is not one of just fueling the body properly; it also imparts that, when endeavoring to build up the body's reserves, overt losses of current gains must be curtailed. Providing the body with some down time and avoiding continuous mental stimulation that leads to the mental fatigue in the first place will allow the brain to recuperate and recover from fatigue.

NUTRIENTS

- Macronutrients
  Ensure adequate consumption of carbohydrates, proteins, and fats in a ratio of 40:30:30 three times daily
- Folate
  1,000 micrograms per day
- Chromium
  200 micrograms per day

BOTANICALS

- *Rhodiola rosea*
  50 milligrams, twice daily
- *Ginkgo biloba*
  60–120 milligrams, twice daily
- Ginseng
  0.25–0.5 grams twice daily

Multiple Sclerosis

A condition that is characterized by demyelinating lesions (loss of the protective layer that surrounds the nerves and allows for efficient nerve signal impulses) in the brain and spinal cord, the symptoms of multiple sclerosis (MS) can include weakness, balance problems, impaired vision, numbness, bladder dysfunction, and sometimes changes in psychological status. A chronic health condition, people with MS often experience variable signs and symptoms, and MS is considered a relapsing/remitting disease, meaning that symptoms come and go over time. In short, symptoms can worsen for a period of time and then suddenly greatly or partially improve. There is little evidence for why this occurs at this time. The name of the disease, multiple sclerosis, exemplifies the disease process as it occurs in the central nervous system (CNS) (composed of the brain and spinal cord), characterized by multiple sclerosed, or scarred, areas throughout the brain and spinal cord. The process involves different components of the immune system that attack and destroy the insulating material surrounding nerve cells (myelin) and in some cases destroy the nerves themselves. Myelin is similar to the insulating material around electrical wires; a wire without this layer will inefficiently transmit electrical potentials.

Often initially appearing in young adults (average age is 30 but peak incidence occurs in the mid-20s), MS symptoms may occur in attacks that are separated by months or years, making it difficult to diagnose. True diagnosis cannot be unequivocally made until symptoms have occurred in separate areas of the nervous system. Statistics concerning MS vary; it affects 250,000 to 350,000 people in the United States and anywhere from 1.1 to 2.5 million people worldwide.[1] These numbers may not be wholly accurate as MS is a disease that is not always reported or caught by physicians. About 1 of every 700 people has MS in the United States, and it is the second most common disease that affects the CNS in young adults. Women are twice as likely to be affected as men, and the disease occurs most commonly in Caucasians of northern European origin, especially Scottish descent. Family history plays a role, although the risk for inheriting the full genetic factors that contribute to MS ranges from 2 percent to 4 percent; but risk among identical twins is nearly 30 percent.[2]

Geographic location and MS have been linked, especially among Caucasians. There is a relationship between where a person lived as a child and his or her risk of developing MS later in life, suggesting an environmental link at work in the disease. The incidence of MS is greater in persons living (as children) in northern areas of Europe and North America.[3] Other evidence suggests that when people move from a high-risk area to a low-risk area, or the reverse, prior to the age of 15, they may acquire the risk associated with the new area, and if they are older than age 15, they retain the same risk associated with the old area.[4] Otherwise, the geographic hypothesis is weakened by the lack of an identifiable infectious agent and weak analysis testing the association between MS and any previous infection in subjects.[5]

As mentioned previously, the causative factors for MS are many, and no one specific causative factor has been identified. Natural therapeutics provide several forms of treatment with established benefits in people with MS and can help reduce the symptoms of this disease. Long-term effects of natural therapeutics are not known at this time; however, this does not imply that these therapies should not be employed. Again, MS is a disease with probably several causes, one of them being biological individuality, and what may provide some benefit in one patient may provide great or little benefit in another.

NUTRITIONAL FACTORS

Interesting research has been done in the area of vitamin D and MS. Researchers have hypothesized that a form of vitamin D, known as 1,25-dihydroxyvitamin D-3, exerts protective effects against MS due to the following: 1. Vitamin D3 fully protects animals from an experimentally induced form of MS, which is widely used as a research model for human MS. 2. Because of the environmental relationship between latitude and MS, it is hypothesized that a crucial factor is lack of ultraviolet light-induced vitamin D-3 synthesis in the skin and that vitamin D-3 acts as a selective immune system regulator that works to inhibit autoimmune disease; therefore in low sunlight conditions, insufficient protective amounts of D-3 are manufactured.[3] Despite the circumstantial nature, this theory may explain the geographical distribution of MS, and two especially interesting geographic examples: MS rates in Switzerland are elevated in low altitudes and depressed at high altitudes, where UV light is more intense, and in Norway, where MS rates are higher inland, but much lower near the cost where vitamin D-3-rich fish is regularly consumed.[6] The authors of this work suggest that further research in this area may approach the possibility that MS could be prevented in genetically susceptible people through the use of supplemental vitamin D-3.

The research implicating deficiency of vitamin D as a causative factor in MS is further evidenced by the fact that most people with MS are affected by this, as shown in their low bone mass and high fracture rates.[7] (Vitamin D plays an integral role in calcium metabolism and thus bone strength.) However, the strongest evidence is the ability of vitamin D to completely inhibit experimental forms of MS in animals; this is carried out by the ability of vitamin D to stimulate the production of two proexperimental MS immune factors (interleukin 4 and transforming growth factor beta-1) in animal models.[8]

In the only study of its kind, a group of young MS patients was supplemented with calcium, magnesium, and vitamin D over a period of one to two years in order to determine the effects of these nutrients on disease course.[9] The patient's own case history served as the control in this study; that is, after the course of supplementation, the number of symptom exacerbations was compared to the number experienced prior to taking the supplement protocol. While supplemented, these MS patients had less than one-half the symptom flares that were expected from prior disease character, and no side effects were reported. This study provides some insight into the usefulness of these nutrients in controlling disease symptoms and their role in stabilizing myelin in MS.

Vitamin B-12, with its many contributory functions to neurologic function, has been studied to some extent in MS. Studies involving vitamin B-12 and MS have demonstrated an association between deficiency of this vitamin and occurrence of the disease. Additionally, other studies have demonstrated an increased risk of red blood cell deformation (macrocytosis), low blood and cerebrospinal fluid levels of B-12, and elevated levels of binding capacity in MS.[10] Investigators are unable to speculate the exact role of B-12 in MS pathology; however, it is hypothesized that binding or transport abilities of B-12 are to blame, and there is a striking similarity in the epidemiologic patterns of MS and pernicious anemia.

Additionally, B-12 deficiency has been shown to contribute to the destruction of myelin and axons in the white matter areas of the central nervous system.[11] A case review of MS and B-12 studies revealed a significant association between MS and dysfunctional B-12 metabolism; cases reported included low serum B-12 levels, elevated saturation capacities, and macrocytosis (blood cell deformity—a sign of insufficient B-12).[12] The authors of this review speculate that B-12 deficiency may further exacerbate MS symptoms or impair patient recovery from symptomatic events. Blood levels of vitamin B-12 and B-12 binding capabilities were measured in a group of people with MS.[13] Although no deficiency was detected in this group of patients, there was a significantly large decrease in the unsaturated B-12 binding capacities, meaning that storage capabilities were reduced in comparisons to healthy subjects. Subsequently, these patients were treated with very large doses (60 milligrams every day) of B-12 for the next six months. Abnormalities in brain stem and visual nerve function (evoked potentials) improved at a greater speed during the supplementation phase than during the presupplement period, indicating that large amounts of B-12 may improve some aspects of MS neurologic function.

In a different type of investigational study, it was revealed that serum B-12 levels in people with MS are related to the age at which the person first begins to experience disease symptoms.[14] The study found that people whose MS appeared prior to age 18 (average age of 10 years) had significantly lower serum B-12 levels than those whose MS appeared after the age of 18 (average age of 35 years). Investigators found that levels of folate were unrelated to these phenomena and suggested that there is a specific association between time of onset of MS and metabolism of B-12. In addition, because of the importance of B-12 in myelin and immune system functions (there is a large body of research concerning viral infection as one cause of MS), the authors of the study suggest that a deficiency of B-12 is a critical factor in the development of MS.

ANTIOXIDATIVE THERAPY

The role of antioxidant status in MS patients has been explored from both a causative and treatment standpoint. Oxidative stress has been implicated in many disease processes, not only MS.[15] Oxidation is a damaging biologic process that occurs basically as a side effect of normal metabolism. Unfortunately, the environment is full of other oxidants (namely pollution and chemicals) that are ingested along with the air we breathe and food we eat. Oxidation damages DNA molecules and fatty acids in the body, making it difficult for genes, and therefore cells, to repair themselves adequately. Continuous damage at these microscopic levels is widely considered to be the root cause of age-related decline.[16]

Levels of vitamins have been measured in MS patients in order to determine if these patients had adequate amounts in their blood. A study determined the amount of antioxidant vitamins (ascorbic acid, beta-carotene, retinol, and alpha-tocopherol) and the level of pro-oxidation that was occurring (as measured by thiobarbituric acid reacting substances [TBARS] generation).[17] The levels of the four vitamins were significantly lower in the MS patients compared to the healthy control subjects (measures of increased oxidation were higher in the MS patients compared to the control subjects also), indicating a possible increased need for antioxidant-type vitamins in people with MS, most notably during an exacerbation of symptoms.

In a separate study, significant increases in the amount of plasma lipid oxidizability and autoantibodies against oxidized low-density lipoproteins, in addition to a measurable decrease in antioxidant capacity of patient plasma, were measured in persons experiencing a flare-up of MS symptoms.[18] These findings highlight the importance of antioxidants in the prevention and treatment of disease conditions, including MS. By supplementing with adequate amounts, one may possibly mitigate the effects of oxidation on lipids, an important step in the prevention of MS.

Supplementation with vitamins C, A, E and the minerals zinc and selenium provide a good antioxidative base therapy. All of these nutrients have proven antioxidative effects and have been widely studied for their efficacy in preventing oxidative damage in the body and restoring antioxidant status in disease states.[19] Recent research has revealed a group of even more powerful antioxidant compounds derived from plant sources. These compounds, known as oligomeric proanthocyanidins, can be found in many plant foods; however, the most abundant sources include green tea, bilberry, grape seed, buckwheat, and red wine. Supplying adequate amounts of these foods in the diet may greatly decrease one's oxidative burden. Providing large amounts (studies of the protective effects of green tea revealed that those who consumed the equivalent of 10 or more cups per day experienced the greatest preventative effect) of these compounds (with the exception of red wine) in food or supplement form (supplements will allow for greater consumption) can provide a proactive and preventative strategy for lessening the severity of the MS disease process.

FATTY ACIDS

Essential fatty acids (EFAs) are needed by humans in order to perform various physiologic functions, including modulation of inflammation and synthesis of immune system factors, and contribute to the formation of cellular membranes throughout the body. Deficiency of the essential fatty acids is a relatively common condition in countries with processed-food diets. It is theorized that humans evolved on a diet consisting of a 1:1 ratio of omega-6 to omega-3 fatty acids, whereas today the typical Western diet consists of a ratio between 10:1 and 25:1, and in some cases, it may be as high as 40:1. It is this imbalanced fatty acid ratio that is linked to chronic inflammatory health problems. A common misconception is that all commonly consumed omega-6 fatty acids (linoleic acid, arachidonic acid, and gamma linolenic acid) are unhealthful, when the reality is that only excessive intake of linoleic and arachidonic acid (combined with decreased omega-3 fatty acids) contribute to chronic inflammation, as these fatty acids are necessary to perform essential functions in the body. Gamma linoleic acid has considerable health benefits and is not linked to the problems associated with an unbalanced fatty-acid profile.

Evidence from both a biochemical and epidemiologic perspective reinforces the beneficial role of EFAs. A review article covering studies that utilized both omega-6 and omega-3 polyunsaturated fatty acids in the treatment of MS suggests a positive tendency in the reduction of the severity and frequency of symptom relapses over a two-year period, providing an overall benefit to the patients.[20] An earlier collective review of three studies using EFAs in the treatment of MS also revealed a positive effect from addition of these fats to the diet.[21] The results from this review combined the data from the studies regarding neurologic assessments that were carried out over a two-and-a-half-year period. Patients who were treated with EFAs experienced less-rapid progression of disability compared to control subjects. In addition, it reduced the severity and duration of MS relapses in all treated patients regardless of disability levels. The benefits of EFA supplementation are demonstrated in several additional studies investigating their use in the treatment of MS. Combined with broad-spectrum nutritional supplementation, this combination provides additional benefits to the MS patient.

A group of recently diagnosed MS patients were studied to determine whether providing EFA supplementation, dietary advice, and a vitamin supplement would influence their clinical course.[22] This group received supplemental EFA and vitamins for two years and experienced a significant reduction in the mean (average) annual rate of symptom flares and experienced less disability as measured on the Expanded Disability Status Scale (EDSS) when compared to prestudy levels. This study provides additional evidence supporting the role of EFA supplementation and nutritional support, even when supplied in a broad manner as a multivitamin. Using essential fatty acids creates a more favorable cellular environment in autoimmune diseases and conditions in which inflammatory processes are at work.

The use of EFAs to treat MS has its origins in the Swank diet, which consists of maintaining a dietary regimen that is nearly devoid of saturated fats (which usually come from processed fatty foods). Evidence shows that long-term adherence to an extremely low amount of saturated fat in the diet tends to slow the progression of the disease, as well as decrease the number of symptom attacks. A large number of MS patients who maintained this diet were followed for 34 years and were then divided into three groups of neurological disability (minimum, moderate, severe); those who followed the diet most closely displayed "significantly" less disease deterioration and death rates than controls. Additionally, the greatest benefits were seen in the "minimum" neurologic disability group, with a 95 percent survival rate (excluding other causes of death) and retainment of high levels of physical activity.[23]

FOOD ALLERGY

Food allergy, a common culprit in many conditions, should be strongly considered in the treatment of MS and all autoimmune conditions. Although clinical evidence for removal of food allergens is difficult to come by, anecdotal evidence does suggest that this approach can help to relieve MS symptoms. Additionally, evidence is accumulating that reflects the intricate relationship between food proteins and perturbations in human immunity.[24] It is important that all persons, regardless of condition, identify foods that may cause negative interactions in their bodies. Food allergies and sensitivities, when identified and removed, result in the alleviation of many patients' symptoms in numerous health conditions.

By removing these foods, the body is able to perform its regular functions with less energy directed at combating and/or dealing with foods that it does not tolerate well. Again, if one is ill, it is most important to identify all factors that distract the body from focusing on complete health and healing.

OTHER LIFESTYLE MODIFICATIONS

Maintenance of physical fitness is important in people with MS. Although becoming fatigued is contraindicated in MS, getting regular, stimulative exercise can be beneficial for preventative maintenance as regular exercise and physical activity can minimize states of decondition and help people with MS to maintain optimal physical function. A study designed to determine the relationship between physical activity and social, mental, and physical health and well-being in people with MS revealed that persons with MS who reported participating in regular exercise scored higher on physical functioning and general health measurements than those who did not exercise at all.[25]

When MS symptoms flare, many patients will attribute this to a recent stress in their life. Stress appears to be one of the hairs that breaks the camel's back when it comes to symptom exacerbation in this condition. Therefore, a person with MS will benefit from stress modulation techniques and lifestyle changes that address the stress. Additionally, botanical medicines can offer support in the form of supporting adrenal gland function. The adrenal glands are responsible for secreting the body's "stress" hormones, catecholamines. These hormones rise as stress levels increase, and their purpose, at least initially, is to help the body adapt to the stress that it experiences. Over time and when exposed to chronic stress, it is theorized that the adrenal glands may not function up to par in this respect, due to over stimulation. This may leave a person with less physiologic capacity to deal with stress.

Cordyceps Sinensis

A fungus harvested in mountainous regions of China, Cordyceps is said to be an adaptogenic agent. An adaptogen is an agent that assists a person in counteracting adverse physical, chemical, or biological stressors by generating nonspecific resistance. More simplified, adaptogens bolster our body's stress defenses. Cordyceps was used to measure the physiologic stress response in animals in one study, utilizing the weight of the adrenal gland as an outcome.[26] After supplementing the animals with Cordyceps and then exposing them to stress, it was found that the animals given the Cordyceps did not have as large adrenal glands as those not supplemented and exposed to stress. (The adrenal glands grow in response to stress in order to compensate for increased demand on this gland.) Cordyceps can be used to assist the body in dealing with stress and its hormonal consequences by supporting the function of the adrenal gland.

Panax Ginseng

This species of ginseng (more popularly known as Asian ginseng) is considered an adaptogenic herb as well, with the ability to stimulate the adrenocortical hormone system of the adrenal gland. Used to combat stress, ginseng can increase the body's resistance to environmental stress and may improve well-being. This herb may increase cortisol (a stress hormone from the adrenal glands) levels in the blood,[27] and it stimulates function of the adrenal gland as well.[28] Supplemental dosing of ginseng at times of stress, as well as in anticipation of stressful life periods, may assist a person with MS in dealing with the stress without suffering as many physical effects. Preemptive stress modulation is ideal, as repeated stresses will serve to undermine any healing progress a person has made since their last symptom episode. Ginseng is well tolerated and has few side effects for stress modulation purposes.

CONCLUSION

A disease with many unknowns, MS has many therapuetic options. Natural therapies for MS are plentiful, with results varying from individual to individual. These therapies work to alleviate the symptoms and, at the same time, provide the body with adequate sources of the materials it needs to stay healthy. Prevention of disease progression is highly important in MS. The key, of course, is to begin therapy early in the disease process, as the further the progression, the more recalcitrant it can be. Nutritional therapies also need time to work, as they are designed to alter patient metabolism over duration of time; simply taking multivitamins for a few weeks will almost certainly provide no lasting benefit. Whether trying to stay healthy or prevent the continuation of disease, it is important to give those therapies with clinical backing a chance to work in treating this disease.

Multiple sclerosis is without question a complex and multifaceted health condition that warrants a holistic look at the factors that contributed to the onset and propagation of the symptoms. With all chronic conditions, looking at the underlying triggers of the symptoms is important. Noteworthy is that the symptoms are not the condition; rather, they serve as benchmarks for successful treatment of the deeper issues of susceptibility. Indeed, there is an age and geographic prevalence for MS, as well as a tendency for females to have MS. Yet, not all young females get MS, regardless of geography or any other factor for that matter. Genetics may load the gun, but diet and lifestyle pull the trigger.

NUTRIENTS

- Vitamin D
  10 micrograms (400 International Unites)
- B-12
  2500 micrograms per day (methylcobalamin preferably)

Antioxidants

- Vitamin A
  2,500 International Units per day
- Vitamin C
  1,000–2,000 milligrams per day
- Vitamin E
  400–800 International Units per day
- Selenium
  200 micrograms per day
- Zinc
  25 milligrams per day

BOTANICALS

- Panax ginseng
  100 milligrams twice per day
- Cordyceps
  2,000 milligrams per day

Oppositional Defiant Disorder

Oppositional Defiant Disorder (ODD) is characterized by a continuous pattern of uncooperative, defiant, and hostile behavior targeted at persons in positions of authority that, as a result, interferes with normal day-to-day functioning. Primarily diagnosed in children, ODD may occur throughout life as well. Nearly all children are oppositional at some time or another, and this is especially true when they are stressed, tired, hungry, or emotionally upset. Considered a normal part of development in two- to three-year-olds and in early adolescence, ODD becomes a concern when hostile and uncooperative behavior is so frequent that it begins to affect the social, family, and academic aspects of the child's life. Additionally, this behavior pattern may be excessive in comparison to other children of similar age and developmental level. Children with ODD will argue, disobey, talk back, and defy anyone who represents authority to them; this can profoundly affect the rest of their development in all areas of life. Other notable symptoms of ODD may include:

- Frequent displays of anger or resentment
- Excessive arguing with adults
- Frequent temper tantrums
- Refusal to comply with requests and rules
- Deliberate attempts to upset others
- Easily annoyed by others, emotionally labile
- Revenge-seeking behavior
- Failure to take responsibility for their own actions

Symptoms are usually displayed in a variety of settings, most notably the home and school environments. It is estimated that 5 percent to 15 percent of school-aged children have ODD.[1] The exact causes of ODD are not fully known and are multiple. Other disorders may be present, such as attention deficit hyperactivity disorder (ADHD); learning disabilities; mood disorders, including depression and bipolar disorder; and anxiety disorders. Treatment of ODD is more successful when the accompanying disorder is treated as well; therefore, a child suspected of having ODD should have a thorough evaluation exploring any other potential coexisting disorders. Additionally, when left untreated, ODD may progress to conduct disorder, and the child will have problems with antisocial behavior and difficulties with relationships and holding a job. Because of the many coexisting factors that can occur with ODD, an adolescent psychiatrist should properly evaluate a child considered to be suffering from this disorder; a more expansive listing of diagnostic criteria can be found in the *Diagnostic and Statistical Manual of Mental Disorders* (DSM-IV).

Standard treatment of ODD involves numerous forms of psychotherapies including counseling, social skills training, and pharmaceutical prescribing. When accompanied by ADHD, ODD is treated with similar stimulant drugs (Ritalin and Adderall) and other medications that may be applicable to any other underlying disorder (depression, anxiety, etc.). Research regarding the use of other psychiatric drugs in the treatment of oppositional defiant disorder is currently available.

Treatment for ODD from a nutritional deficiency standpoint utilizes similar foci that were explored in the previous chapters: ADHD, Anxiety, Bipolar disorder, Depression, and Learning Disability. There are few solitary studies on nutritional influence in ODD; the large majority of this research focuses on ODD that is coexistent with ADHD, which is appropriate from a clinical standpoint in that ODD is, in one sense, a subcategory of ADHD. The division of diseases and their symptoms in medicine is at times an interesting phenomenon; a cluster of symptoms, and in this case of behaviors, is sometimes placed into a category in which it best fits. ODD is more than likely a variant of the same pathologies that occur in those with ADHD; the next section will highlight the nutritional factors that are important in ODD.

NUTRITION

The importance of nutrition in all neurologic disorders is paramount; science continues to discover the many ways that nutritional factors are incorporated into physiologic reactions and the effect that their absence has on proper function. With ODD, as with other neurologic conditions, it is essential that the brain is supplied with optimal nutrition in hopes that by fueling this organ correctly (the brain consumes nearly 20 percent of the total caloric intake per day) we can avert or absolve symptoms, which are signs that something is not well, whether physically or mentally.

A study investigating the use of two different nutritional products on children with ODD and ADHD revealed interesting results in regard to the importance of nutrition in these children.[2] The children in this study were supplemented with a simple carbohydrate-based product and another derived from fruits and vegetables. Based on a six-week time frame, a decrease in the severity and number of ODD, conduct disorder, and ADHD symptoms were noted within the first two weeks of the study. These researchers suggest that symptoms of the mentioned disorders might be further attenuated when specific carbohydrates (saccharides used in glycoconjugate synthesis) are incorporated into the diets of these children.

The brain is, in some people with a particular susceptibility quite sensitive to inadequate or imbalanced intake of nutrients. Some children have exhibited a decline in behavioral and academic performance when not thoroughly nourished. These same children, when supplemented with a vitamin and mineral combination, experienced improved academic and behavioral outcomes in comparison to others.[3] In another study of children and vitamin supplementation, researchers found that a vitamin and mineral supplement led to fewer incidences of antisocial behavior and better cognitive performance in school in the children who received it.[4] These two examples illustrate the importance of and a connection between adequate nutritional factors in children and their performance on a social and educational basis. Because ODD has no definitive causes, it makes sense to at least provide optimal nutrition to children at risk or with this disorder. Positive research regarding the role of nearly every nutrient can be found in relation to childhood development and performance; therefore, it stands to reason that in a disorder with no real etiology, nutrition will play an increasingly important role.

There is a collection of research that focuses on zinc as a potential nutritive agent that has been found in low supply in children with ADHD,[3] and a separate study has found lower levels of zinc in children with ADHD in comparison to those without.[5] Because zinc has been identified as a factor in each type of ADHD, it is assumed that children with ODD will benefit from zinc supplementation as well. Zinc is a cofactor in the synthesis of neurotransmitters and has an indirect role in the synthesis of dopamine metabolism. This is important as low levels of zinc are associated with ADHD and ODD, and supplementation with zinc has alleviated some of these symptoms in clinical studies.[6]

Magnesium is commonly deficient in the general population, and symptoms can range from insomnia to agitation and muscle cramps. A group of children with symptoms of ODD were treated for six months with supplemental magnesium in order to determine its effectiveness.[7] A significant decrease in hyperactivity was noted in this treatment group; magnesium is useful in providing a calming effect, something that is rarely attained in children with ODD symptoms. Magnesium supplementation when used appropriately has very few side effects and serves to decrease symptom intensity.

The identification of solitary nutrient deficiencies in behavioral disorders such as ODD and ADHD implies that if one nutrient is deficient, there is a high probability that more are in short supply as well. Acting synergistically, multiple nutrient inadequacies present a greater problem for the child with a behavioral disorder. In one study, the most common nutrient deficiencies found in children with ODD and ADHD symptoms were magnesium, copper, zinc, calcium, and iron.[8] These finding were apparent in children who were hyperactive more so than in children without behavioral symptoms. Upon noting the deficiencies, the subjects in this study were supplemented with magnesium, zinc, and calcium, which led to a decrease in hyperactivity. When treated without magnesium, the hyperactive behavior returned, demonstrating a clear link between magnesium and behavior.

Another interesting approach in behavioral disorders such as ODD and ADHD is the use of phosphatidylserine. A biological molecule known as a phospholipid, phosphatidylserine serves as a main component of cellular membranes in the human body and acts to stabilize the other constituents that make up the cellular membranes. Found in large amounts in the human brain, phosphatidylserine serves to regulate cellular communication and membrane metabolism.[9] As a nutritional supplement, phosphatidylserine serves to increase neurologic energy mechanisms via increased synaptic communications as well as increased production, release, and effectiveness of the neurotransmitter dopamine.[10] Phosphatidylserine supplementation in patients with behavioral disorders resulted in a slightly greater than 90 percent improvement, with doses of 200 to 300 milligrams per day for up to four months providing the greatest absolution of symptoms.[11] Supplemental administration of phosphatidylserine is thought to normalize brain lipid content, thereby assisting the return of normalized function of neuronal cells.[12]

These few studies implicate the important role of nutrients in managing behavioral disorders; some symptoms are resolved with the addition of simple nutritional supplements. ODD and related disorders such as ADHD carry a similar theme in that individuals may have unique biologic weaknesses that do not allow them to function optimally in the face of one or more nutrient deficiencies. When supplied in adequate amounts, supplemental nutritional factors will diminish symptoms, and may lead to complete resolution over time. A full spectrum of nutrients is indicated when treating behavioral disorders, as the research points to several different possible causes. An individualized approach is important; each person with ODD may react differently to various nutritional factors and current dietary habits are important to consider. The development of physiologic systems depends on varying levels and types of nutrients at different periods during the course of development.

CONCLUSION

As with many conditions affecting the presentation of psychologically driven behavior, ODD can be challenging for those hoping to intervene on behalf of the individual exhibiting the symptoms. Compliance can be particularly difficult for the individual expressing ODD behavior and is a unique hurdle.

Noteworthy is that food allergy testing, and subsequent elimination of the foods from the diet, can be an excellent place to start. The avoidance of substances can occur relatively passively and, when done correctly, does not have to become a focal point for the ODD tendencies. Once the alleviation of symptoms begins to become notable, other interventions to enhance biochemical functioning become significantly easier to implement.

NUTRIENTS

In addition to the recommendations in the chapter on ADHD, the following nutrients may be used.

- Diet
  A balanced diet that includes carbohydrates, proteins, and fats in a ratio of 40:30:30 percent each day, three times per day
- Zinc
  25 milligrams per day
- Magnesium
  5 milligrams per kilogram body weight per day
- Calcium
  5 milligrams per kilogram body weight per day
- Phosphatidylserine
  200–300 milligrams per day

Parkinson's Disease

Parkinson's disease (PD) is a disorder that progressively affects the brain; it is characterized by a decreased ability to elicit spontaneous movements, difficulty walking, postural instability, and rigidity and tremor. PD is caused by a degeneration of a particular group of nerve cells in a part of the brain known as the substantia nigra. Degeneration of these nerve cells causes a scarcity of dopamine, a vital neurotransmitter. The shortage of dopamine is what leads to the characteristic impairments of movement in PD.

Men and women are both affected by PD, with slightly higher occurrences in men. The frequency of the disease is higher in people over the age of 60, and although not a new disease (Parkinson's symptoms are mentioned in ancient medical texts), there has recently been an astounding increase of younger people diagnosed with this disease. In the United States, it is estimated that approximately 500,000 people have Parkinson's, with 50,000 new cases diagnosed per year.[1] Both the prevalence and incidence of PD is expected to increase as the general population ages. The average age of onset is 60, with peak incidence in the late 70s and early 80s age group. Parkinson's is found throughout the world, and disease rates differ from country to country.

The cause of Parkinson's disease is not definitively known, although several promising theories exist. Parkinson's has been shown to be an inherited disease based on twin and family studies, and some environmental factors may contribute as well. PD has been reported in people that at one time took an illegal street drug that was contaminated with a substance known as MPTP (1-methyl-4-phenyl-1,2,3,6-tetrahydropyridine). In addition, there is strong evidence that an alteration of a gene on chromosome 4 may lead to PD as well. The most accepted theory suggests that some people probably have an inherited susceptibility to the disease that is affected by certain environmental factors.

Symptoms of PD most often begin with a tremor of a person's limb while at rest, which often starts on one side of the body, usually a hand. As the disease progresses, it becomes more difficult for the person to move (akinesia); the limbs move rigidly, the gait is described as "shuffling," and posture becomes more stooped. The ability to create facial expressions is limited, and people with PD may experience depression, personality changes, dementia, sleep difficulty, and speech impairments. The disease is progressive and typically continues to worsen over time.

PD is diagnosed based on patient symptoms. There is no specific laboratory test that can diagnose it; a neurologist will typically evaluate the patient and their symptoms and make a diagnosis based on the findings. Sometimes, a specific type of brain scan may help doctors identify PD; other times, a patient with suspected PD will be given anti-Parkinson's drugs to determine if they benefit from them. Absolute diagnosis of Parkinson's is achieved by identification of microscopic Lewy bodies, which are found in the cells of the brain. A hallmark of PD, Lewy bodies have been found in a large number of people that were never diagnosed with the disease. Because of this, some researchers feel that if everyone lived long enough, most people would develop the disease.

Standard treatment of PD involves the use of drugs that are converted into dopamine in the brain, which allows for replacement of the lost dopamine that is normally synthesized within the brain. This drug, known as levodopa, does not prevent progressive changes of PD and causes side effects because it is converted into dopamine before it reaches the brain. Levodopa can be taken with another medication (carbidopa, or Sinemet) that will prevent its conversion to dopamine prior to reaching the brain; this serves to "conserve" the levodopa so its full potential is used in the brain.

NUTRITIONAL FACTORS

Parkinson's disease is essentially a neurodegenerative disease. When viewed in this sense, the importance of nutrition is highlighted, as the brain requires a large amount of energy to maintain not only its function, but its structural integrity as well. Because of the increased appearance of PD at older ages, it makes sense that nutritional support plays a role in the prevention of this disease, as chronic insufficient nutrition may lead to the appearance of several disease states, especially those of degenerative nature. The role of nutrition in PD appears throughout the literature; the following is a brief overview of some of the most salient information.

Vitamin C

In one study investigating the role of oxidation and antioxidant levels in the brains of patients with PD, ascorbic acid was found to be deficient.[2] And in another trial investigating the use of vitamin C in the treatment of Parkinson's disease symptoms, supplementation was found to cause modest improvements in the functional performance of people with PD.[3] In a trial using both alpha-tocopherol (a form of vitamin E) and ascorbic acid, both vitamins were given to people with early forms of PD.[4] The purpose of this study was to determine the preventative effects of high-dose antioxidants on the progression of PD. Compared to other patients (study subjects were limited to those patients taking anticholinergic medications only, as a marker for Parkinson's disease that had not advanced to a stage requiring dopamine agonists), those receiving the mixed antioxidant therapy of alpha tocopherol and vitamin C did not require levodopa treatment for two and a half years after those who received no antioxidant therapy did. This study suggests that antioxidant therapy in the form of vitamin C and alpha tocopherol may slow the progress of PD. And in an older study utilizing vitamin C for the treatment of levodopa side effects, 4 grams per day of the vitamin were able to reduce nausea and other levodopa side effects in a patient with PD.[5]

Vitamin E

This vitamin may serve as a potential preventive therapeutic as well in the development of PD. A survey conducted in the late 1980s concerning the dietary habits of Parkinson's patients before the age of 40 revealed that increased intakes of foods high in vitamin E were associated with lower incidence of PD.[3] Because of the widespread evidence that oxidative stress in the substantia nigra plays a role in the pathogenesis of PD, the role of vitamin E in preventing this type of damage was investigated.[6] Researchers propose that chronic high-dose vitamin E may serve as beneficial therapy in the prevention and treatment of PD (through protection of the substantia nigra cells from oxidative damage).

B Vitamins

B vitamins are particularly important in PD, specifically folate and B-12 in their role in the synthesis of neurotransmitters. Additionally, there is evidence that a standard medication for PD, levodopa, may contribute to deficiency of folic acid and B-12 therefore perpetuating the disease cycle.[7] Niacin may become deficient in patients who are treated with levodopa and other PD medications (benserazide and carbidopa, decarboxylase inhibitors).[8] Supplementing niacin concomitantly with standard PD treatment may serve to prevent deficiency and may actually assist in maintaining elevated brain levels of levodopa, thereby increasing therapeutic value of the drug by elevating levels of dopamine in the brain.[9] Vitamin B-6 may become deficient when patients are treated with a combination of levodopa and carbidopa, and treatment with vitamin B-6 was shown to be beneficial in some patients in two older studies.[10] B-6, in addition to thiamine (B-1), was shown to provide symptomatic relief of PD when it was injected intraspinally in one case study.[3] Although this is not a standard mode of supplementation, it demonstrates the efficacy of vitamins as medicine and their effectiveness when used to treat symptoms of this disease. It is also important to point out that B-6, when administered with levodopa, enhances the metabolism of this drug, hastening its conversion to dopamine outside of the brain, which leads to decreased drug efficacy. This does not occur, however, when a person is taking levodopa with carbidopa.

ANTIOXIDANTS

The role of oxidative processes continues to dominate some of the causative research in PD. Increasing evidence implicates the oxidative process and inflammation in impairment of mitochondrial function (the mitochondria is considered the "powerhouse" of the cell).[11] Studies reviewing the benefits of nutritional antioxidants have demonstrated a neuroprotective effect from vitamin E and polyphenols (phytochemicals derived from green tea and other plants), which may serve to protect against neurodegenerative diseases such as Parkinson's.[12]

Glutathione is a small protein composed of three amino acids: cysteine, glutamic acid, and glycine. Synthesized in the liver and found throughout the body, glutathione is a potent antioxidant.[13] It is involved in DNA synthesis and repair, protein synthesis, amino acid transport, immune system function, and prevention of oxidative cellular damage.[14] Glutathione is thought to play a major role in protecting cells from oxidative damage and is known to become more depleted in the substantia nigra as PD progresses.[15] Because of the degree of glutathione depletion in the substantia nigra is so evident as disease progresses, researchers advocate the supplementation with glutathione be a high therapeutic priority for PD patients.[16] The use of glutathione as an adjunctive treatment for PD was shown to provide much benefit when administered intravenously as well.[17] As a supplement that is normally synthesized within the cells of the body, replacing it in people with PD may serve to slow the progression of this disease; it is not known exactly what leads to the deficiency of this protein in the cells of people with PD, but replacement may be provide benefit in these patients.

Coenzyme Q10

Coenzyme Q10 (CoQ-10) is a compound found within every cell of the body; it is found in the greatest concentrations in the most metabolically active organs. An essential cofactor of the electron transport chain as well as an important antioxidant, nearly 30 percent of the body's CoQ-10 is found in the nucleus, and nearly 50 percent is found within the mitochondria. CoQ-10 is soluble in fat and acts as an antioxidant and membrane stabilizer in the cells, and perhaps the most important function of CoQ-10 is its role in the generation of adenosine triphosphate (ATP) in oxidative respiration.[18] CoQ-10 is a vital part of cellular energy production and because of this it has several therapuetic uses.

Regarding its role in PD, research has found that CoQ-10 may play an important part in disease modification. Some of the main features of PD are associated with CoQ-10 deficiency, and a study that supplemented subjects with 360 milligrams of CoQ-10 for four weeks found that it was able to provide significant mild symptom improvement of PD symptoms including visual function, which itself is a PD symptom.[19] In a multicenter trial investigating the use of CoQ-10 and its effect on slowing the progression of PD, CoQ-10 was supplied in doses of 300, 600, or 1,200 milligrams per day in 80 subjects with early PD who were not undergoing any other treatment.[20] The study subjects were followed for a period of 16 months and were evaluated using the Unified Parkinson Disease Rating Scale (UPDRS) at follow-up visits occurring at the first-, fourth-, eighth-, twelfth-, and sixteenth-month visits. Researchers concluded that based on their findings, CoQ-10 was safe and well tolerated by the patients at all doses, and less development of disability was noted in the CoQ-10 supplemented group than the placebo group; the most benefit occurred in the 1,200 milligram per day dose group. From these studies, the effectiveness of CoQ-10 in treating the symptoms and in slowing progressive deterioration in PD is quite apparent.

PROTEIN

The evidence surrounding specific dietary changes in PD is compelling, focusing on macronutrients such as protein. An effect that is associated with patients taking levodopa for symptom management, a high-protein diet is known to interfere with the availability of levodopa in the brain and can lead to recurrent loss of symptom control, known as the "off-on" phoenmenon.[21] Subsequent studies were performed to determine the effects of low- versus high-protein intakes in PD patients. A low intake of 0.5 grams protein per kilogram per day appeared to improve symptom control during the course of the day in comparison to a high-protein diet of 10 grams per kilogram body weight per day, which actually increased the symptom periodicity.[22] Another study that evenly divided low-protein (0.8 g/kg) intake throughout the day revealed that the amount and distribution of dietary protein could affect response to levodopa treatment; it is thought that levodopa is affected by protein not by absorption but through a variation in plasma amino acids.[23]

Other interesting studies of dietary protein and PD include one in which a low-protein diet of 50 gram per day for men and 40 grams per day for women was compared to a high-protein diet of 80 grams per day for men and 70 grams per day for women.[24] The patients on the low-protein diet experienced greater performance, decreased tremor, and better hand agility and movement capabilities in comparison to the high-protein group. Researchers in this study suggest that protein may affect levodopa efficacy in the brain, rather than in the blood stream. The results of these studies suggest an important role for the modification of diet, especially in regard to protein intake. By simply altering protein levels, patients may experience fewer symptoms that may even allow them to use less of their medications at times.

Amino Acids in Parkinson's Disease

Amino acids are the individual building blocks of proteins. Proteins are widely used throughout the body; to say they are essential to proper function is an understatement, as proteins (and their constituent amino acids) are used in nearly every metabolic reaction in the body and are incorporated into nearly every structure from bone to cellular membranes. More specifically, neurotransmitters are composed of the very amino acids that may be prohibited from absorption by the pharmaceutical drug levodopa.

L-tyrosine

L-tyrosine is a precursor of dopamine and may be insufficiently utilized in PD patients due to altered biopterin levels (biopterin serves as a cofactor in tyrosine hydroxylase) in their blood.[25] Tyrosine was compared to levodopa for its effects on symptom management in a group of PD patients.[26] During the course of treatment (for three years), patients taking L-tyrosine experienced better clinical results with fewer side effects than those patients taking levodopa or other dopamine agonist drugs.

D-phenylalanine

A single study of this amino acid revealed that use of the D form (amino acids appear in two main forms known as L and D, which refers to their structural arrangement) improved symptoms of rigidity, speech, walking, and depression, but did not relieve tremor symptoms.[27] However, some evidence suggests that amino acids such as phenylalanine may aggravate the "on-off" effect in patients taking levodopa.

L-tryptophan

L-tryptophan is useful in PD for two reasons. First, it is found in lower levels in PD patients who are treated with levodopa (L-tryptophan and levodopa compete with each other for absorption);[28] second, it is useful in the treatment of PD-associated depression.[29] In one study, the use of L-tryptophan in PD patients improved factors such as mood and motivational drive in comparison to a placebo, and it improved functional ability more so than when compared to levodopa.[30]

All three of these amino acids may be prevented from being completely absorbed by levodopa, leading to insufficient supply in the body. From the cited studies, it appears to be important that these amino acids are supplied to the PD patient due their positive effects on symptoms and mood.

OTHER FACTORS: GINKGO AND MAGNESIUM

In addition to the earlier suggestions, the addition of other substances such as magnesium and ginkgo may possibly serve to further enhance the bioavailablity and absorption in the brain when using these addiotnal substances. Both ginkgo and magnesium are known to dilate blood vessels in the body, under different mechanisms. Ginkgo works specifically on the vasculature of the brain to dilate the vessels and is well documented in the literature to provide increased blood flow to the brain, increasing oxygenation.[31] Additionally, when combined with phosphatidylcholine, a phospholipid molecule, ginkgo is more readily absorbed into the tissues. This allows even greater efficacy for this herb to work on the brain. Magnesium works as a smooth muscle relaxant (calcium channel blocker) and can dilate blood vessels because of this. Some evidence exists that magnesium dilates blood vessels in the central nervous system (CNS) to reduce ischemia.[32] Because of the actions of ginkgo and magnesium, we theorize that by increasing oxygenation and blood flow to the brain, this organ will be better conditioned to avoid continued degenerative changes. Blood flow to areas of injury is vital, as evidenced by an uncontrolled diabetic, who may begin to lose toes due to insufficient vascular nutrition when blood flow is compromised. Therefore, people with PD may benefit from ginkgo and magnesium as added cerebral blood flow enhancing agents.

CONCLUSION

Parkinson's disease is a terribly debilitating illness with no real standard treatment other than symptom management. Characterized by degeneration of specialized dopamine-producing neurons in the substantia nigra, there are many theorized causes of this destruction. Foremost among them is an acceleration of or a susceptibility to oxidative damage in this area; supplementation with common vitamins supports the production of neurotransmitters and acts as antioxidants. Providing the PD patient with extra antioxidants, regardless of form, can serve to benefit them in hopes of delaying or preventing the cumulative neurodegenerative damage from oxidative stress. Nutritional supplements that are normally produced in the body can provide additional support for symptoms of PD and act as buffers against disease progression. Regulation of dietary protein is a relatively simple step to be taken that can attenuate the symptoms of PD, especially in those being treated with levodopa. Finally, a few key amino acids, when provided in supplemental form, can help to offset symptoms that may be induced by standard pharmaceutical treatment of PD.

PD, as a condition, reflects the vulnerability of the central nervous system, which is often compared to a mainframe computer that is amazingly able to juggle countless functions and tasks with ease. Indeed, just as the rest of our bodies are not impervious to assaults from the environment, our brains likewise can become susceptible. Addressing the issue of susceptibility at the earliest sign of symptoms or potential symptoms is essential. The adage "an ounce of prevention is worth a pound of cure" is important. Likewise, it is important to realize that the best offense is a good defense and that upon fueling the body optimally, one is most able to succeed in the ultimate of target goals: maintaining function and alleviating symptoms within the confines of current knowledge. Indeed, the incorporation of natural medicine interventions are a must when it comes to this health issue.

NUTRIENTS

- Vitamin C
  1,000–2,000 milligrams per day
- Vitamin E
  400–800 International Units per day
- B vitamins
  A B-complex vitamin should be taken to avoid pharmaceutical-induced deficiency of B-12, folate, and B-6
- Glutathione
  250 milligrams per day
- Coenzyme Q10
  1,200 milligrams daily in 4 divided doses
- L-tyrosine*
  1,500 milligrams per day, divided doses
- D-phenylalanine*
  500 milligrams per day
- L-tryptophan*
  500 milligrams per day or 50 milligrams 5-HTP 2 times per day
- Dietary Protein
  Limit to 0.5–1.0 grams per kilogram body weight if taking levodopa
- Magnesium
  300–400 milligrams per day, divided doses

*All amino acids should be taken 30 minutes away from protein meals. Consult your doctor prior to taking these amino acids.

BOTANICALS

- *Ginkgo biloba*
  120–240 milligrams per day, divided doses

Schizophrenia

A chronic, severe, and disabling disease of the brain, schizophrenia is marked by symptoms such as hearing internal voices and believing that others may be reading their minds, controlling their thoughts, or plotting against them. Terrifying to the person experiencing them, these symptoms often cause people with schizophrenia to be fearful and withdrawn, and their speech and behavior often appear disorganized and incomprehensible. Often, the first signs of schizophrenia appear as troubling changes in behavior, and coping with these changes is incredibly difficult for people who know the patient. The change in behavior, when people cannot tell the difference between reality and illusion, is known as psychosis, or a psychotic episode. In order for a person to have a diagnosis of schizophrenia, the person must experience two or more of the following symptoms for at least one month's duration:

- Delusions: These are bizarre, false beliefs that may include paranoid thoughts (someone is "out to get them") or grandiose thoughts (believing they are a president, etc.).
- Hallucinations: These are unreal perceptions of the environment, which may affect auditory (hearing voices), visual (seeing faces or lights), olfactory (smelling), and tactile (touch, as if something is crawling on or touching them) senses.
- Disorganized thinking/speech: Abnormal thoughts are usually measured by disorganized speech, which can be disjointed, or very little speech.
- Negative symptoms: The other symptoms note the presence of abnormal behavior, whereas negative symptoms include flat affect (no emotion or expression, low energy), social withdrawal, and even poor hygiene and grooming habits.

- Catatonia: This is characterized by "waxy flexibility." People may become fixed in a certain position for extended periods of time, and if moved by another person, they will continue to stay fixed in that position.

A display of any of these systems indicates an active phase of schizophrenia; however, schizophrenics oftentimes will have milder symptoms both before and after the active phase. There are three basic types of schizophrenia, including

1. Disorganized schizophrenia, which is marked by lack of emotion and disorganized speech.
2. Catatonic schizophrenia, which is marked by waxy flexibility and rigid posture, but sometimes excessive movement.
3. Paranoid schizophrenia, which is marked by strong delusions or hallucinations.

Some people may only have one psychotic episode, whereas others may have many of them throughout their lives and may be able to function relatively well in between episodes. A person with more chronic schizophrenia may never fully recover from episodes and requires continuous treatment to control symptoms. Most people with schizophrenia will have symptoms throughout their lives; only one in five people with schizophrenia will recover completely. (It is notable that many statistics shared regarding recovery from any given health condition is based on conventional treatments only and does not reflect the appropriate addition of natural medicine supportive therapies targeted at supporting healthy function.) A complete diagnostic evaluation is available in the *Diagnostic and Statistical Manual of Mental Disorders*, Fourth Edition (*DSM-IV*).

Schizophrenia is one of the most common mental illnesses; one estimate figures that about 1 of every 100 people is affected by schizophrenia, which equates to 1 percent of the population.[1] It is estimated that over 2 million Americans suffer from this illness in a given year. Found throughout the world, schizophrenia affects men and women equally. Schizophrenia seems to appear earlier in men than women (men usually develop signs in their early 20s whereas women develop signs in their late 20s to early 30s). It is estimated that the cost of schizophrenia to society approaches $32.5 billion dollars per year in the United States alone.[1]

CAUSES OF SCHIZOPHRENIA

There are several contributing factors to schizophrenia, ranging from brain anatomy to genetics to nutrition.

Anatomy

Recent research has placed an emphasis on brain structures as part of the puzzle in finding the cause of this disease. The brains of schizophrenics commonly have larger lateral ventricles (part of series of spaces within the brain that contain cerebrospinal fluid). The exact significance of this is not fully understood at this time, but provides an interesting link between brain structure and proper function. Additionally, other brain structures have been noted to be of abnormal size as well. A reduced size of the hippocampus, increased size of the basal ganglia, and abnormalities in the shape of the prefrontal cortex have been somewhat consistently noted in people with schizophrenia (however, these changes have been seen in people without schizophrenia as well).

Genetics

Schizophrenia is known to be more common in families who have one or more members with the disease, indicating a genetic component to the passing of this disease from one generation to another. Utilizing studies of twins, researchers have shown that the tendency for both identical twins to develop schizophrenia is around 30 percent to 50 percent, and the tendency for fraternal twins (they share only one half the same genes as the other twin, whereas identical twins have the exact same genetic makeup) is approximately 15 percent. This is the same percentage for nontwins as well.

Environment

Other factors that may contribute to the development of schizophrenia include family stress, poor social skills and interactions, infections at an early age, or mental emotional trauma early in life.

Neurotransmitters

One popular theory of schizophrenia focuses on the possibility that an overactive dopamine neurotransmitter system may be part of the cause. Strong evidence in the literature supports this theory; yet at the same time, there is other evidence that does not provide strong support for this theory and serves to refute it.

There are many factors that contribute to the development of this disease. Intensely studied, science continues to uncover interesting factors that relate to the causes of this disease, many of which focus on the role of nutrition as a causative and curative factor for schizophrenia. Schizophrenia causes a high degree of disability in those affected by it, and current medications are not greatly effective at controlling its symptoms and do not endorse a curative effect by treating the underlying cause. When used continuously, patients are often troubled by the side effects of the medication and symptoms that are refractory to treatment by medication.

NUTRITION

Folic Acid

Several nutrients have been studied in relation to their effects in schizophrenia. Folic acid continues to be implicated in many of the diseases covered in this book, and schizophrenia is not an exception. Specifically, folate deficiency has been attributed to symptoms of several neuropsychiatric diseases, including schizophrenia symptoms. For example, folic acid deficiency has been shown to be high in patients with schizophrenia, and psychiatric symptoms are known to occur with greater frequency and severity in those patients with a deficiency of this vitamin.[2] Additionally, other researchers have indicated that schizophrenic-like symptoms are a secondary effect of folate deficiency.[3] Deficiency of folate is known to exacerbate symptoms associated with declining cognitive function as well, demonstrating the integral role of this vitamin in maintaining healthy neurologic status.[4] In a study of 123 patients with psychiatric disorders, including schizophrenia, it was found that 33 percent of these patients were either borderline or clearly deficient in red blood cell levels of folate.[5] These patients were supplemented with 15 milligrams of methylfolate per day for six months in addition to their normally prescribed medications. At the end of the trial, the patients receiving the methylfolate treatment experienced a significant improvement in clinical and social outcomes, and these improved over time. In one particular case of folate-responsive schizophrenic-like symptoms, a mildly retarded adolescent girl was, after considerable testing of blood amino acids and their enzymes (defect in N5-10-methylenetetrahydrofolate reductase, also known as methylene reductase), determined to have an inability to properly metabolize folic acid. This was speculated to be the cause of the schizophrenic symptoms, which was treated by dosing the patient with folate.[6] Following up on this study, another group of investigators examined whether abnormally low levels of the aforementioned enzyme might contribute to schizophrenia pathology.[7] They did not find a statisically significant difference in the activity of the enzyme between healthy, nonschizophrenics and schizophrenic patients. The investigators did, however, proclaim that their findings did not rule out that abnormal methylene reducatase activity might be present in an as yet undiscovered subgroup of schizophrenic patients. All of these studies point to the importance of folate in schizophrenia and symptom control. The importance of methylation reactions and folate, which serves as a cofactor in these reactions, is highlighted in these studies. A low-cost and low-risk therapy, supplementation of schizophrenic patients with folate may assist in providing a therapeutic response.

Pyridoxine

Pyridoxine, or vitamin B-6, plays an important role in the synthesis of neuro-transmitters that are involved in the development of psychotic states. There are many reports of supplemental B-6 alleviating psychotic symptoms in schizo-phrenia and other mental disorders.[8] A study that utilized supplemental B-6 in the treatment of schizophrenic patients with comorbid minor depression pro-duced positive results.[9] Patients were supplemented with 150 milligrams per day, in addition to their standard medications, for four weeks. A small percentage (22 percent) of the patients experienced significant improvement in depressive symptoms as well as schizophrenic symptom scores, indicating that a portion of schizophrenics with depression may benefit from supplemental pyridoxine.

Vitamin B-6 was used to ameliorate symptoms in a schizophrenic patient with drug-induced Parkinsonism (this occurs as a side effect of some schizophrenic medications) using 100 milligrams per day. This treatment resulted in a dramatic and persistent decrease in the Parkinson's-like symptoms as well as a reduction in psychotic behavior.[10] The investigators in the trial attribute the effectiveness of B-6 in this case to several reasons. Pyridoxine deficiency is associated with decreased brain serotonin concentrations as well as melatonin production in animal studies, suggesting that the movement disorders and psychosis symptoms may have been ameliorated simply by enhancing the functions of those two neurotransmitters; an effect of pyridoxine on GABA and dopamine activities was suggested as well. Deficiency of pyridoxine in schizophrenic patients may contribute to additionally psychotic behavior and seems to increase the risk of drug-induced movement disorders in some schizophrenics. Another inexpensive and simple treatment, B-6 supplementation should not be overlooked in the treatment of schizophrenics.

Vitamin C

Low levels of vitamin C, or ascorbic acid, has been implicate in schizophre-nia. This common vitamin has multiple indications for health and is probably the most researched vitamin throughout the literature. Interestingly, it may play a role in schizophrenia as well. In a study designed to determine the utilization of vitamin C in hospitalized schizophrenics, it was revealed that schizophrenic patients might require higher levels of vitamin C than the suggested optimal intake required for healthy people in comparison to other patients; this was de-termined after analyzing intake, plasma, and urinary excretion levels of both schizophrenic and nonschizophrenic patients.[11] Another study investigating simi-lar vitamin C parameters in a different group of schizophrenics revealed similar results, suggesting impairment in the metabolism of vitamin C in people with schizophrenia.[12] These studies, performed on different groups of patients with schizophrenia, provide interesting insight into the role of vitamin C in this dis-ease; if these patients do not metabolize vitamin C as well as nonschizophrenics, this must be taken into account when considering nutritional treatments and supplementation therapies. Applying this to patients, one case study involved a 37-year-old schizophrenic who benefited substantially from the addition of supplemental vitamin C to his standard medical treatment, demonstrating the possible usefulness of this vitamin when applied to schizoprhenia.[13]

Niacin

Niacin, and its other form, niacinamide (Both are forms of vitamin B-3) is one of the longest-used vitamins in the treatment of schizophrenia, having been employed since the 1940s to treat psychiatric conditions. In a large clinical trial, over 1,000 schizophrenics were treated with either niacin or niacinamide at doses of 1.5 to 6 grams per day for a duration of three months to five years.[14] The treating physician in these cases proclaimed that this treatment was most effective in patients with early and acute schizophrenia and not effective in those with a chronic condition.

In another study, niacinamide was found to produce antianxiety effects equivalent to benzodiazepine medications; niacin is thought to stimulate, without binding to, the same neurotransmitter receptor sites (GABA) as benzodiazapenes.[15] Other research regarding treatment with niacin and niacinamide is both positive and negative; more investigations into its use are needed to fully elucidate its utility in schizophrenia.

Fatty Acids

Fatty acids, which occupy many central physiologic functions throughout the body, play several important roles, especially in the area of cellular membrane function. A highly interactive portion of the cell, the cellular membrane is the final factor that determines what enters and leaves the cell, and newer research is uncovering the role of the cellular membrane in regulation of other bodily functions (i.e., cellular signaling). Much evidence is indicative of the role of disordered membrane phospholipid metabolism in schizophrenia. A new theory of schizophrenia is that it is a disorder of membrane phospholipid metabolism that is associated with an increased loss of polyunsaturated fatty acids from the cellular membrane, through enhanced activity of phospholipase A2.[16] Membrane changes that result from this process occur throughout the body, leading to physical abnormalities; these membrane abnormalities may stand to have highly adverse effects on the brain, where sequential coordination of millions of neurons are dependent on cohesive functioning on the cellular membrane.

Additional evidence of the fatty acid link to schizophrenia includes the theory of abnormal brain turnover of phospholipids detected by magnetic resonance imaging and reduced cellular membrane levels of omega 3 and 6 polyunsaturated fatty acids. Additionally, four out of five trials using eicosapentaenoic acid (EPA) in the treatment of schizophrenia provided positive results.[17] Increased phospholipid breakdown and decreased levels of polyunsaturated fatty acids (PUFAs), especially arachidonic acid (AA), have been demonstrated throughout the literature in other studies.[18] Research is currently delving into the various physiologic functions of membrane phospholipids and PUFAs and their role in schizophrenia. Most of this research hints at altered cellular signaling and how it relates to neurobiological manifestations of schizophrenia and therapeutics. Supplementation of schizophrenic patients with a mixture of PUFAs (EPA/DHA at 180:120 milligrams) and antioxidant vitamins (vitamin E/C, 400 IU: 500 milligrams) twice daily for four months produced significant reductions in psychopathology based on the outcome scores of several psychiatric rating scales.[19] Interestingly, PUFA levels returned to pretreatment levels four months after the conclusion of the study, yet the previously experienced clinical improvements remained in effect for the study subjects. In a comprehensive review of the scientific databases containing descriptions of clinical trials utilizing PUFAs to treat symptoms of schizophrenia, it was determined that the use of PUFAs produced favorable results in the subjects, with little or no side effects.[20] Many studies performed using this treatment were carried out for relatively short periods of time in which to expect physiologic changes to occur. It is estimated that every cell in the human body is replaced within 120 days; if there is merit to this theory, it makes sense to determine the results of fatty acid supplementation and its effects on membrane phospholipid content after enough of a time period to allow for complete replacement with these fatty acids. Given the already positive results of these studies, it stands to reason that a longer study period may affect better outcomes using PUFAs for symptom management.

CONCLUSION

Schizophrenia, like other disease involving the brain, has numerous contributing factors, none of which has been shown to be 100 percent causative. In all reality, this will continue be the case, but examining potential therapies provides medicine with additional therapies that work to avert symptoms, without further contributing to side effects. From the brief studies included in this chapter, it has been shown that supplementation with even solitary vitamins can attenuate symptoms, and, in some cases, can quite drastically avert them. The role of fatty acids in schizophrenia adds more fuel to the importance of a proper diet containing these essential fats. PUFAs continue to appear throughout the literature as an important preventive therapeutic for a number of diseases; schizophrenia is yet another. The importance of proper cell membrane function continues to appear in the research as a prevention for many of these diseases, and alteration of the cell membrane fatty acid content is relatively easily achieved utilizing dietary modifications and supplementation.

Clinically notable benefits have been seen among individuals suffering from schizophrenia when adjunctive natural medicines therapies have been used. The mentioned nutrient-based interventions are by no means the only therapies that assist a patient to reestablish improved quality of cognitive processes. Indeed, the support of proper biochemical pathways regardless of the ultimate diagnosed condition, whether it is psychological or physical, creates a foundation for improved health outcomes. Added benefits include support of neurological and overall body tissues that endure significant stress from schizophrenia.

NUTRIENTS

- Folic Acid*
  10–15 milligrams per day
- Pyridoxine
  100–150 milligrams per day
- Vitamin C
  1,000–2,000 milligrams per day, divided doses
- Niacin**
  3–5 grams per day, divided doses
- Essential Fatty Acids
  Eicosapentaenoic Acid/Docosahexaenoic Acid (EPA/DHA) at 150 milligrams, two to three times daily

*Folic acid should not be supplemented without concurrent B-12 to prevent masking adverse neurological pathology.
**Under close medical supervision due to niacin flushing and potential liver toxicity.

PART II

Most Common Brain-Targeted Nutra-Botanicals

B-1

MECHANISM OF ACTION

Vitamin B-1, also known as thiamine, has several uses in the body. Thiamine is primarily used in the metabolism of carbohydrates, one of the three main food constituents. In carbohydrate metabolism, thiamine is used in the formation of thiamine diphosphate, which serves as a coenzyme in the process of carbohydrate processing. Thiamine is therefore necessary for energy production and assists in proper nerve cell function. Additionally, thiamine serves as a cofactor in the hexose monophosphate shunt, in the processing of pentose. A deficiency of thiamine can result in increased pyruvic acid in the blood, which is then converted into lactic acid; elevated levels may be used to diagnose thiamine deficiency.

DEFICIENCY

Classic clinical symptoms of B-1 deficiency include beriberi and Wernicke-Korsakoff syndrome.[1] Beriberi affects the body in general, with symptoms of peripheral nerve damage, sleep disturbances, poor memory, and lack of appetite. When excessive, beriberi may affect the heart (known as wet beriberi) and may cause palpitations, difficulty breathing, edema, and cardiac failure if left untreated. Wernicke-Korsakoff syndrome generally is the result of excessive alcohol intake in combination with little or no dietary B-1. Primarily affecting the brain, Wernicke-Korsakoff is marked by confusion, lying (confabulation), inability to speak, and difficulty in using the muscles of the eyes, and it may lead to coma when untreated. Severe deficiency of thiamine is relatively rare in the general population; however, many people do not consume on a continual basis the recommended dietary allowance of thiamine of 1.5 milligrams. Other symptoms associated with a mild thiamine deficiency include fatigue, depression, constipation, and nerve paresthesias.[2]

USES

Thiamine is useful in the treatment of beriberi and Wernicke-Korsakoff syndrome as well as several other conditions. It is used to prevent deficiency in conditions such as Crohn's disease, multiple sclerosis, diabetes, and other neurological disorders. Thiamine is used to treat impaired mental function in the aged, as well as people with Alzheimer's disease, and in epileptics who are treated with a particular pharmaceutical (Dilantin).

Considered essential for energy production in the brain, a deficiency of thiamine may be charachterized by impaired mental function and psychosis if severe enough. A previously mentioned study indicated that nearly 30 percent of all people who entered psychiatric wards were deficient in thiamine.[3] Women experiencing neuritis during pregnancy and people with peripheral neuritis can be treated with oral thiamine to assist in resolving symptoms involving nerve pain. Insufficient intake of thiamin may occur in conditions in which absorption is a problem, such as diarrhea, alcoholism, liver cirrhosis, and other gastrointestinal diseases. Others may have inadequate intakes, such as anorexics or bulimics, and those who experience extended nausea and vomiting. Increased intake of thiamin is necessary in other conditions, and when not supplemented, may lead to a deficiency state. These conditions include pregnancy, increased physical activity, and increased carbohydrate consumption.[4] Thiamine is used in the treatment of metabolic disorders such as subacute necrotizing encephalopathy (SNE or Leigh's disease), lactic acidosis due to pyruvate carboxlase deficiency, hyperalaninemia, and branched chain aminoacidopathy (maple syrup urine disease).

Thiamine has specific effects on brain function in addition to its role as a nutrient. Thiamine may mimic the effects of the neurotransmitter acethycholine.[5] When used to treat people with Alzheimer's disease (in which patients suffer from reduced levels of acetylcholine), thiamine, in doses from 3 to 8 grams per day, was able to potentiate and mimic the actions of acetylcholine and improved mental function.[6] In patients with epilepsy, thiamine was able to improve mental function in those patients taking Dilantin (also known as phenytoin).[7]

DOSING REVIEW

Common supplementation amounts are generally 1–2 milligrams per day.

For mild thiamine deficiency, 5–30 milligrams per day in divided doses can be used.

For states of frank thiamine deficiency, up to 300 milligrams per day in divided doses can be used.

Genetic enzyme deficiency disorders are typically treated with 10–20 milligrams per day; SNE can benefit from up to 4,000 milligrams per day in divided doses of thiamin. In Alzheimer's disease or age-related dementia, doses of 3–8 grams per day have been used, and in epileptics taking Dilantin, a dose of 50–100 milligrams may be used.

No toxicity is observed with proper thiamine use. Thiamine is intricately involved in energy production with the other B vitamins, and magnesium is needed in order to convert thiamine into its active coenzyme form.

B-2

MECHANISM OF ACTION

Vitamin B-2, known as riboflavin, is converted in the body into the coenzymes riboflavin 5-phosphate (flavin mononucleotide or FMN) and flavin adenine dinucleotide (FAD). These enzymes work to transport hydrogen in the body and are active in oxidation-reduction reactions and in intermediary metabolism.[1] Simply put, riboflavin plays an active role in energy production. Additionally, riboflavin serves as a cofactor in several other enzymes involved in cellular respiration and indirectly supports red blood cell integrity.[2]

DEFICIENCY

A frank deficiency of riboflavin results in angular stomatitis, glossitis, neuropathy, keratitis, sore throat, and seborrheic dermatitis, and severe cases may manifest as normocytic and normochromic anemia. Riboflavin may be involved in the mobilization of iron from its storage form, ferritin, for its production of heme and globin synthesis.[3]

Other signs of deficiency include visual disturbances including light sensitivity and loss of visual acuity; burning and itching of the eyes, mouth, lips and tongue; and mucous membrane irritation. Deficiency of riboflavin can occur in conditions of chronic infectious processes, liver disease, cancer, and alcoholism. Deficiency is more common in the elderly.

USES

Riboflavin, in addition to treating frank deficiency, is effective in preventing migraine headaches[4] and cataracts.[5] Other uses include treating acne, carpal tunnel syndrome, and some forms of peripheral neuropathy. Additionally, ribo-flavin is used to treat sickle cell anemia.[6] Riboflavin plays a very important role in energy production and is needed for cellular regeneration of the powerful antioxidant glutathione. Glutathione serves as one of the cells' most important antioxidants.

DOSING REVIEW

The Recommended Dietary Allowance for riboflavin is 1.7 milligrams for males and 1.3 milligrams for females. Riboflavin is available in two forms: the first is simple riboflavin and the second is an activated form known as riboflavin-5-phosphate.[7]

Standard daily doses of riboflavin range from 1 to 4 milligrams per day. Deficiency symptoms are treated with 5–30 milligrams daily in divided doses.

To prevent migraines, 400 milligrams per day may be used. Reduced cataract formation is associated with using 2–3 milligrams per day. Studies of riboflavin absorption reveal that the maximum amount that can be absorbed from a single dose is 27 milligrams in adults.[8] No side effects or toxicity are noted with ribo-flavin, with the exception that riboflavin may be photosensitizing in some people.

B-3

MECHANISM OF ACTION

Vitamin B-3 includes niacin (nicotinic acid) and niacinamide (nicotinamide). Niacin specifically refers to nicotinic acid; however, both forms are often referred to as niacin; this is inaccurate as both have different actions when taken in large amounts. Niacin is converted into niacinamide when taken in small doses, and both agents have identical pharmacologic actions in the body when taken in smaller doses (around 20 milligrams). When taken in larger doses (greater than 50 milligrams per day), the two forms have distinct pharmacologic properties. Niacin is needed for metabolism of lipids, glycogenolysis, and tissue respiration. Incorporated into the coenzymes nicotinamide adenine dinucleotide (NAD) and nicotinamide adenine dinucleotide phosphate (NADP), niacin assists in the function of these coenzymes as hydrogen carrier molecules in cellular respiration.

At doses close to 1,000 milligrams per day, niacin can lower total blood cholesterol levels by 8 to 21 percent, low-density lipoprotein (LDL) cholesterol by 8 to 25 percent, increase high-density lipoprotein (HDL) cholesterol by 15 to 35 percent, and lower triglycerides by 20 to 50 percent.[1] Niacin is thought to exert this effect by slowing the release of free fatty acids from fat tissue as well as by inhibiting one enzymatic control (cyclic AMP) of triglyceride lipase, resulting in a slowing of lipolysis in the body.[2] Niacin is also able to decrease the synthesis of LDL and VLDL by the liver and enhances the removal rate of triglyceride-containing chylomicrons in the bloodstream by increasing lipoprotein lipase activity.[3] Niacin causes vasodilation of the surface blood vessels leading to flushing that is most likely mediated by prostaglandin molecules; tolerance usually develops after a few weeks of supplementation. Some clinical research has shown that schizophrenics do not demonstrate the characteristic blood vessel dilation when taking niacin, suggesting a faulty cellular phospholipid-dependent signaling response.[4] However, doses of niacin over 50 milligrams can potentially cause side effects such as gastric upset, nausea, and liver damage. Because of the flushing reaction, several manufacturers produce a delayed-release form of niacin; this type of niacin is apparently no safer than standard niacin as this form may cause liver damage as well.[5]

Niacinamide does not affect blood lipids and does not cause the typical vasodilation associated with niacin.[3] Large doses of niacinamide are used to prevent the progression of type 1 diabetes (insulin dependent)[6] and may protect the cells that manufacture insulin (pancreatic islet cells) from further cellular damage.[7] Niacinamide acts as an antioxidant as well, adding to further cellular protection in the body.

DEFICIENCY

Deficiency of niacin leads to pellagra, a disease characterized by dermatitis, dementia, and diarrhea; the skin becomes dry and scaly, dementia becomes prominent, and the gastrointestinal tract mucous lining is not as well formed, leading to diarrhea. Common at the turn of the nineteenth century, pellagra is not as common today because many foods are fortified with small amounts of the vitamin. In chronic alcoholism, however, pellagra may be seen. Other causes of niacin deficiency include suboptimal dietary intake or supplementation, the pharmaceutical drug isoniazid, certain tumors (carcinoid), and Hartnup disease, which leads to an inability to absorb tryptophan, an amino acid that is essential for the endogenous formation of niacin. Other conditions such as diabetes, hyperthyroidism, lactation, liver cirrhosis, and pregnancy may contribute to a frank niacin deficiency.

USES

Niacin is used to treat hyperlipoproteinemia, peripheral vascular disease, pellagra, schizophrenia, depression, ADHD, and diabetes, among others.

Niacin is manufactured in the body from the amino acid tryptophan, and because of this, niacin is sometimes viewed as a nonessential nutrient. However, if dietary intake of tryptophan is insufficient, niacin production is affected.

Necessary for the production of energy, niacin is primarily used for treating elevated cholesterol and triglycerides, assisting in healthy mental function (conditions like schizophrenia), Raynaud's syndrome (painful blood vessel constriction in the hands or feet when exposed to the cold), and intermittent claudication (cramping in the calf from inadequate oxygen supply), and it may assist in helping with blood sugar control.

DOSING REVIEW

The Recommended Dietary Allowances (RDAs) of niacin are 16 milligrams per day for men and 14 milligrams per day for women. For pregnant or lactating women the RDA is 17–18 milligrams per day.

Standard doses of niacin as a supplement are typically 10–20 milligrams per day.

In cases of deficiency, doses range from 50 to 100 milligrams per day.

For hyperlipoproteinemia, doses start at 125 milligrams two times per day and may be increased gradually to 1.5–3 grams per day.

Because of the side effects of niacin in large doses (over 50 milligrams), a form known as inositol hexaniacinate can be taken; this form is virtually free from side effects when taken in large doses. Patients taking large doses of niacin, regardless of form, should have their liver enzymes screened every three months to monitor for safety.

If using inositol hexaniacinate, start with 500 milligrams three times daily for two weeks and then increase to 1 gram per day.

Take all forms with food.

B-5

MECHANISM OF ACTION

B-5, also known as pantothenic acid, is involved in the metabolism of carbohydrates, proteins, and lipids and thereby contributes to energy production in the body. Coenzyme A is derived from pantothenic acid, and this important enzyme is needed for the production and metabolism of fatty acids, for acetylation reactions in gluconeogenesis (the creation of glucose in the body), as well as for the manufacture of acetylcholine and steroid hormones. Some research shows that B-5 may stimulate the production of acetylcholine in the gut and a precursor form of B-5, dexpanthenol, may stimulate fibroblast growth thereby benefiting the epithelium.[1]

The active form of pantothenic acid is known as pantetheine; in its stable form, known as pantethine, it can significantly lower cholesterol and triglycerides.[2] Pantothenic acid itself does not have these effects. Pantethine appears to inhibit the synthesis of cholesterol and assist in the metabolism of fats.[3] There are no known side effects or toxicity from pantethine.[4]

DEFICIENCY

Severe deficiency of B-5 leads to burning, numbness, and shooting pains in the feet, as well as fatigue.[5] Other signs of deficiency include sleepiness, headaches, muscle weakness in the legs, and possible changes in mental disposition. B-5 production can become compromised with the use of antibiotic medications, as antibiotics destroy some of the gastrointestinal microbes that are responsible for producing B-5.[6]

USES

B-5 contributes to energy metabolism as well as the production of adrenal hormones and red blood cells through its form in coenzyme A. B-5 levels are related to rheumatoid arthritis. Research shows that blood levels of B-5 are lower in people with rheumatoid arthritis in comparison to those without, and the severity of disease symptoms increased with lower blood levels of the vitamin.[7]

DOSING REVIEW

The recommended daily intake for B-5 is 5 milligrams per day for men and women, and 6–7 milligrams per day for pregnant or lactating women.

Standard supplemental dosing of B-5 is 250 milligrams two times per day.

For arthritis, 2 grams of B-5 per day can be used, and for lowering cholesterol and triglycerides, 300 milligrams three times per day can be used.

B-6

MECHANISM OF ACTION

Vitamin B-6, known as pyridoxine, is necessary for the metabolism of amino acids, lipids, and carbohydrates in the body. Converted into the coenzymes pyridoxal phosphate and pyridoxamine phosphate, B-6 is involved in the function of approximately 60 enzyme systems, including transamination of amino acids; the synthesis of gamma-aminobutyric acid (GABA) in the brain; the conversion of tryptophan to niacin; metabolism of serotonin, dopamine, and norepinephrine; the synthesis of heme in hemoglobin; and the metabolism of phospholipids and polyunsaturated fatty acids.[1] B-6 plays a highly important role in healthy brain function due to its role in the production of the amino-acid based neurotransmitters (serotonin, dopamine, melatonin, epinephrine, and norepinephrine). B-6 is needed for the metabolism of the amino acid homocysteine, which at high levels is an independent risk factor for cardiovascular disease.[2] Pyridoxine acts as an antioxidant as well.[3]

DEFICIENCY

A deficiency state of pyridoxine manifests as symptoms in the peripheral nerves, skin, and mucous membranes, as well as the hematopoietic system (development of red blood cells). In children, a deficiency of B-6 can affect the development of the central nervous system.

Deficiency can occur from several disease states, such as alcoholism, congestive heart failure, hyperthyroidism, liver cirrhosis, and gut malabsorption conditions,[1] and in people taking pharmaceutical drugs such as oral birth control pills[4] and theophylline.[5] The food coloring FD&C yellow #5 is a known antagonist of B-6 in the body.[6]

Decreased levels of pyridoxine are associated with increased blood levels of C-reactive protein (C RP), a nonspecific marker of inflammation that is associated with increased cardiovascular disease.[7]

USES

B-6 has been shown to assist many health conditions in addition to its benefits to neurologic function. Some of these conditions include asthma, cardiovascular disease, carpal tunnel syndrome, diabetes symptom prevention, kidney stones, pregnancy-associated nausea, and PMS.[6] B-6 is helpful in autism,[8] depression,[9] epilepsy,[10] and ADHD levels.[11]

DOSING REVIEW

The Recommended Daily Allowances (RDAs) of vitamin B-6 for men is 1.3 to 1.7 milligrams per day and 1.3 to 1.5 milligrams per day for women. Pregnant or lactating women require 1.9–2.0 milligrams per day.

The standard supplemental dose is 2 milligrams per day. Various treatment regimens suggest dosing from 25 to 100 milligrams per day for specific symptom treatment. Women taking oral contraceptives should take 25 to 30 milligrams per day, and for the treatment of PMS, 50 to 100 milligrams per day is suggested.

Doses larger than 50 milligrams in one day should be divided into separate doses due to the water-soluble nature of the vitamin. Long-term dosing of B-6 over 500 milligrams per day is associated with toxicity when taken over several months or years.[12] Signs of toxicity include tingling in the feet and decreased coordination.

B-12

MECHANISM OF ACTION

Vitamin B-12, known as methylcobalamin, is available in two synthetic forms: cyanocobalamin and hydroxycobalamin. Required for the production of nucleic acids, myelin sheath syntheis, production of cells, red blood cell manufacture, and normal growth, B-12 is a highly important vitamin. B-12 is needed to maintain certain enzymes (involved in protein synthesis, fat and carbohydrate metabolism) in their reduced state, maintaining their effectiveness. B-12 is necessary for the body to utilize another important vitamin, folate. Insufficient amounts of B-12 lead to a functional deficiency of folate.[1] B-12 is absorbed in the small intestine (terminal ileum) bound to intrinsic factor. B-12 absorption is greatly reduced in the absence of this glycoprotein that is secreted by the stomach, although approximately 1 percent of orally dosed B-12 can be absorbed without intrinsic factor or sufficient stomach acid.[2] B-12 deficiency is associated with increased levels of homocysteine, an independent risk factor for cardiovascular disease.[3]

DEFICIENCY

B-12 can be stored in large amounts in the body; however, deficiency states are not rare. Frank deficiency of B-12 can lead to megaloblastic anemia and neurologic damage when severe. Neurologic damage occurs because B-12 is necessary for the production of the myelin sheath that encapsulates nerves, and the absence of this protein can progress to nerve degeneration. Deficiency of B-12 can also cause neurologic symptoms such as depression,[4] paresthesias (nerve tingling and numbness), ataxia (movement difficulty), weakness, memory loss, and personality and mood irregularities.[5] These symptoms can occur in the absence of B-12 deficiency anemia, which is often considered the first sign of deficiency.[6]

Risk of B-12 deficiency increases with age and is more common in men as well as Caucasians and Latin Americans.[7] Deficiency can result from decreased intake, malabsorption syndromes, and pernicious anemia (an autoimmune condition in which the body is unable to produce intrinsic factor). Other causes of insufficient absorption include atrophic gastritis (accompanied by an increased stomach pH), acid-blocking pharmaceuticals, and certain gastrectomy surgeries (removal of part of the stomach).

USES

B-12 is necessary for healthy neurologic function, as deficiency results in brain and nervous system symptoms. Deficiency in the elderly can mimic Alzheimer's disease symptoms and is relatively common in this age group. Additionally, it is thought that B-12 deficiency is a major cause of depression in the elderly.[8] Deficiency of B-12 can be the cause of psychological disturbances in the elderly, prior to manifesting as anemia.[9]

The activation of enzymes that manufacture certain neurotransmitters such as serotonin and dopamine is dependent on a brain compound known as tetrahydrobiopterin (BH4). BH4 synthesis is in turn stimulated by both vitamin B-12 and folate. BH4 levels have been found to be deficient in people with depression, and studies implicate that supplemental B-12 and folate may increase brain levels of BH4, thereby alleviating the depression.[10]

Because of the necessity of B-12 in the production of myelin, this vitamin is used in the treatment of multiple sclerosis (MS). Although MS is theorized to have many causes, B-12 deficiency can aggravate the disease and contribute to continued demyelination.

B-12 is also used for other conditions such as AIDS, asthma, diabetic neuropathy, decreased sperm counts, and tinnitus.[9]

DOSING REVIEW

The recommended dietary allowance of B-12 is 2.4 micrograms for adults, and 2.6 to 2.8 micrograms for pregnant and lactating women. The standard supplemental dose is 100 micrograms per day to ensure adequate oral absorption and to maintain tissue storage.

For people with absorption problems, intramuscular administration is used at doses of 30 micrograms per day for 5 to 10 days, and maintenance doses of 100–200 micrograms one time per month are recommended.

Note: Folate may mask B-12 deficiency. Folate will improve vitamin B-12 associated anemia, but will not affect B-12-related neurologic degeneration. For this reason, B-12 and folate should always be supplemented together.

Dimethylglycine (DMG)

MECHANISM OF ACTION

Dimethylglycine (DMG) is a methylated form of the amino acid glycine. DMG is produced in the body, but it exists for only a few seconds before being converted; it is also formed from betaine during the course of homocysteine methylation.[1] Acting as a methyl group donor, DMG has a reputation for benefiting children with autism, with results becoming noticeable within days of taking the supplement. Research shows an immune enhancing effect from DMG, as humoral and cell mediated immune responses are increased with supplementation.[2] DMG is absorbed in the small intestine and metabolized in the liver to monomethylglycine or sacrosine, which is then converted into glycine. DMG has been shown to have anticonvulsant effects in mixed complex partial and grand mal seizures.[3]

USES

DMG has been used to improve autism symptoms such as speech and behavior[4] and to improve behavior in ADHD. Additionally, it is used to enhance neurologic function as a treatment for epilepsy. Some research has investigated DMG for improvement of oxygen utilization, liver function, and athletic performance. DMG is used to enhance immune function and to treat conditions such as alcoholism, addiction, and chronic fatigue syndrome.

DEFICIENCY

Formed in the body, deficiency states of DMG are not known to exist.

DOSING REVIEW

There is no RDA for DMG. For treatment of autism, a starting dose of 60 milligrams per day is recommended, working up to 500 milligrams per day. A typical dose for treatment of other conditions is 125 milligrams per day, with food.

Docosahexaenoic Acid (DHA)

MECHANISM OF ACTION

Docosahexaenoic acid (DHA) is a long chain polyunsaturated fatty acid derived from the tissues of fish and other marine animals as well as microalgae. An omega-3 fatty acid, DHA is a competitive precursor in the cyclooxygenase and lipoxygenase pathways with arachidonic acid.[1] DHA is converted into eicosapentaenoic acid, another essential polyunsaturated fatty acid in humans,[2] and along with other long chain polyunsaturated fatty acids, it is incorporated into the gray matter of the brain.[3]

DHA plays a highly important role in brain function and is thought to contribute to proper structural, neurologic, and synaptic membrane development.[4] Additional research shows that DHA exerts a positive effect on retinal function and development, visual function, learning ability, and memory.[5] DHA is incorporated into the brain in large amounts throughout the third trimester of pregnancy as well as in the first few months of life.[6] Further evidence for the importance of DHA in human development is its presence in breast milk; children who are fed solitarily with DHA-devoid formula have lower levels of DHA in the brain and throughout the body. Clinical studies are ongoing to determine what effect this may have on neurologic development and outcomes.

DHA has beneficial effects in cardiovascular disease; supplementation with DHA results in elevated HDL and reduced serum triglycerides.[7] It also, however, elevates LDL cholesterol and particle size, but does not appear to elevate total cholesterol.[8] DHA exerts slight effects on blood viscosity by increasing the ability of red blood cells to deform, which allows them to travel with greater ease through narrow spaces (thus decreasing potential clots in narrowed arteries).[9]

DEFICIENCY

Insufficient amounts of DHA are found in diets that do not contain any cold-water marine animal food sources. It is also hypothesized that pregnancy may deplete DHA stores in women over the long term.[10] Infants who are not breast-fed have lower amounts of DHA in their bodies than those who are, and as mentioned previously, this may have an effect on neurologic development.

USES

DHA as a supplement has been shown to decrease stress-related aggression.[11] When given to premature infants, DHA was shown to improve visual function,[12] and it decreases the severity of movement disorders in children with dyspraxia.[13] Supplementation seems to improve the development of neurologic structures, as this fatty acid is incorporated into the gray matter of the brain, one-third of which is composed of long chain polyunsaturated fatty acids.[14]

Diets rich in DHA may also decrease mortality in people with coronary artery disease.[15]

DOSING REVIEW

There is no established RDA for DHA. It is typically supplemented with other polyunsaturated fatty acids, such as eicosapentaenoic acid. The majority of research utilizes 1–3 grams of DHA per day; most fish oil supplements contain roughly 12 percent DHA. Five grams of supplemental fish oil will usually contain 72–312 milligrams of DHA. No side effects are currently recognized with supplementation.

Eicosapentaenoic Acid (EPA)

MECHANISM OF ACTION

Eicosapentaenoic acid (EPA) is a long chain polyunsaturated fatty acid that is derived from mainly cold-water fish and other marine animals. An omega-3 fatty acid, EPA is a competitive inhibitor of arachidonic acid in the cyclooxygenase and lipoxygenase pathways.[1] EPA is considered an essential fatty acid and is incorporated into cellular membranes, having an effect on membrane fluidity and intercellular signaling.

Research shows a beneficial effect of EPA on schizophrenic and depressive disorders; much research is continuing in these areas, as well as the effects of essential fatty acids in other neurologic diseases.[2] Supplementation with EPA can reduce triglyceride levels and increase fasting levels of blood glucose and insulin,[3] and it has been shown to increase HDL cholesterol by nearly 12 percent in some studies.[4] EPA is shown to decrease platelet aggregation and increase red blood cell deformability, allowing erythrocytes to travel with greater ease through narrowed arteries thereby decreasing the likelihood of clotting.[5]

USES

In the treatment of depression, EPA used as an adjunctive treatment to standard antidepressant pharmaceuticals was shown to decrease symptoms of guilt, low self-esteem, insomnia, and depressed mood.[2] Used in the treatment of borderline personality disorder, EPA modestly improved symptoms of aggression and depression.[6] In the treatment of cardiovascular disease, EPA was shown to decrease mortality.[7] EPA has antiinflammatory activity and is used to treat various diseases in which inflammation is problematic.[8]

DEFICIENCY

The standard American diet is typically low in essential fatty acids; the lack of omega-3 and omega-6 fatty acids in cellular membranes is theorized to be a contributing factor to several disease states. Some vegetable oils can be converted in small amounts in the body into EPA, but a person eating a typical modern diet is more than likely consuming insufficient amounts of these nutrients.

Several studies of people with depression indicate that omega-3 fatty acids are deficient in this population.

DOSING REVIEW

There is no RDA for EPA. Typically, EPA supplements contain 169–563 milligrams of EPA in 5 grams of fish oils. Most fish oil supplements contain roughly 18 percent EPA.

As an adjunctive antidepressant treatment, 1 gram twice daily is used. As an adjunctive treatment for schizophrenia, 3 grams in divided doses per day has been used.

In borderline personality disorder, 1 gram per day is used.

5

Hydroxytryptophan (5-HTP)

MECHANISM OF ACTION

Commonly referred to as 5-HTP, this compound is closely related to the amino acid L-tryptophan and the neurotransmitter serotonin. L-tryptophan undergoes transformation in the body into 5-HTP, which is then converted into serotonin. 5-HTP is an intermediary metabolite of L-tryptophan in the synthesis of serotonin. 5-HTP's main mechanism of action is to increase the levels of serotonin in the central nervous system; other neurotransmitters (such as dopamine and norepinephrine) and other brain chemicals (such as melatonin and beta-endorphin) are increased following supplementation with 5-HTP.[1]

Supplemental 5-HTP surpasses the conversion of L-tryptophan into 5-HTP by tryptophan hydrolase, which is the limiting step in the production of serotonin. This enzyme may be inhibited or decreased by stress and vitamin B-6 and/or magnesium deficiencies. 5-HTP can function as an antioxidant as well.[2] Absorption of 5-HTP in the intestine occurs without a transport molecule and is not affected by the presence of other amino acids or proteins. Because of this, 5-HTP can be taken with food without any effect on bioavailablity.

5-HTP, when taken orally, can enter the brain and enhance production of the neurotransmitter serotonin.[3] Because of this effect, 5-HTP is used to treat conditions in which serotonin may play a role; these include depression, insomnia, and others. Serotonin itself modulates appetite, depression and mood, anxiety, and aggressive behavior.[4] Supplemental 5-HTP is commercially derived from the plant Griffonia simplicifolia found on the African continent.

USES

5-HTP is effective for treating depression,[5] and it appears to provide significant improvement of depressive symptoms, even in patients with depression that was previously resistant to standard treatment.[6] 5-HTP may be as effective as standard pharmaceutical antidepressants such as fluvoxamine and imipramine.[7] Other uses of 5-HTP include treatment for ADHD, anxiety, cerebellar ataxia, fibromyalgia, sleep disorders, some forms of epilepsy, migraines, obesity, and Parkinson's disease.

DEFICIENCY

There is no RDA for 5-HTP; however, certain diets that are deficient in protein with low amounts of the amino acid tryptophan may predispose a person to low states.

DOSING REVIEW

Initial dosing of 5-HTP typically starts at 50 milligrams, three times per day with meals. If, after two weeks of supplementation, the desired response is not yet achieved, the dose may be increased to 100 milligrams three times per day. When using this supplement, it is best to use the smallest possible dose to achieve the greatest clinical effect.

The standard dose of 5-HTP for depression is 150–300 milligrams per day.

For treatment of insomnia, a dose of 100–300 milligrams prior to bedtime is used.

Note: Prior to supplementation checking with one's physician and pharmacist to avoid potential drug-natural medicine interactions is imperative.

Folate

The term "folate" refers to a grouping of several forms of folic acid. Synthetic folic acid is nearly 100 percent bioavailable, whereas folic acid found in foods is roughly 40 percent to 50 percent bioavailable. Folic acid has a side chain, polyglutamate, which must be enzymatically cleaved away prior to its absorption in the small intestine.[1] Once absorbed, folic acid is reduced to tetrahydrofolate before entering various metabolic cylces.[2] Folic acid works intimately with vitamin B-12 in the body. Folic acid is vital for synthesis of DNA; without folate, cells cannot divide properly. The development of the nervous system is dependent on folic acid as well; deficiency of folate is linked to several birth defects including neural tube defects. Folic acid plays a role in the metabolism of homocysteine; low levels of folate in the blood are associated with increased levels of this amino acid. Folic acid is necessary for the metabolism of homocysteine into methionine and for the conversion of s-adenosylmethionine (SAMe).[3] Elevated homocysteine is considered a risk factor for atherosclerosis, thromboembolism, deep vein thrombosis, ischemic stroke, and heart attack.[4]

USES

Insufficient folic acid is thought to contribute to the development of Alzheimer's disease; research shows that low levels of folic acid may be related to degeneration of the outer layers of the brain (cerebral cortex),[5] and decreased blood levels of folic acid are associated with brain degeneration that has been noted at autopsy as well. Elevated levels of homocysteine contribute to DNA damage and cell death in the brain, and are therefore considered to be neurotoxic.[6] Both physical and mental dysfunction can occur in the elderly with low blood levels and dietary intake of folic acid.[7]

Folic acid has also been noted to be low in people suffering from depression,[8] and low levels are associated with a decreased clinical response to antidepressant therapy as well.[9] Population studies indicate that people who do not consume enough dietary folic acid or those with low blood levels are at an increased risk of having depression.[10]

Additionally, folate is needed for the metabolism of tetrahydrobiopterin, which is a necessary enzymatic cofactor for the enzymes that produce the neurotransmitter serotonin.

DEFICIENCY

Folic acid deficiency is the most common type of vitamin deficiency. Folic acid is widely available in plant sources of foods but is quite low in animal sources, except liver. Alcohol and several prescription drugs affect the metabolism of folic acid as well, limiting the use of the vitamin in the body. Deficiency of folic acid leads to decreased cellular replication and increases the rate of cellular death.[11] Other symptoms of folic acid deficiency include delayed growth, anemia, gingivitis, diarrhea, abnormal pap smears, depression, insomnia, fatigue, irritability, and forgetfulness.[12]

DOSING REVIEW

The Recommended Dietary Allowances (RDAs) for folate in adults are 400 micrograms per day and in pregnant and lactating women 500–600 micrograms per day.

A typical supplemental dosage is 400 micrograms per day; treatment for other conditions can range up to 10 milligrams per day.

Note: When taking supplemental folic acid, it is necessary to take B-12 as well because folic acid can mask a B-12 deficiency by reversing anemia but will not treat B-12 deficiency–induced neurologic symptoms.

Ginkgo biloba

MECHANISM OF ACTION

Ginkgo leaf contains several active constituents and is typically standardized to contain 24 percent flavonoid glycosides, which are the main active ingredients. Ginkgo's constituents have their own pharmacologic actions; however, it appears that many of these compounds are more potent when acting synergistically.[1] Ginkgo is thought to exert several effects; it protects tissues from oxidative damage, protecting cell membranes from lipid peroxidation,[2] and it can protect neurons specifically from oxidative damage following episodes of ischemia.[3] By protecting tissues from oxidative damage, ginkgo is thought to protect the central nervous system (CNS) from degeneration that is linked to dementia. Ginkgo inhibits platelet activating factor (PAF) from binding to various cells, which has the effect of decreasing platelet aggregation, smooth muscle contraction, neutrophil degranulation, and free radical production. This effect serves to protect tissue from injury-related damage.[4]

Ginkgo benefits the CNS and other vascular conditions through its circulatory enhancing effects; it increases blood delivery to the brain and eyes specifically. This effect appears to be mediated through decreased blood viscosity and smooth muscle contraction.

Ginkgo benefits Alzheimer's disease by protecting cells from toxicity produced by beta amyloid peptides,[5] and it appears to enhance the cholinergic neurotransmitter system.[6] Other evidence suggests that ginkgo limits the enzyme catechol-O-methyltransferase (COMT), thereby preventing the breakdown of adrenergic neurotransmitters, and increases the amount of alpha adrenoreceptors in the brain that are reduced as part of the aging process.[7]

USES

Ginkgo is primarily used in the treatment of Alzheimer's disease, vascular, and mixed dementias. Ginkgo stabilizes and improves some aspects of cognitive and social function in patients with dementia,[8] Some evidence suggests ginkgo leaf extract might modestly improve some measures of cognitive function, particularly short-term visual memory and possibly speed of cognitive processing, in nondemented patients with age-related memory impairment.[9] Ginkgo leaf extract might modestly improve cognitive function, such as memory and speed of cognitive processing in people with no complaints of memory impairment.[10] Ginkgo is able to increase pain-free walking distance in people with intermittent claudication,[11] and it is effective at improving memory.[12]

DEFICIENCY

There is no RDA for *Ginkgo biloba*.

DOSING REVIEW

For treatment of dementia, doses of 120 to 240 milligrams per day in divided doses are used. For improvement of cognitive function in healthy people, a dose of 120 to 600 milligrams per day is used.* Higher doses may have pronounced blood thinning effects and warrants medical supervision. For treatment of ADHD, 50 milligrams ginkgo extract can be taken in combination with 200 milligrams American ginseng twice daily.

*The majority of research shows that lower doses of 120 to 240 milligrams are more effective than higher doses up to 600 milligrams per day. Ginkgo supplements should be taken in a form standardized to contain 24 percent glycosides.

Ginseng

There are three main types of ginseng used: American (referred to as Panax quinquefolius), Asian (referred to as Panax ginseng), and Siberian (referred to as Eleutherococcus senticosus).

AMERICAN

Mechanism of Action

The root of American ginseng is the medicinally used part of the plant. The active components are the ginsenosides, panaxosides, and saponins.[1] There are thought to be at least 11 different forms of the ginsenosides in various ginseng species.[2] American ginseng is used medicinally as an agent to lower blood pressure, an antispychotic, a central nervous system depressant, and an ulcer protectant. Other activities include increased gastrointestinal motility and fever-lowering effects.[3] Some ginsenosides may improve memory function by acting on acetylcholine in the brain in an as of yet unknown mechanism; they do not seem to affect the metabolism and release or reuptake of this neurotransmitter.[4] American ginseng stimulates parts of the immune system; monocytes and tumor necrosis factor alpha are enhanced by this herb.[5]

Uses

American ginseng is used for decreasing postprandial (following meals) blood sugar in patients with type 2 diabetes; 3 grams of the herb prior to meals can effectively decrease blood sugar levels following a meal.[6] The ability of ginseng to lower blood sugar is attributed to the level of ginsenosides in the herbal preparation. The mechanism of action is unknown at this time.

American ginseng taken with the herb ginkgo may decrease ADHD symptoms in children. Studies are underway to further evaluate these findings.[7]

American ginseng is considered an adaptogen, or a substance that can non-specifically increase the body's resistance to various environmental stresses. In this capacity, American ginseng is used for insomnia, ADHD, stress, improving stamina, loss of appetite, loss of memory, dizziness, headache, convulsions, and for improving immune function.

Deficiency

There is no RDA for American ginseng.

Dosing Review

The standard does of American ginseng ranges from 0.25 to 0.5 grams of the herb root twice daily. In conditions of extreme debilitation, doses of 0.8 grams are taken twice daily. For ADHD symptoms, 200 milligrams of American ginseng twice daily is used.

For type 2 diabetes, doses range from 3 to 9 grams; caution should be used when taking any glucose-lowering herb in addition to diabetes pharmaceuticals.

ASIAN

Mechanism of Action

The root is the medicinally used part of Panax ginseng. The active constituents are referred to as both ginsenosides and panaxosides.[8] Ginsenosides also potentiate nerve growth factor and might confer neuroprotection through nicotinic activity.[9] Panax ginseng is considered to be an adaptogenic herb, which can increase the body's nonspecific responses to stress; research indicates that Panax ginseng has an effect on the hypothalamic-pituitary-adrenal (HPA) axis, stimulating increased cortisol secretion by the adrenal glands.[10] Panax ginseng also increases levels of the hormone dehydroepiandrosterone sulfate (DHEA-S) in women.[11]

Uses

Panax ginseng is effective at improving cognitive function by enhancing mental arithmetic skills, abstract memory, and reaction times.[12] Its combination with the herb ginkgo has been shown to improve memory in middle-aged people.[13] Panax ginseng is effective at lowering fasting blood glucose levels and reducing hemoglobin A1c in type 2 diabetics.[14] Supplementation with the influenza vaccine during flu season for 12 weeks decreases the risk of catching both colds and flu viruses.[15]

Deficiency

There is no RDA for Panax ginseng.

Dosing Review

Typical doses of Panax ginseng are 100 milligrams twice per day. For treatment of diabetes, 200 milligrams twice per day has been used.

SIBERIAN

Mechanism of Action

The root and leaves of Siberian ginseng are used medicinally. The active constituents are the eleutherosides A through M.[16] Siberian ginseng has antioxidant effects and can prevent brain damage resulting from ischemic stroke.[17] It acts as an immune stimulant and anti-inflammatory and can stimulate the pituitary-adrenocortical system.[18]

Uses

Siberian ginseng can improve memory and mood in middle-aged people.[19] It is also used for Alzheimer's disease, ADHD, diabetes, appetite stimulation, and chronic fatigue syndrome. As an adaptogen, Siberian ginseng is used to enhance the body's response to environmental stress. The herb is also used for treating elevated blood lipids,[20] ischemic stroke,[21] and heart arrythmias.[22]

Deficiency

There is no RDA for Siberian ginseng.

Dosing Review

Standard dosing of Siberian ginseng is 200 to 400 milligrams per day.

Huperzine A

MECHANISM OF ACTION

Derived from the Chinese club moss Huperzia serrata and from Lycopodium selago, Huperzine A is an alkaloid constituent. Huperzine A is a reversible acetycholinesterase inhibitor that can cross the blood-brain barrier.[1] This constituent can inhibit the activity of acetycholinesterase in the brain for several hours, which allows for increased levels of acetylcholine in different areas of the brain.[2] Because of its effects on acetylcholine, Huperzine A is considered a beneficial therapuetic agent in the treatment of memory impairment, myasthenia gravis, and dementia.[3]

Compared to pharmaceutical anticholinesterase inhibitors (tacrine, donepezil), Huperzine A is thought be a more specific and longer-acting acetylcholinesterase inhibitor.[4] Huperzine A is more bioavailable than tacrine and allows for greater physiologic efficacy because it crosses the blood-brain barrier.[5] Additionally, Huperzine A can protect neurons from toxins (glutamate), is thought to prevent seizures, and may protect acetylcholine stores (peripheral and central) against certain nerve agents that affect the physiology of the neuron.[6]

USES

Huperzine A, because of its specific effects on the neurotransmitter acetylcholine, is used effectively in the treatment of senile, infarct-induced, and Alzheimer's dementias and for improving memory and cognitive function.[7]

In Alzheimer's disease, Huperzine A leads to significant improvements in memory and cognitive and behavioral function.

Myasthenia gravis patients were able to prevent muscle weakness using an intramuscular injectable form of Huperzine A. The time of prevention was greater in comparison to the drug neostigmine.

Improvement in memory function was noted in healthy adolescent students, and another group of students that complained of poor memory had improved memory scores after taking Huperzine A.[8]

DEFICIENCY

There is no RDA for Huperzine A.

DOSING REVIEW

For memory improvement: 100 micrograms two times per day. For Alzheimer's and infarct-induced dementia: 50–200 micrograms two times per day. For age-related dementia: 30 micrograms two times per day. Huperzine A is available in an injectable form as well; 400 micrograms per day can be used for myasthenia gravis.

Magnesium

MECHANISM OF ACTION

The most abundant positive ion in the body and the second most abundant positive ion inside of cells, magnesium maintains several important uses in the body. Magnesium is thought to contribute to over 300 enzymatic reactions[1]; some of which include the formation of cyclic AMP, ion movement across cell membranes, and both protein and carbohydrate metabolism. Magnesium is necessary to maintain the electrical potentials of nerves and muscles and for the transmission of these impulses across the neuromuscular junction.[2] The tissues in the body with the highest amount of magnesium are the brain, heart, liver, and kidneys—the most metabolically active organs—which underlines the essential role of magnesium in the production of energy. The human body is thought to contain roughly 25 grams of magnesium, with 50 percent to 60 percent found in the bones and the rest inside of the cells throughout the body. Noteworthy is that only 1 percent of magnesium can be found in the serum, thus standard testing is not an accurate reflection of functional levels.

The relaxing effect of magnesium on smooth muscles (blood vessels-hypertension, bronchioles-asthma, and uterus-preterm contractions) is thought to be caused by the antagonistic effect of magnesium on calcium-directed muscle contractions.[3] In other words, magnesium can act as a mild calcium channel blocker. Some research shows that magnesium may dilate blood vessels in the brain, thereby reducing ischemia as well.

USES

Magnesium is used for many disease conditions; the following is only a partial listing for conditions that benefit from magnesium supplementation.

Hypertension: Low levels of magnesium allow for increased peripheral vascular resistance and spasm of blood vessels, which leads to increased pressure.[4]

Ischemia and stroke: Magnesium may protect neurons through a variety of mechanisms.[5]

Congestive heart failure: Magnesium serves to increase coronary blood flow, is antiarrhythmic, and improves other indices of cardiovascular health.[6]

Migraines: These headaches may be the result of decreased magnesium levels.[7]

Type 2 diabetes: This may be partially the result of decreased magnesium intake.[8]

Asthma: Symptoms from asthma benefit from magnesium administration.[9]

Magnesium is crucial for the production of energy systems throughout the body and for maintaining nerve conduction. It is required for the sodium and potassium pump that regulates the amounts of these electrolytes in and out of the cells. When these become unbalanced in the cell, energy production is disrupted.

DEFICIENCY

Magnesium is thought to be deficient throughout the U.S. population; this is attributed to decreased intake and absorption.[10] In particular, the elderly and those with high-stress lifestyles are at the most at risk for deficiency. Other factors that contribute to decreased magnesium stores are poor dietary intake, oral contraceptive use, excessive intake of calcium (this opposes the body's ability to absorb magnesium), alcohol, injury (surgery), and liver and kidney diseases.

Testing serum levels of magnesium is thought to provide an inaccurate picture; because the majority of the body's magnesium stores are inside of the cells, a low serum level of magnesium may indicate the end stage of deficiency. More accurate magnesium test levels can be found by testing red blood cell levels of magnesium.

Magnesium deficiency is thought to be contributory to a number of disease conditions, such as high blood pressure, insomnia, premenstrual syndrome, mental confusion, irritability, weakness, insomnia, increased stress, loss of appetite, diabetes, and cardiovascular disease.[11]

DOSING REVIEW

The RDA for magnesium is 350 milligrams per day for men and 280 milligrams per day for women. Most often, the ideal intake of magnesium is based on a person's body weight; the formula is 6 milligrams per 2.2 pounds of body weight for standard supplementation purposes. When treating certain disease conditions in which low magnesium levels are thought to be contributory, up to 12 milligrams per 2.2 pounds of body weight is used. Therefore, a 150-pound person may be supplemented with 409 to 818 milligrams of magnesium per day. At higher dosing levels the potential for loose stools or diarrhea must be monitored.

N-Acetyl-Carnitine

MECHANISM OF ACTION

Also known as acetyl-L-carnitine, this compound is mainly derived from the amino acid carnitine; it is an ester form and is structurally similar to the neurotransmitter acetylcholine. It is formed in some amount in the body inside of the cellular mitochondria. N-acetyl-carnitine is thought to enhance the activity of the cholinergic nervous system by serving as a precursor molecule to acetyl coenzyme A, making up a structural segment of acetylcholine.[1] Additionally, it acts to assist in the transport of acetyl groups into the mitochondria and promotes the production (increased choline acetyltransferase activity) and release of acetylcholine.[2] N-acetyl-carnitine is also thought to have neuroprotective effects, assist in the serotonin neurotransmitter pathways, enhance the transmission of nerve impulses in the brain, and decrease the age-related loss of glucocorticoid receptors in the hippocampus. Research has shown that N-acetyl-carnitine may increase blood flow to the brain in patients with cerebrovascular disease.[3] Because of the many effects of acetyl-L-carnitine, this compound has been studied for the treatment of Alzheimer's disease (which is accompanied by significant decreases in acetylcholine and cholinergic neurons).[4]

USES

N-acetyl-carnitine is used to improve cognitive function and memory in people with age-related cognitive decline and memory impairment.[5] It is also beneficial for people with cerebrovascular insufficiency (decreased or impaired blood flow to the brain), vascular dementia, and those recovering from stokes.[6] N-acetyl-carnitine was shown to improve cerebral blood flow in people with chronic brain ischemia after only one dose,[7] and it can improve memory and visual-space orientation skills in recovering alcoholics with cognitive impairment.[8]

N-acetyl-carnitine is also used in the treatment of AIDS, where it may slow the decline of CD4 lymphocytes.[9] It is also used for the treatment of HIV medication-related neuropathy.[10]

N-acetyl-carnitine is used for improving energy and is a part of formulas designed for weight loss, as this compound assist in the transport of long chain fatty acids into the mitochondria where they are used for energy production.[11] N-acetyl-carnitine is also used to improve sperm motility; this compound is present in sperm and seminal fluid and has been found to be low in infertile and low-motility sperm samples.[12]

DEFICIENCY

There is no RDA for N-acetyl-carnitine.

DOSING REVIEW

For the treatment of Alzheimer's disease: 1,500–4,000 milligrams in divided doses per day. Age-related memory impairment: 1,500–2,000 milligrams per day. Stroke recovery: 1,500 milligrams per day. Age-related depression: 1,500–3,000 milligrams in divided doses per day. Best taken 30–60 minutes away from meals.

Phosphatidylserine

MECHANISM OF ACTION

Phosphatidylserine is a type of phospholipid that is manufactured in the human body. Phosphatidylserine is also obtained from most foods.[1] It is the most plentiful phospholipid found in the brain and plays a vital role in maintaining the structural and functional integrity of the nerve cell membrane. It assists in these functions by regulating the internal cellular environment, release of secretory vessicles, intercellular communication, regulation of cell growth, and signal transduction.[2]

The mechanism of action of phosphatidylserine in the treatment of Alzheimer's disease and age-related memory impairment is not clearly elucidated at this time; however, one theory suggests that those with dementia or age-related memory impairment have abnormalities in their neuronal membranes, which leads to structural and functional neurotransmitter abnormalities. Additionally, this population often has changes in the levels of the neurotransmitters serotonin, norepinephrine, and acetylcholine, and researchers believe that these changes may be the result of an alteration in brain phospholipid content. By supplementing with an external source of phospholipids, in the form of phosphatidylserine, this may normalize brain phospholipid functions.[3] Phosphatidylserine can increase the levels of serotonin, dopamine, norepinephrine, and acetylcholine in people with Alzheimer's disease and may decrease age-related dendritic loss as and cholinergic neuron loss.[4]

Phosphatidylserine can decrease the cortisol and adrenocorticotropin elevation that follows strenuous exercise. This may serve to attenuate some forms of exercise-induced physiologic stress.[5]

USES

Phosphatidylserine is used in the treatment of Alzheimer's disease and for senile dementia. It can increase cognitive function, behavioral ratings, and global improvement scales in the short term.[6] In people with age-related cognitive decline and memory impairment, phosphatidylserine can improve attention, arousal, memory, and verbal fluency.[7] Some research shows that phosphatidylserine may improve depression in the elderly as well.[8] Highly trained athletes had an increased sense of well-being and decreased postexercise muscle soreness when taking phosphatidylserine.[9]

DEFICIENCY

Low levels of phosphatidylserine are associated with impaired mental function and depression in the elderly.[10] Under regular circumstances, the brain manufactures its own phosphatidylserine; however, this process is compromised when nutrients such as folic acid, vitamin B-12, and essential fatty acids are in short supply in the body.

DOSING REVIEW

There is no RDA for phosphatidylserine. The standard supplemental dose is 100 milligrams three times a day. Some research shows the use of 200–300 milligrams per day for the treatment of ADHD.[11]

The essential fatty acid docosahexaenoic acid (DHA) seems to enhance the ability of phosphatidylserine to accumulate in neuron cell membranes. Therefore, these two nutrients should be taken concomitantly.

Vitamin C

MECHANISM OF ACTION

Vitamin C, also known as ascorbic acid, is a water-soluble vitamin that must be obtained from food sources for human health. Vitamin C has multiple physiologic effects in the body, namely in oxidation-reduction reactions as an antioxidant. It is also necessary for the metabolism of carnitine and tryptophan (amino acids), thyroxin (a thyroid hormone), and the neurotransmitters dopamine and norepinephrine.[1] It is used in the process of cellular respiration, metabolism of carbohydrates, conversion of cholesterol into bile acids, the synthesis of proteins and lipids used in the body, metabolism of iron, and the conversion of folic acid to folinic acid.[2] Vitamin C is also needed for optimal function of the immune system.[3]

USES

The use of vitamin C for multiple conditions is backed by several clinical and population studies that illustrate its benefits in human health. Vitamin C's status as an excellent (relating to efficacy and cost) antioxidant may be the primary purpose of its widespread use in disease. Some of the most often treated diseases using vitamin C include: asthma, cancer, colds, coronary artery disease, fatigue, infections, menopause, multiple sclerosis, Parkinson's disease, and wound healing.[4] The antioxidant effect of vitamin C is important in regard to protecting the brain and its function from the ravages of oxidative processes in the body.

DEFICIENCY

The RDA for vitamin C is only 90 milligrams per day for men and 75 milligrams per day for women; for pregnant and lactating women, 120 milligrams per day is recommended. Because vitamin C is not produced in the human body, it can become easily deficient in a diet void of fruits and vegetables, which are the richest sources of the vitamin. Although not as commonly deficient as it was in the past, some research suggests that vitamin C levels can be insufficient prior to signs of deficiency.[5] One of the first signs of vitamin C deficiency is fatigue, but it may go unnoticed for some time due to the many other causes of fatigue.[6] If deficient for three to five months, a person will develop scurvy, which is marked by gum swelling and bleeding, hyperkeratosis, and small hemorrhages in the viscera (internal organs) and the muscles.[7] Wound healing is much slower in states of deficiency.

DOSING REVIEW

There is a wide range of doses suggested for vitamin C, the lowest being the RDA of 75–90 milligrams per day. However, Linus Pauling recommended doses ranging from 2 to 9 grams during normal health and even higher doses during illness.

For optimal use of the vitamin, a dose of 500 to 1,000 milligrams per day is recommended. Higher doses may be considered for disease conditions in which a high amount of oxidative stress is present.

Vitamin E

MECHANISM OF ACTION

Also known as alpha-tocopherol, vitamin E is a fat-soluble vitamin derived from many sources outside of the human body. The main function of vitamin E in the body is as an antioxidant and the benefits of this vitamin are primarily attributed to this effect. There are eight different forms of vitamin E; however, the only biologically active form is alpha-tocopherol. In order to become biologically active, alpha-tocopherol is dependent on the alpha-tocopherol transfer protein that is found in the liver. Alpha-tocopherol binds to this protein and is then transported throughout the body.[1] Vitamin E primarily works in the lipids of the body as an antioxidant. It is incorporated into the lipid layers of cell membranes and works to stabilize and protect them from various environmental assaults, such as heavy metals, chemical toxins (benzene, solvents), drugs, and free radicals.

Vitamin E is also very important for immune function; it serves to protect the cells of the immune system from oxidative damage and during times of chronic viral illnesses.

USES

Vitamin E's effects on human health lay primarily in its role as an antioxidant. As mentioned previously, vitamin E is protective of the fatty aspects of the body, primarily the lipid-containing cellular membrane. Lipid peroxidation is one of the main causes of cellular damage in the body, and nerve cells are some of the most susceptible cells to this type of damage. Because of this, vitamin E is used primarily in atherosclerosis, alcohol-induced liver disease, epilepsy, infections, inflammation, menopause, multiple sclerosis, neuralgia, neuromuscular degeneration, Parkinson's disease, premenstrual syndrome, and several other conditions.[2]

DEFICIENCY

Deficiency of vitamin E can be difficult to achieve in the short term primarily because it is a fat-soluble vitamin that is stored in the body. However, vitamin E can become depleted in certain conditions such as fat malabsorption (celiac disease, cystic fibrosis), in premature infants, in genetic diseases of red blood cells that do not allow for maintenance of normal blood levels, and in patients undergoing dialysis. Signs of deficiency include muscle weakness, damage to nerves, loss of coordination, and red blood cell damage leading to decreased lifespan of these cells.[3]

DOSING REVIEW

The RDA for vitamin E is 15 milligrams for both men and women, which is equivalent to 22 International Units of natural vitamin E or 33 International Units of synthetic vitamin E. Standard therapeutic doses range from 400 International Units to 800 International Units.

Vitamin C assists in regenerating vitamin E that has become oxidized in the body and potentiates its antioxidant effects; therefore these two supplements should be taken together to maximize their effects.

Zinc

MECHANISM OF ACTION

Zinc is the second most abundant trace element in the body, totaling nearly 2 grams.[1] During periods of increased zinc demand in the body, zinc absorption is increased and zinc already within the body is conserved.[2] Zinc serves as a cofactor in protein synthesis, including that of DNA and RNA, and is used in more enzymatic reactions that any other mineral. Zinc is contained in over 300 enzymes that are thought to have a hand in genetic expression in the body and is a direct catalyst for over 100 enzymes.[3] Zinc is needed for growth and development, behavior and learning, proper immune function, healing of tissue damage, reproduction, taste and smell, and the function of the insulin and thyroid hormones.[4] The majority of zinc is absorbed from foods (which is only 40 percent) in the small intestine, and absorption increases during times of zinc deficiency.[5]

Zinc serves as a cofactor in the synthesis of several neurotransmitters and some research demonstrates low levels of zinc in children with ADHD in comparison to children without.[6] Additionally, low serum levels of zinc in people with ADHD may not respond as well to standard medical therapy.[7]

Zinc plays a large role in the function of several immune cells,[8] and deficiency seems to negatively affect the function of T cells.[9] Zinc is thought to inhibit viral replication in the common cold as well.[10]

USES

Zinc has several uses; however, the most common include treatment of ADHD, anorexia nervosa, alcoholism, alcoholic cirrhosis, infection and inflammation, and situations of trauma and starvation. Decreased zinc absorption is associated with conditions such asdiabetes mellitus, liver disease, celiac disease, chronic diarrhea, and pancreatic insufficiency.[11] Therefore, zinc supplementation should be included in the treatment of these conditions as well.

DEFICIENCY

Frank zinc deficiency is not as common in the United States in comparison to other parts of the world because the majority of Americans consume at least the RDA in zinc each day.[12] However, zinc may easily become deficient as the result of many conditions of decreased intake due to poor diet and several disease conditions.[13]

A truly reliable test for zinc deficiency does not exist; current testing methods are not efficient at determining zinc status. (They are neither sensitive nor specific.) Zinc deficiency is best evaluated by a positive response in symptoms from supplementation.

Conditions that may require the supplementation of zinc include chronic diarrhea; gastrointestinal diseases or conditions in which malabsorption is evident; alcoholism and liver disease; and trauma or infections. Symptoms of zinc deficiency include slow growth, mental lethargy, irritability, low thyroid function, decreased taste and smell, nausea, diarrhea, poor healing of wounds, rough or dry skin, and decreased sperm count.[14]

DOSING REVIEW

The RDA for zinc is 11 milligrams per day for men and 8 milligrams per day for women. Pregnant and lactating women should have 12 milligrams per day. It is estimated that the typical male consumes roughly 13 milligrams per day and the typical female consumes roughly 9 milligrams per day in North America.[3] For general supplementation, doses of 15 to 20 milligrams per day are recommended.

It is often best tolerated when taken with a meal.

Nutrient Deficiency Signs and Symptoms

There is great controversy over the use of the term "deficiency" when it comes to vitamins, minerals, and other nutrients. In the most formal sense, a nutrient deficiency officially occurs when a nutrient's absence results in an overt disease state. The most classic and best known of the vitamin deficiencies arises when vitamin C becomes deficient and results in a condition called scurvy. Without sufficient vitamin C levels, the human body begins to literally fall apart—the connective tissues, like skin, hair, nails, and gum, and even the circulatory system begin to fail. The treatment, of course, is replacement of the nutrient, in this case vitamin C.

Scurvy was prevalent in the days of Christopher Columbus and other seagoing pioneers. However, the sailors didn't become deficient overnight, nor did their symptoms immediately present as the worst-case scenario. Instead, the nutrient deficiency led to progressive changes within the body. So, looking for changes in one's health may offer insights about deficits that may be arising, which need to be confirmed by a qualified medical professional.

Essential to success when working on fueling the human body properly is to avoid getting either too little or too much of a nutrient. Just as insufficient nutrient levels can cause problems, so can excess amounts. There is a saying that we use when lecturing to the public and healthcare professional communities, and if one remembers the essence of the message it can save a lot of unnecessary suffering: "Just because it's Natural doesn't make it Safe." After all, one can get too much of anything: medication, sun, water, and even chocolate. Also important to remember, "natural medicines" are still medicines and they do have the potential to interact with prescription and over-the-counter medications, thus having a strong relationship between the patient and healthcare provider is essential.

This appendix is divided into two alphabetical listings, one for minerals and the other for vitamins/nutrients. This appendix is intended to offer clues that, when confirmed through appropriate testing, will allow for the potential of greater success in achieving optimized health.

MINERALS

Suboptimal levels of the following minerals may be linked in part to the symptoms listed. Important to note, though, is that once symptoms begin to appear, other biochemical changes also begin to manifest within the body and a full and comprehensive physical exam and laboratory testing is indicated. It is important to remember that many of the listed health conditions can also present with symptoms that need medical attention without being associated with nutrient deficiencies. For example: Numbness and tingling in the legs may also be a sign of a back injury, neurological disease, or diabetes.

Calcium Deficits May Lead to One or More of the Following Symptoms

Brittle/Weakened Nails
Cramps
Depression
Dermatitis (eczema)
Gum and Tooth Disease
Heart Palpitations
High Blood Pressure
Hyperactivity
Insomnia
Irritability
Mental Performance Diminishment
Muscular Twitches
Nervous Aggitation
Numbness/Tingling in Limbs
Osteomalacia
Osteoporosis
Retarded Growth
Rickets

Note: Excess calcium intake can lead to numerous health conditions as well.

Chromium Deficits May Lead to One or More
of the Following Symptoms

Anxiousness
Blood Sugar Dysregulation
Diabetes
Elevated Cholesterol
Fatigue
Hypoglycemia
Irritability
Retarded Growth

Note: Excess chromium intake can lead to kidney and liver damage.

Copper Deficits May Lead to One or More
of the Following Symptoms

Anemia (microcytic and hypochromic)
Depression
Diarrhea
Fatigue
Hair Loss
Heart Muscle Weakening
High Cholesterol
Increased Frequency/Severity of Infections
Lowered White Blood Cell Count
Osteoporosis

Note: Excess copper intake can also cause numerous health conditions, including hyper-activity, immune suppression, and lowered zinc levels.

Iodine Deficits May Lead to One or More
of the Following Symptoms

Constipation
Decreased Body Temperature
Decreased Mental Function
Diminished Reflexes
Fatigue
Impaired Childhood Development
Weight Gain (unexplainable)

Note: Inadequate amounts of iodine lead to mental and physical growth impairment; this, along with the prevention of thyroid goiters, is why salt is iodized. Avoidance of salt, especially by children, may contribute to iodine deficits. Iodine is essential for thyroid hormone production, thus getting a laboratory test to measure thyroid function when weight gain is notable is worthwhile.

Iron Deficits May Lead to One or More of the Following Symptoms

Anemia (microcytic and hypochromic)
Confusion and Weakness
Cracks at the Corner of Mouth
Depression
Dizziness
Fatigue
Headaches
Inflamed Tongue
Lack of Appetite
Trouble Swallowing
Weakened Bones

Note: Iron overload/excess is a leading cause of poisoning in the United States. Adults need to be very cautious in regard to supplementing and should only do so with clear guidance and monitoring by their healthcare provider. Excess iron also leads to several disease states, including increased cardiovascular disease. Insufficient iron, though, leads to diminished capacity to deliver optimal levels of oxygen and certain nutrients to target tissues throughout the body.

Magnesium Deficits May Lead to One or More of the Following Symptoms

Altered Coordination
Anxiety
Cold Hands and Feet
Eclampsia
Edema (swelling)
Hallucinations
Heart Arrhythmias
High Blood Pressure
Hyperactivity
Impaired Concentration
Increased Heart Beat
Insomnia
Kidney Stones
Loss of Appetite
Muscle Twitching/Spasms
Muscle Weakness

Nausea
Nystagmus
Oversensitivity to Sounds
Restlessness
Startling Readily and Dramatically
Seizures
Vomiting

Note: Excess magnesium can lead to numerous symptoms, including low blood pressure and flushing, and can also cause heart arrhythmias and muscle weakness. The latter two symptoms appear in both the deficiency and excess categories, pointing to the importance of balance when supplementing.

Manganese Deficits May Lead to One or More of the Following Symptoms

Dermatitis
Diminished Ovarian Functioning
Diminished Testicular Functioning
Low Cholesterol
Weight Loss (unintended)

Note: Intriguing is that excess amounts can lead to impairment in judgment, hallucinations, insomnia, and symptoms that mimic Parkinson's disease.

Phosphorus Deficits May Lead to One or More of the Following Symptoms

Anxiety
Bone Pain
Irritability
Lack of Appetite
Muscle Weakness
Numbness and Tingling in Limbs
Tremors

Note: Bone pain can also be a sign of very serious disease and needs to be discussed immediately with your healthcare provider.

Potassium Deficits May Lead to One or More of the Following Symptoms

Blood Sugar Dysregulation
Constipation

Decreased Reflexes
Depression
Dry Eyes
Edema (swelling)
Fatigue
Heartbeat Irregularities
Impaired Cognitive Functioning
Insomnia
Muscle Weakness

Note: Though potassium can help with heart problems when appropriate, supplementing without careful blood monitoring and review of current medications can be very dangerous.

Selenium Deficits May Lead to One or More of the Following Symptoms

Elevated Cholesterol
Increased Frequency of Infections
Male Infertility

Note: The toxicity associated with selenium is very serious and supplementation should not exceed 200 micrograms per day.

Sodium Deficits May Lead to One or More of the Following Symptoms

Confusion
Depression
Dermatitis
Disorientation
Dizziness
Fatigue
Headache
Irritability and Mood Changes
Lack of Coordination
Lethargy
Low Blood Pressure
Memory Impairment
Seizures

Note: Sodium chloride, also commonly known as table salt, often may be actively avoided for individuals trying to control elevated blood pressure. Yet, sodium is a very important electrolyte and excess restriction can lead to deficit states. A simple blood test can determine if you have overrestricted.

Zinc Deficits May Lead to One or More
of the Following Symptoms

Acne
Brittle Nails
Depression
Dermatitis (eczema)
Diminished Taste Sense
Elevated Cholesterol
Fatigue
Forgetfulness
Hair Loss
Impaired Wound Healing
Increased Frequency of Infections
Irritability
Male Infertility
Night Blindness
Paranoid Tendencies
White Spots on Nails

Note: Excess intake of zinc can lead to a copper deficiency and numerous symptoms. In order to decrease stomach irritation, zinc is typically taken with food.

VITAMINS

Suboptimal levels of the following vitamins and nutrients may be linked in part to the symptoms listed. Important to note, though, is that once symptoms begin to appear, other biochemical changes have also begun to manifest within the body, and a full and comprehensive physical exam and laboratory testing are indicated. It is also important to remember that many of the listed health conditions can also present with symptoms that need medical attention without being associated with nutrient deficiencies. For example: numbness and tingling in the legs may also be a sign of a back injury, neurological disease, or diabetes.

Biotin Deficits May Lead to One or More
of the Following Symptoms

Anemia
Decreased Appetite
Elevated Blood Sugars
Elevated Cholesterol

Fatigue
Hair Loss
Insomnia
Muscle Weakness
Smooth Tongue

Note: Biotin is considered water soluble and thus routine intake in the diet is important to maintain adequate levels. Typically biotin is found in B-complex vitamins.

Choline Deficits May Lead to One or More of the Following Symptoms

Altered Liver Function
Elevated Cholesterol
Maldigestion of Dietary Fats
Neurological Deficits
Stomach Ulcers

Note: Choline is crucial for neurotransmitter and cellular functioning. Many nutritionally oriented physicians believe that choline deficiency is significantly underdiagnosed.

Essential Fatty Acids Deficits May Lead to One or More of the Following Symptoms

Acne
Behavior Disturbances
Bumps on Back of Upper Arm (fine raised)
Cognitive Development
Dermatitis
Dry Hair and Skin
Fatty Liver
Hair Loss
Hormonal Dysregulation
Hyperactivity
Increased Frequency of Infections
Infertility
Inflammation
Lack of Concentration (ability)
Lack of Coordination
Learning Disability

Note: There are many sources of essential fatty acids, particularly vegetables, seeds, nuts, and fish. It is estimated that, largely due to processed foods and a carbohydrate-dependent diet, only one in six individuals in the United States consume optimal levels of essential fatty acids. Neurological treatments frequently focus on EPA/DHA derived from cold deep-watered fish.

Folic Acid Deficits May Lead to One or More of the Following Symptoms

Anemia (megaloblastic)
Changes in Memory
Decreased Appetite
Decrease Sensations (feet/legs)
Flattened Mood
Elevated Homocysteine
Headache
Inflammed Tongue
Insomnia
Muscle Weakness
Restless Leg Syndrome

Note: It is very important that folic acid supplementation not be pursued without additional supplementation with B-12. Folic acid supplementation has been shown to mask B-12 deficiency, which ultimately leads to serious health issues.

Inositol Deficits May Lead to One or More of the Following Symptoms

Anxiety
Dermatitis (eczema)
Elevated Cholesterol
Hair Loss

Note: Inositol and choline are commonly taken together to support liver functioning and are sometimes referred to as lipotropic factors.

Niacin (Vitamin B-3) Deficits May Lead to One or More of the Following Symptoms

Bad Breath
Canker Sores
Confusion
Dementia
Depression
Dermatitis
Diarrhea
Disorientation

Headaches
Irritability
Lack of Appetite
Limb Pain
Memory Impairment
Mood Instability
Muscle Weakness
Skin Changes (inflammatory eruptions)

Note: Large doses of vitamin B-3 in the form of niacin can cause flushing and liver en-zyme elevation and needs to be done under close supervision. Overt niacin deficiency is called Pellagra and is classically called the disease of the 4 Ds: Depression, Dementia, Diarrhea, and Dermatitis.

Pantothenic Acid (Vitamin B-5) Deficits May Lead to One or More of the Following Symptoms

Depression
Dermatitis
Diminished Coordination
Fatigue
Feet Burning Sensation
Hair Loss
Increased Heart Rate
Irritability
Lack of Appetite
Low Blood Pressure
Muscle Weakness

Note: Actual deficiencies are uncommon among individuals eating a broad and healthy diet.

Pyridoxine (Vitamin B-6) Deficits May Lead to One or More of the Following Symptoms

Acne
Altered Hormone Metabolism
Anemia
Carpal Tunnel Symptoms
Depression
Dizziness
Hair Loss
Inflamed Eye (conjunctivitis)
Inflamed Mouth/Tongue

Irritability
Lack of Appetite
Muscle Weakness
Numbness/Tingling of Extremities
Seizures

Note: Supplementation with vitamin B-6 can often offer significant relief from neurological symptoms when dosed correctly and in balance with the other B vitamins. It should be noted that certain antiseizure medications can be made less effective with supplemental B-6 added to one's regime and careful consultation with a healthcare provider is critical.

Riboflavin (Vitamin B-2) Deficits May Lead to One or More of the Following Symptoms

Altered Vision (blurred)
Cataracts
Depression
Dermatitis
Fissures of Tongue/Mouth
Hair Loss
Inflammation of Tongue
Irritation by Light
Itchy Red Eyes

Note: Typically, riboflavin is supplemented with vitamin B-1 (thiamine) and the other B vitamins in order to support the biochemical synergy within the body.

Thiamine (Vitamin B-1) Deficits May Lead to One or More of the Following Symptoms

Cardiac Diminished Function
Confusion
Depression
Diminished Coordination
Diminished Memory
Irritation by Sound
Lack of Appetite
Nervous Irritability
Numbness of Extremities

Note: Overt B-1 deficiency leads to a disease state called beriberi, which manifests with both cardiovascular and neurological problems. Alcoholics and individuals who have been on diuretics for prolonged periods of time are especially likely to present with signs and symptoms.

Vitamin A Deficits May Lead to One or More of the Following Symptoms

Acne
Blindness
Bumps (fine raised on back of arms and along hair follicles)
Dry Eyes and Skin
Fatigue
Hair (dry)
Increased Frequency of Infections
Insomnia
Loss of Sense of Smell
Night Blindness

Note: Vitamin A supplementation needs to occur under close supervision. As a fat-soluble vitamin, the body is able to store it and very serious side effects can arise, including liver problems, fatigue, and many of the symptoms that it is used to treat. Vitamin A toxicity can be fatal.

Vitamin B-1: See entry for Thiamine

Vitamin B-2: See entry for Riboflavin

Vitamin B-3: See entry for Niacin

Vitamin B-5: See entry for Pantothenic Acid

Vitamin B-6: See entry for Pyridoxine

Vitamin B-12 Deficits May Lead to One or More of the Following Symptoms

Anemia (macrocytic)
Depression
Dizziness
Fatigue
Headaches
Inflamed Tongue
Irritability
Mood Instability
Numbness of Limbs
Spinal Cord Function Deterioration

Note: Individuals who are vegetarians are even more prone than the average individual for B-12 deficiency. The elderly are also at a particularly high risk of deficiency due both to dietary changes and also diminished digestion tract function, including changes in stomach acidity.

Vitamin C Deficits May Lead to One or More of the Following Symptoms

Bleeding Gums
Bruising (overly)
Dental Problems (loose teeth)
Depression
Edema
Fatigue
Increased Susceptibility to Infection
Irritability
Muscle Weakness
Poor Wound Healing

Note: Vitamin C supplementation is most effective when taken with bioflavonoids. Many nutritionally oriented physicians believe that if dietary intake is inadequate, supplementation with 1,000 to 2,000 milligrams per day in divided doses can be health promoting and can help patients cope with both physical and mental stressors.

Vitamin D Deficits May Lead to One or More of the Following Symptoms

Increased Risk of Fractures
Increased Risk of Multiple Sclerosis (proposed)
Insomnia
Irritability
Osteomalacia
Osteoporosis
Rickets

Note: Vitamin D is frequently at suboptimal levels in the elderly, particularly those who don't consume fortified dairy products or spend sufficient time in sunlight. Supplementation needs to be done under close supervision because vitamin D is fat soluble and is stored within the body.

Vitamin E Deficits May Lead to One or More of the Following Symptoms

Anemia (megaloblastic)
Decreased Red Blood Cell Production (from destruction)

Infertility
Muscular Weakness
Neuromuscular Degeneration

Note: Vitamin E possesses its broadest therapeutic range when taken in its natural, mixed tocopherol/tocotrienol form. Noteworthy is that excess amounts of vitamin E have a blood-thinning effect and should not be taken in combination with other blood thinners without consultation with a qualified healthcare provider.

Vitamin K Deficits May Lead to One or More of the Following Symptoms

Excess Bruising
Hemorrhage
Osteoporosis

Note: Use of antibiotics without adequate replacement of gastrointestinal flora can lead to a vitamin K deficiency when combined with a diet low in dark leafy green vegetables.

Toxic Substances and Related Brain and Body Health Changes

The following lists of toxicity syndromes and their symptoms, although not exhaustive, offer insight into potential contributing factors that may or may not be significant in preventing optimal brain function. This information is not intended to be diagnostic of isolated disease states. Rather, the sole purpose is to provide a focus of potential factors that contribute to underlying health conditions. One or more symptoms may be present; one does not need to have all symptoms in order to be suffering from a toxicity syndrome. It is important to remember: "When in doubt, test don't guess." Thus, follow-up testing is absolutely essential to definitively identify the presence or lack of a toxicity factor.

ALUMINUM TOXICITY

Altered Coordination (including walking)
Dementia/Memory Loss
Encephalopathy
GI Pain and Irritation
Kidney Disease
Liver Dysfunction

ARSENIC TOXICITY

Burning Sensation of Arms and Legs
Confusion
Dermatitis
Fatigue
Hair loss
Headaches

Itchy Skin
Muscle Pain
Nerve Pain (Neuropathy)
Poor Wound Healing
Seizures
Tingling of Hands and Feet

CADMIUM TOXICITY

Anemia
Fatigue
Hair Loss
Kidney Dysfunction
Lack of Appetite
Liver Dysfunction

CALCIUM TOXICITY

Altered Coordination
Altered Memory Capacity
Depression
Irritability
Muscle Weakness
Psychosis

COPPER TOXICITY

Depression
Irritability
Muscle Pain
Nervousness

FOLIC ACID TOXICITY

Euphoria
Hyperactivity

LEAD TOXICITY

Altered Coordination
Anemia
Anxiety
Confusion
Depression
Fatigue

Headaches
GI Pain
Lack of Concentration
Loss of Appetite
Malaise
Restlessness
Sleepiness

MANGANESE TOXICITY

Altered Judgment
Decreased Memory
Lack of Appetite
Parkinson's-like Symptoms

MERCURY TOXICITY

Altered Coordination
Altered Memory
Anemia
Autism (possible)
Depression
Dizziness
Impaired Hearing and Vision
Insomnia
Irritability
Lack of Appetite
Metallic Taste
Numbness
Psychosis
Sleepiness

POTASSIUM TOXICITY

Altered Cognitive Function
Muscle Weakness

SELENIUM TOXICITY

Fatigue
Garlic-like Breath
Hair Loss
Irritability
Metallic Taste
Muscle Pain
Yellow Skin

APPENDIX C

Selecting the Right Food for You— Avoiding Food Allergies

The incidence of food allergies is vastly underestimated. Some may argue that as many as 50 million people in America alone suffer from an allergy-based illness. That is virtually one in five with standard diagnosable allergies. Yet, clinically it is likely even close to one in two, which is 50 percent, and this number, from what is seen in clinical practice, is growing.

FOOD ALLERGY AND FOOD INTOLERANCES

A food allergy is defined as an immune reaction to some foods and not others and is unique to the affected individual. Conversely, food intolerance, unlike a food allergy, does not mount an immune reaction. Food intolerance may be due to a number of factors, including an enzymatic defect inherent in some people or a chemical component—either an additive or a naturally occurring compound in the food—that the body may be unable to handle.

A common food intolerance is lactose intolerance. People with lactose intolerance cannot digest milk products because they lack the enzyme to do so. The enzyme lactase is usually present in our gut and is responsible for breaking down the milk sugar, lactose. An inability to do this may cause cramping and diarrhea from eating milk products. This is the body's way of saying, "I can't eat this, don't give it to me!" In the case of food allergies, your body may send you similar messages; but they are due to an immune reaction that can lead to cramping, diarrhea, headache, changes in brain function, fatigue, and aching joints.

SYMPTOMS ARE THE CLUES OF A HEALTH CHALLENGE

Symptoms associated with food allergies can vary from person to person, affecting how you function and feel. One person may get headaches, another irritation of the bowel, and yet another fatigue, joint problems, attention deficit, depression, or myriad other symptoms. Symptoms may range from mild discomforts to incapacitating illness, with etiology to specific foods that are unique to each individual. Symptoms may cause you to feel sick and tired day in and day out and thus begin to blend into daily reality (it can be like walking around with a black cloud over your head, and many times you, your friends, and your loved ones will simply assume that these less-than-optimal feelings are due to "just getting old").

Realize that any food can cause a food allergy in the susceptible individual, and symptoms can happen immediately or several days after. It is virtually impossible to identify these delayed food reactions without scientific testing. After all, when was the last time you felt crummy and thought, "I wonder what food I ate two or three days ago that caused me to feel this way?" Yet delayed reactions happen frequently. It is not surprising that without high-tech testing, which is now available and very affordable, identifying cause and effect may become a challenge. Symptoms of delayed food allergies are diverse and may affect any system in the body.

The ELISA method of food allergy testing is a highly sensitive and reliable test that can detect delayed food allergies happening in your body. Now this testing can be done in the comfort of one's home with no physician order required. A small finger stick with a high-tech auto-lancet allows for the collection of a few drops of blood, which are then placed on absorbent strips and mailed to a lab. The lab generates a report and mails it back to the sender.

The ELISA test measures antibodies, or immunoglobulins, which are important proteins that your immune system makes in an effort to defend itself from noxious elements. This is a good thing when kept in check. However, an overzealous immune system can lead to excess inflammation and destruction of tissues. These Immunoglobulin G (IgG) food-mediated immune reactions can have long-standing health consequences, primarily because IgG antibodies can remain active for months at a time, promoting a state of chronic inflammation and degenerative sequelae.

COMMON SYMPTOMS LISTING

Please note that these symptoms can also be due to other underlying health issues, thus working with one's physician or healthcare provider is essential.

The Digestive System

Abdominal Cramping	Coated Tongue
Abdominal Pain	Colitis

Anal Itching
Aphthous Ulcers/Canker Sores
Bad Breath
Belching
Bloating after Meals
Canker Sores
Gagging
Gallbladder Disease
Infantile Colic
Irritable Bowel Syndrome
Itching on Roof of the Mouth

Constipation
Crohn's Disease
Diarrhea
Failure to Thrive
Feeling of Fullness in Stomach
Flatulence
Mucus in Stools
Ulcerative Colitis
Undigested Food in Stools
Vomiting

Nervous System

Aggressive Behavior
Anxiety
Confusion
Depression
Excessive Daydreaming
Hyperactivity
Inability to Concentrate
Indifference
Irritability

Learning Disabilities
Mental Dullness
Mental Lethargy
Numbness
Poor Work Habits
Restlessness
Slurred Speech
Stuttering

Musculoskeletal System

Arthritis
Growing Pains
Joint Aches and Pains
Muscle Aches and Pains

Osteoarthritis
Rheumatoid Arthritis
Muscle Weakness

Genitourinary System

Bed Wetting
Premenstrual Syndrome
Urinary Frequency

Urinary Urgency
Vaginal Discharge
Vaginal Itching

Respiratory System

Asthma
Chest Congestion
Chronic Cough
Chronic Nasal Congestion
Excessive Mucus Formation

Hoarseness
Horizontal Crease across the Nose
Persistent Nose Picking
Postnasal Drip
Recurrent Sinusitis

Exercise-Induced Anaphylaxis   Runny Nose
Exercise-Induced Asthma   Sore Throat
Gagging   Stuffy Nose

Cardiovascular System

Angina   Palpitations
Arrhythmias   Rapid Heart Rate
High Blood Pressure   Vascular Headaches

Skin, Hair, Nails

Acne   Eczema
Brittle Nails and Hair   Hives
Dandruff   Paleness
Dark Circles Under Eyes   Psoriasis
Dermatitis Herpetiformis   Rashes
Dry Skin   Swelling and Wrinkles under Eyes

Ears and Eyes

Blurry Vision   Itchy Ears
Ear Drainage   Meniere's Syndrome
Earache   Motion Sickness
Fluid in the Middle Ear   Recurrent Ear Infections
Fullness in the Ears   Tinnitus
Hearing Loss   Watery Eyes

Miscellaneous

Food Cravings   Insomnia
Chronic Fatigue   Nausea
Dizziness   Nightmares
Excessive Drowsiness after Eating   Obesity
Faintness   Rapid Weight Fluctuation
Fatigue   Swelling of Hands, Feet, or Ankles
Feeling of Fullness in the Head   Teeth Grinding
Headaches   Water Retention
Frequent Awakenings during
   the Night

WHAT HAPPENS WHEN A FOOD ALLERGY OCCURS IN MY BODY?

Under food antigen attack, IgG forms food antigen-antibody complexes in blood circulation. An antigen is simply anything taken in that isn't naturally part of the body. An apple or a virus for example, under certain circumstances, may induce a reaction in the body and cause symptoms.

Workings of an Immune Attack

These food antigen-antibody complexes may deposit in various organs and tissues where they may trigger inflammatory reactions. Delayed-onset food allergies are much more common than immediate hypersensitivity reactions mediated through Immunoglobulin E (IgE) antibodies. It can be argued that IgG-mediated food allergies account for a variety of chronic health conditions that have been unresponsive to conventional medical care. Fatigue, irritability, aching joints, cognitive dysfunction, and chronic migraines are a few known complications due to delayed-onset food allergies.

There is no argument that there is a clear and definite relationship between what you eat and how you feel. Knowing this, the first order of business in promoting your health is to avoid the foods that are making you sick! Not providing your body with the proper fuel is like getting out of the car and trying to push it up the hill; it merely defeats the purpose.

IT'S NOT ALL IN YOUR HEAD

Countless scientific studies have shown the link between food allergies and symptoms. For example, milk-specific IgG, in particular, IgG to the milk protein casein, is diagnostic of milk allergy causing eczema in adults. IgG-mediated allergy to casein and other milk proteins has also been implicated in the development and progression of infantile autism.

IgG antibodies to gluten, a protein fraction of wheat, has been implicated in aggravation of symptoms of rheumatoid arthritis. In one study, a decrease in gluten-specific IgG serum levels correlated with an improvement in the symptoms of rheumatoid arthritis in 40 percent of subjects placed on a gluten-free diet, compared to a 4 percent improvement in a control group, over a one-year period. Gluten allergy is also a well-established etiology to Celiac's disease of the bowel. In addition, casein, as well as gluten, has been implicated in cases of idiopathic schizophrenia. These are prime examples of how fueling the body with the wrong foods can have grave consequences.

WHAT SHOULD I DO IF I HAVE A FOOD ALLERGY?

Treatment is simple: identify and eliminate food allergens and implement a rotation-style diet. These two simple measures can have profound effects on one's health. Realize that mucosal immunity, the Gut Associated Lymphoid Tissue (GALT), plays an integral part in systemic immunity and health. GALT is the largest immune organ of the body and represents our first line of defense against foreign agents such as foods, microbes, and other substances. The quality of our mucosal immunity is influenced by our genetics, dietary and lifestyle habits, and microbial colonization of the gut. Manipulation of these factors offers interesting possibilities for the prevention of chronic degenerative conditions as well as autoimmune diseases.

CASE STUDIES (COURTESY OF US BIOTEK LABORATORIES)

1. A 10-year-old boy with autism presented with a positive stool culture for Candida albicans. Also, food allergy testing revealed elevated antibody levels to dairy, egg, and gluten. The child was advised to avoid all allergenic foods and supplemented with essential fatty acids (EFAs) and CELLULARFood, a gastrointestinal restoration product. After two months, the child's practitioner reported great improvement in this young boy's mental condition from following the Elimination and Rotation Diet Plan through US BioTek Laboratories.
2. A 35-year-old gentleman suffered from constipation, muscle pain, continual infection, nasosinusitis, and chronic fatigue. A blood test through US BioTek Laboratories revealed elevated antibodies to egg. After two months of avoiding egg, and following the dietary recommendations from US BioTek, he reported considerable improvement and relief from his symptoms.
3. The parents of one-year-old Matthias sought help for their son who had the problem of waking every two hours since moving to a new town a few months earlier. Both parents leave for work in the morning and are exhausted having to care for Matthias throughout the night. Physical examination of the child revealed a normal, healthy little boy. A food allergy panel was ordered through US BioTek to rule out food allergies as a possible etiology to Matthias's problem. The results showed a strong delayed-type hypersensitivity to dairy products. Upon withdrawal of dairy products from his diet, Matthias was able to sleep throughout the night in less than a week's time. A few weeks later when Matthias was accidentally exposed to dairy products, he again woke repeatedly throughout the night.

ONCE YOU HAVE YOUR TEST RESULTS—
IT'S A MATTER OF KNOWING THE NEXT STEP

A favorite saying of Dr. Chris Meletis sums up the nature of any of life's projects, including food allergies: "In order to achieve a goal, one must first understand the nature of the goal." The following pages have been created to help you successfully avoid your IgG food sensitivities that differ from an IgE or immediate reaction. IgG reactions are also commonly known as delayed reactions, meaning that it can take upward of 72 hours to fully react to a food consumed. Thus, for illustration purposes, a food consumed on Monday may not present with overt symptoms until Wednesday or possibly Thursday. One can easily see how important getting tested for IgG reactions can be, for we all typically look at what we have just eaten within a given day as the source of troublesome symptoms.

You can think of the "G" in IgG as standing for "gradual," because the symptoms arising typically take a while to manifest. Therefore, you will want to make sure that you don't eat any foods scoring low more than once every four days. Otherwise, clinically it has been observed that you can experience a "stacking effect." Low scores are like small steps making up a staircase. No single step results in much effect, yet if you consistently add your steps together the stacking effect is gaining momentum of upward movement. Stacking the effect of allergic responses is detrimental. Thus, eating a food, even one with a low score, three days in a row that you have an IgG reaction to will lead to a cumulative reaction that is potentially greater than any of the three previous days by themselves. Eating "moderate" foods more than once every four days adds larger steps than if low-reacting foods are consumed over the same period of time and thus leads to a higher level of reactivity more quickly. This is clinically what patients report and it makes sense relative to the scientific and medical literature.

READING YOUR REPORT

There are four general categories of reactions: No Reaction, Low, Moderate, and High. You can think of these as the size of the "reaction stairs"; the bigger the reaction the higher the level of reactivity. Consuming a food frequently increases the chance of having a negative reaction.

WHAT SHOULD I DO ABOUT MY RESULTS?

All results and medical information you have regarding your health is always important to share with your primary healthcare provider. So, sharing these results with your physician or other provider is a wise choice. With that said, here are some general guidelines that many patients have chosen to follow to maximize the benefits of the test results.

- High-Reacting Foods
  Totally avoid these foods for three to six months. Read labels and actively avoiding coming in contact with them. This includes in processed foods as well.
- Moderate-Reacting Foods
  It is best to also totally avoid these foods. If you don't have many reactions, this will not be too hard. If you eat a food that is moderate reacting too often, it is possible to further exacerbate the reactions, which can ultimately yield a high reaction occurring for a given food.
- Low-Reacting Foods
  For most individuals, these foods can be eaten freely once every four days to start with. After the first three months, they can be eaten more

often, depending on the symptoms and the individual's overall sense of well-being. Clinically, if an individual has few or no moderate or high reactions, then the low scores can be considered as a person's high scores, and the foods should be avoided to see if symptoms abate.

- No-Reaction Foods
  These foods are just as the name sounds, nonreactors at this time. "At this time" can't be emphasized enough if you decided to start eating a food that otherwise was never or rarely in your diet and now due to other food reactivity levels are being avoided and another nonreactor is being substituted routinely a level of reactivity can arise. Overeating a certain food can become problematic, so variety is important. This typically is where the traditional rotation diet is recommended.

ROTATION DIET

The standard rotation diet is enough to make a person lose their mind, figuratively, of course. In the past, a rotation diet would allow a patient to eat only specified foods each day for four days, after which the menu would start over again. This works well for the small percentage of the population that tolerates strict guidelines and a rigid regime.

Clinically, following a rotation diet food list works better from a compliance perspective. It is important to consistently look at the lists of your no-reaction, lows, moderates, and highs and review your options on a daily basis. Remember, if you eat a low food on Monday and the same food again on Wednesday before the 72-hour full window is gone, you will have the potential of initiating a "stacking event," thus amplifying the effect of the low-reaction food. Put another way, a Low + Low is more than a Low Burden on your body.

THE BAR GRAPHS

You will notice that the bar graphs on your reactions don't end exactly in the middle of each category. No-reaction, low, moderate, or high, each has a degree of severity. So, one food may be a low-moderate whereas another may be a high-moderate. Take this into consideration as well. Try to pick the lower-reacting food in a given category of reactivity. The only exception to that rule is that if you have indulged already with that specific food within 72 hours.

RETESTING

There are two types of food reactions that can be well described clinically: fixed and variable allergies. Reactive foods are lifelong problems and will always be present to a degree regardless of your active avoidance of them. Although you may tolerate them better, the fact is that they never totally go away. But, some foods react on a variable level and are found to be high because you were eating them too often for your body's unique biochemistry. The only way to know which case you are dealing with is through retesting to see how your IgG reactions have changed. Also by building up your body and giving it a rest you can improve levels of reactivity as well. In fact, specific supplements can be used to aid in the allergy reactivity.

SUMMARY

Your body can only operate as well as it is fueled. Just as a car can't operate on the wrong fuel, neither can one's body. Identifying potential culprits, and thus alleviating obstacles that may be preventing increased success and wellness, makes good sense.

Clinically, the outcomes often are astounding for those suffering from allergies who so often are not even aware of level of impact.

Note: IgG Food Allergy testing is now available without a physician's order and the sample can be collected in the comfort of your own home. The sample is then sent into a licensed laboratory and the results are returned to the sender. If you would like to order this test for yourself, a friend, or a family member, you can call 503-656-1993 for more information or visit the following Web site: www.vitamedics.com.

Notes

Sources are listed in numerical order of their first citation. Sources are sometimes cited multiple times in a chapter; similarly, more than one source is sometimes cited for a given fact or theory.

PART I: BRAIN AILMENTS AND NUTRA-BOTANICAL INTERVENTIONS

ADD/ADHD

1. National Institute of Health, Publication No. 96-3572 (1994; repr. 1996). Booklet. p. 44.

2. Centers for Disease Control and Prevention, "Prevalence of Attention Deficit Disorder and Learning Disability," *Attention Deficit Disorder and Learning Disability: United States, 1997–98*, Series 10, No. 206. 18 pp. (PHS) 20021534.

3. E. Galili-Weisstub and R. H. Segman, "Attention Deficit and Hyperactivity Disorder: Review of Genetic Association Studies," *Isr J Psychiatry Relat Sci.* 40, no. 1 (2003): 57–66.

4. J. Smidt, P. Heiser, A. Dempfle, K. Konrad, U. Hemminger, A. Kathofer, A. Halbach, et al., "Formal Genetic Findings in Attention-Deficit/Hyperactivity-Disorder," *Fortschr Neurol Psychiatry* 71, no. 7 (July 2003): 366–77.

5. K. M. Linnet, S. Dalsgaard, C. Obel, K. Wisborg, T. B. Henriksen, A. Rodriguez, A. Kotimaa, et al., "Maternal Lifestyle Factors in Pregnancy Risk of Attention Deficit Hyperactivity Disorder and Associated Behaviors: Review of the Current Evidence," *Am J Psychiatry* 160, no. 6 (June 2003): 1028–40.

6. F. Brucker-Davis, "Effects of Environmental Synthetic Chemicals on Thyroid Function," *Thyroid* 8 (1998): 827–56.

7. L. Galland, "Nutritional Supplementation for ADHD" in *Attention Deficit Hyperactivity Disorder: Causes and Possible Solutions*, ed. J. A. Bellanti, W. G. Crook, and R. E. Layton (Jackson, TN: International Health Foundation, 1999).

8. S. J. Schoenthaler, "Nutritional Deficiencies and Behavior" in *Attention Deficit Hyperactivity Disorder: Causes and Possible Solutions*, ed. J. A. Bellanti, W. G. Crook, and R. E. Layton (Jackson, TN: International Health Foundation, 1999).

9. A. Brenner, "The Effects of Megadoses of Selected B Complex Vitamins on Children with Hyperkinesis: Controlled Studies with Long-Term Follow-Up," *J Learn Disabil* 15 (1982): 258–64.

10. M. Coleman, G. Steinberg, J. Tippett, et al., "A Preliminary Study of the Effect of Pyridoxine," *Biol Psychiatry* 14 (1979): 741–51.

11. N. S. Lee, G. Muhs, G. C. Wagner, R. D. Reynolds, and H. Fisher, "Dietary Pyridoxine Interaction with Tryptophan or Histidine on Brain Serotonin and Histamine Metabolism," *Pharmacol Biochem Behav.* 29, no. 3 (Mar. 1988): 559–64.

12. A. Blokland, W. Honig, F. Brouns, and J. Jolles. "Cognition-Enhancing Properties of Subchronic Phosphatidylserine (PS) Treatment in Middle-Aged Rats: Comparison of Bovine Cortex PS with Egg PS and Soybean PS," *Nutrition* 15 (1999): 778–83.

13. P. M. Kidd, "A Review of Five Nutrients and Botanicals in the Integrative Management of Cognitive Dysfunction," *Altern Med Rev* 4 (1999): 144–61.

14. P. M. Kidd, "Attention Deficit/Hyperactivity Disorder (ADHD) in Children: Rationale for Its Integrative Management," *Altern Med Rev* 5, no. 5 (Oct. 2000): 402–28.

15. T. H. Crook et al., "Effects of Phosphatidylserine in Age-Associated Memory Impairment," *Neurology* 41, no. 5 (1991): 644–49.

16. M. T. Murray and J. T. Pizzorno, *Encyclopedia of Natural Medicine* (Rocklin, CA: Prima Publishing, 1998).

17. Y. Sever, A. Ashkenazi, S. Tyano, and A. Weizman, "Iron Treatment in Children with Attention Deficit Hyperactivity Disorder: A Preliminary Report," *Neuropsychobiology* 35, no. 4 (1997): 178–80.

18. J. Beard, "Iron Deficiency Alters Brain Development and Functioning," *J Nutr* 133 (2003): 1468S–72S.

19. B. Starobrat-Hermelin and T. Kozielec, "The Effects of Magnesium Physiological Supplementation on Hyperactivity in Children with Attention Deficit Hyperactivity Disorder (ADHD): Positive Response to Magnesium Oral Loading Test," *Magnes Res.* 10, no. 2 (June 1997): 149–56.

20. T. Kozielec and B. Starobrat-Hermelin, "Assessment of Magnesium Levels in Children with Attention Deficit Hyperactivity Disorder (ADHD)," *Magnes Res.* 10, no. 2 (June 1997): 143–48.

21. L. Galland, "Nutritional Supplementation for ADHD" in *Attention Deficit Hyperactivity Disorder: Causes and Possible Solutions*, ed. J. A. Bellanti, W. G. Crook, and R. E. Layton (Jackson, TN: International Health Foundation, 1999).

22. P. Toren, S. Eldar, B. A. Sela, et al., "Zinc Deficiency in Attention-Deficit Hyperactivity Disorder," *Biol Psychiatry* 40 (1996): 1308–10.

23. M. Bekaroglu, Y. Aslan, Y. Gedik, O. Deger, H. Mocan, E. Erduran, and C. Karahan, "Relationships Between Serum Free Fatty Acids and Zinc, and Attention Deficit Hyperactivity Disorder: A Research Note," *J Child Psychol Psychiatry* 37, no. 2 (Feb. 1996): 225–27.

24. L. E. Arnold, S. M. Pinkham, and N. Votolato, "Does Zinc Moderate Essential Fatty Acid and Amphetamine Treatment of Attention-Deficit/Hyperactivity Disorder?" *J Child Adolesc Psychopharmacol* 10, no. 2 (Summer 2000): 111–17.

25. J. A. Cocores, R. K. Davies, P. S. Mueller, and M. S. Gold, "Cocaine Abuse and Adult Attention Deficit Disorder," *J Clin Psychiatry* 48, no. 9 (Sept. 1987): 376–77.

26. B. Starobrat-Hermelin, "The Effect of Deficiency of Selected Bioelements on Hyperactivity in Children with Certain Specified Mental Disorders," *Ann Acad Med Stetin* 44 (1998): 297–314.

27. R. Schnoll, D. Burshteyn, and J. Cea-Aravena, "Nutrition in the Treatment of Attention-Deficit Hyperactivity Disorder: A Neglected but Important Aspect." *Appl Psychophysiol Biofeedback* 28, no. 1 (Mar. 2003): 63–75.

28. B. F. Feingold, *Why Your Child Is Hyperactive* (New York: Random House, 1975).

29. C. M. Carter, M. Urbanowicz, R. Hemsley, L. Mantilla, S. Strobel, P. J. Graham, and E. Taylor, "Effects of a Few Food Diet in Attention Deficit Disorder," *Arch Dis Child.* 69, no. 5 (Nov. 1993): 564–68.

30. D. Schardt, "Diet and Behavior in Children," *Nutrition Action Healthletter* (Washington, DC: Center for Science in the Public Interest, 2000), 10–11.

31. M. Boris and F. S. Mandel, "Foods and Additives Are Common Causes of the Attention Deficit Hyperactive Disorder in Children," *Ann Allergy* 72, no. 5 (May 1994): 462–68.

32. L. M. Pelsser and J. K. Buitelaar, "Favourable Effect of a Standard Elimination Diet on the Behavior of Young Children with Attention Deficit Hyperactivity Disorder (ADHD): A Pilot Study," *Ned Tijdschr Geneeskd* 146, no. 52 (Dec. 2002): 2543–47.

Alcoholism (Alcohol Abuse/Dependence)

1. M. A. Enoch, "Pharmacogenomics of Alcohol Response and Addiction," *Am J Pharmacogenomics* 3, no.4 (2003): 217–32.

2. *National Vital Statistics Reports* 50, no.15.

3. J. I. Nurnberger Jr, T. Foroud, L. Flury, E. T. Meyer, and R. Wiegand, "Is There a Genetic Relationship Between Alcoholism and Depression?" *Alcohol Res Health*, 26 no. 3 (2002): 233–40.

4. M. A. Carai, R. Agabio, E. Bombardelli, I. Bourov, G. L. Gessa, C. Lobina, P. Morazzoni, et al., "Potential Use of Medicinal Plants in the Treatment of Alcoholism," *Fitoterapia* 71, Suppl. 1 (Aug. 2000): S38–42.

5. G. Brunetti, S. Serra, G. Vacca, C. Lobina, P. Morazzoni, E. Bombardelli, G. Colombo, G. L. Gessa, and M. A. Carai, "IDN 5082, a Standardized Extract of Salvia Miltiorrhiza, Delays Acquisition of Alcohol Drinking Behavior in Rats," *J Ethnopharmacol* 85, no. 1 (Mar. 2003): 93–97.

6. G. Colombo, R. Agabio, C. Lobina, R. Reali, P. Morazzoni, E. Bombardelli, and G. L. Gessa, "Salvia Miltiorrhiza Extract Inhibits Alcohol Absorption, Preference, and Discrimination in sP Rats," *Alcohol* 18, no. 1 (May 1999): 65–70.

7. S. Serra, G. Vacca, S. Tumatis, A. Carrucciu, P. Morazzoni, E. Bombardelli, G. Colombo, G. L. Gessa, and M. A. Carai, "Anti-Relapse Properties of IDN 5082, a Standardized Extract of Salvia Miltiorrhiza, in Alcohol-Preferring Rats," *J Ethnopharmaco* 88, no. 2–3 (Oct. 2003): 249–52.

8. A. H. Rezvani, D. H. Overstreet, Y. Yang, and E. Clark Jr, "Attenuation of Alcohol Intake by Extract of Hypericum Perforatum (St. John's Wort) in Two Different Strains of Alcohol-Preferring Rats," *Alcohol* 34, no. 5 (Sept.–Oct. 1999): 699–705.

9. M. Perfumi, R. Ciccocioppo, S. Angeletti, M. Cucculelli, and M. Massi, "Effects of Hypericum Perforatum Extraction on Alcohol Intake in Marchigian Sardinian Alcohol-Preferring Rats," *Alcohol Alcohol* 34, no. 5 (Sept.–Oct. 1999): 690–98.

10. R. C. Lin and T. K. Li, "Effects of Isoflavones on Alcohol Pharmacokinetics and Alcohol-Drinking Behavior in Rats," *Am J Clin Nutr* 68 (1998): 1512S–5S.

11. A. Y. Leung and S. Foster, *Encyclopedia of Common Natural Ingredients Used in Food, Drugs and Cosmetics*, 2nd ed. (New York: John Wiley & Sons, 1996).

12. W. M. Keung and B. L. Vallee, "Kudzu Root: An Ancient Chinese Source of Modern Antidipsotropic Agents," *Phytochemistry* 47, no. 4 (Feb. 1998): 499–506.

13. W. M. Keung, "Biogenic Aldehyde(s) Derived from the Action of Monoamine Oxidase May Mediate the Antidipsotropic Effect of Daidzin," *Chem Biol Interact* 130–132, no. 1–3 (Jan. 30, 2001): 919–30.

14. J. Bruneton, *Pharmacognosy, Phytochemistry, Medicinal Plants* (Paris: Lavoisier Publishing, 1995).

15. D. C. Mash, C. A. Kovera, B. E. Buck, et al., "Medication Development of Ibogaine as a Pharmacotherapy for Drug Dependence," *Ann N Y Acad Sci.* 844 (1998): 274–92.

16. S. D. Glick and I. S. Maisonneuve, "Mechanisms of Antiaddictive Actions of Ibogaine," *Ann N Y Acad Sci.* 844 (May 30, 1998): 214–26.

17. J. Caballeria, A. Gimenez, H. Andreu, R. Deulofeu, A. Pares, L. Caballeria, A. M. Ballesta, and J. Rodes, "Zinc Administration Improves Gastric Alcohol Dehydrogenase Activity and First-Pass Metabolism of Ethanol in Alcohol-Fed Rats," *Alcohol Clin Exp Res.* 21, no. 9 (Dec. 1997): 1619–22.

18. V. D. Bovt, V. A. Ieshchenko, M. M. Mal'ko, O. M. Kuchkovs'kyi, and N. V. Hryhorova, "Study on the Connection of Alcohol Motivation with Zinc Content Changes in the Hippocampus," *Fiziol Zh* 47, no. 3 (2001): 54–57.

19. A. V. Skal'nyi, E. N. Kukhtina, I. P. Ol'khovskaia, and N. N. Glushchenko, "Reduction of Voluntary Alcohol Consumption Under the Effects of Prolonged-Action Zinc," *Biull Eksp Biol Med* 113, no. 4 (Apr. 1992): 383–85.

Alzheimer's Disease

1. V. Solfrizzi, F. Panza, and A. Capurso, "The Role of Diet in Cognitive Decline," *J Neural Transm.* 110, no. 1 (Jan. 2003): 95–110.

2. F. Berrino, "Western Diet and Alzheimer's Disease," *Epidemiol Prev* 26, no. 3 (May–June 2002): 107–15.

3. E. K. Perry, A. T. Pickering, W. W. Wang, P. J. Houghton, and N. S. Perry, "Medicinal Plants and Alzheimer's Disease: From Ethnobotany to Phytotherapy," *J Pharm Pharmacol.* 51, no. 5 (May 1999): 527–34.

4. M. Zimmermann, F. Colciaghi, F. Cattabeni, and M. Di Luca, "Ginkgo biloba Extract: From Molecular Mechanisms to the Treatment of Alzhelmer's Disease," *Cell Mol Biol (Noisy-le-grand)* 48, no. 6 (Sept. 2002): 613–23.

5. D. Loew, "Value of Ginkgo biloba in Treatment of Alzheimer Dementia," *Wien Med Wochenschr.* 152, no. 15–16 (2002): 418–22.

6. Y. Luo J. V. Smith, V. Paramasivam, A. Burdick, K. J. Curry, J. P. Buford, I. Khan, W. J. Netzer, H. Xu, and P. Butko, "Inhibition of Amyloid-Beta Aggregation and Caspase-3 Activation by the Ginkgo biloba Extract EGb761," *Proc Natl Acad Sci USA* 99, no. 19 (Sept. 17, 2002): 12197–202. Epub 2002 Sep 04.

7. Center for Public Service, "Alzheimer's Disease: Statistics," 2003. http://www.cps.unt.edu/alzheimers/disease_statistics.htm.

8. A. S. Rigaud, "Epidemiology of Depression in Patients with Alzheimer's Disease and in Their Caregivers," *Presse Med.* 32, Suppl. 24 (July 2003): S5–S8.

9. I. McDowell, "Alzheimer's Disease: Insights from Epidemiology," *Aging* (Milano) 13, no. 3 (June 2001): 143–62.

10. A. L. Miller, "The Methionine-Homocysteine Cycle and Its Effects on Cognitive Diseases," *Altern Med Rev.* 8, no. 1 (Feb. 2003): 7–19.

11. N. Seshadri and K. Robinson, "Homocysteine, B Vitamins, and Coronary Artery Disease," *Med Clin North Am.* 84, no. 1 (Jan. 2000): 215–37, x.

12. D. A. Butterfield, "Amyloid Beta-Peptide (1–42)-Induced Oxidative Stress and Neurotoxicity: Implications for Neurodegeneration in Alzheimer's Disease Brain, a Review," *Free Radic Res.* 36, no. 12 (Dec. 2002): 1307–13.

13. C. Behl and B. Moosmann, "Oxidative Nerve Cell Death in Alzheimer's Disease and Stroke: Antioxidants as Neuroprotective Compounds," *Biol Chem.* 383, no. 3–4 (Mar.–Apr. 2002): 521–36.

14. C. Cecchi, C. Fiorillo, S. Sorbi, S. Latorraca, B. Nacmias, S. Bagnoli, P. Nassi, and G. Liguri, "Oxidative Stress and Reduced Antioxidant Defenses in Peripheral Cells from Familial Alzheimer's Patients," *Free Radic Biol Med.* 33, no. 10 (Nov. 15, 2002): 1372–79.

15. B. P. Rutten, H. W. Steinbusch, H. Korr, and C. Schmitz, "Antioxidants and Alzheimer's Disease: From Bench to Bedside (and Back Again)" *Curr Opin Clin Nutr Metab Care* 5, no. 6 (Nov. 2002): 645–51.

16. A. Y. Leung and S. Foster, *Encyclopedia of Common Natural Ingredients Used in Foods, Drugs, and Cosmetics,* 2d ed. (New York: John Wiley & Sons, 1996), 446–48.

17. M. Blumenthal, W. R. Busse, A. Goldberg, et al., eds., *The Complete Commission E Monographs: Therapeutic Guide to Herbal Medicines* (Boston: Integrative Medicine Communications, 1998), 197.

18. C. A. Newall, L. A. Anderson, and J. D. Phillipson, Herbal Medicine: A Guide for Health-Care Professionals (London: Pharmaceutical Press, 1996), 229–30.

19. S. Akhondzadeh, M. Noroozian, M. Mohammadi, S. Ohadinia, A. H. Jamshidi, and M. Khani, "Melissa Officinalis Extract in the Treatment of Patients with Mild to Moderate Alzheimer's Disease: A Double Blind, Randomised, Placebo controlled Trial," *J Neurol Neurosurg Psychiatry* 74, no. 7 (July 2003): 863–66.

20. C. G. Ballard, J. T. O'Brien, K. Reichelt, and E. K. Perry, "Aromatherapy as a Safe and Effective Treatment for the Management of Agitation in Severe Dementia: The Results of a Double Blind, Placebo-Controlled Trial with Melissa," *J Clin Psychiatry* 63, no. 7 (July 2002): 553–58.

21. S. Akhondzadeh, M. Noroozian, M. Mohammadi, S. Ohadinia, A. H. Jamshidi, and M. Khani, "Salvia Officinalis Extract in the Treatment of Patients with Mild to Moderate Alzheimer's Disease: A Double Blind, Randomized and Placebo-Controlled Trial," *J Clin Pharm Ther.* 28, no. 1 (Feb. 2003): 53–59.

22. N. S. Perry, C. Bollen, E. K. Perry, and C. Ballard, "Salvia for Dementia Therapy: Review of Pharmacological Activity and Pilot Tolerability Clinical Trial," *Pharmacol Biochem Behav.* 75, no. 3 (June 2003): 651–59.

23. J. W. Pettegrew, J. Levine, and R. J. McClure, "Acetyl-L-Carnitine Physical-Chemical, Metabolic, and Therapeutic Properties: Relevance for Its Mode of Action in Alzheimer's Disease and Geriatric Depression," *Mol Psychiatry* 5 (2000): 616–32.

24. R. Mayeux and M. San, "Treatment of Alzheimer's Disease," *N Engl J Med* 341, no. 22 (1999): 1670–79.

25. L. J. Thal, A. Carta, W. R. Clarke, et al., "A 1-year Multicenter Placebo-Controlled Study of Acetyl-L-Carnitine in Patients with Alzheimer's Disease," *Neurology* 47 (1996): 705–11.

26. M. Sano, K. Bell, and L. Cote, "Double-Blind Parallel Design Pilot Study of Acetyl Levocarnitine in Patients with Alzheimer's Disease," *Arch Neurol* 49 (1992): 1137–41.

27. B. Seltzer and I. Sherwin, "Fingerprint Pattern Differences in Early- and Late-onset Primary Degenerative Dementia," *Arch Neurol.* 43, no. 7 (July 1986): 665–68.

28. H. J. Weinreb, "Dermatoglyphic Patterns in Alzheimer's Disease," *J Neurogenet.* 3, no. 4 (July 1986): 233–46; H. J. Weinreb, "Fingerprint Patterns in Alzheimer's Disease," *Arch Neurol.* 42, no. 1 (Jan. 1985): 50–54.

Anorexia

1. F. Rybakowski, A. Slopien, P. Czerski, A. Rajewski, and J. Hauser, "Genetic Factors in the Etiology of Anorexia Nervosa," *Psychiatr Pol.* 35, no. 1 (Jan.–Feb. 2001): 71–80.

2. R. C. Casper, "Depression and Eating Disorders," *Depress Anxiety.* 8, Suppl. 1 (1998): 96–104.

3. A. S. Prasad, "Clinical, Endocrinological and Biochemical Effects of Zinc Deficiency," *Clin Endocrinol Metab.* 14, no. 3 (Aug. 1985): 567–89.

4. C. L. Birmingham, E. M. Goldner, and R. Bakan, "Controlled Trial of Zinc Supplementation in Anorexia Nervosa," *Int J Eat Disord.* 15, no. 3 (Apr. 1994): 251–55.

5. S. Safai-Kutti, "Oral Zinc Supplementation in Anorexia Nervosa," *Acta Psychiatr Scand Suppl.* 361 (1990): 14–17.

6. K. L. Katz, C. L. Keen, I. F. Litt, L. S. Hurley, K. M. Kellams-Harrison, and L. J. Glader, "Zinc Deficiency in Anorexia Nervosa," *J Adolesc Health Care* 8 (1987): 400–406.

7. M. A. Brown, J. Goldstein-Shirley, J. Robinson, and S. Casey, "The Effects of a Multi-Modal Intervention Trial of Light, Exercise, and Vitamins on Women's Mood," *Women & Health* 34, no. 3 (2001): 93–112.

8. L. Patrick, "Eating Disorders: A Review of the Literature with Emphasis on Medical Complications and Cinical Nutrition," *Altern Med Rev.* 7 no. 3 (June 2002): 184–202.

9. R. T. Holman, C. E. Adams, R. A. Nelson, S. J. Grater, J. A. Jaskiewicz, S. B. Johnson, and J. W. Erdman Jr., "Patients with Anorexia Nervosa Demonstrate Deficiencies of Selected Essential Fatty Acids, Compensatory Changes in Nonessential Fatty Acids and Decreased Fluidity of Plasma Lipids," *J Nutr.* 125, no. 4 (Apr. 1995): 901–7.

10. A. P. Simopoulos, "Omega-3 Fatty Acids in Inflammation and Autoimmune Diseases," *J Am Coll Nutr.* 21, no. 6 (Dec. 2002): 495–505.

11. Y. Naisberg, I. Modai, and A. Weizman, "Metabolic Bioenergy Homeostatic Disruption: A Cause of Anorexia Nervosa," *Med Hypotheses* 56, no. 4 (Apr. 2001): 454–61.

Anxiety

1. P. E. Greenberg, T. Sisitsky, R. C. Kessler, S. N. Finkelstein, E. R. Berndt, J. R. Davidson, J. C. Ballenger, and A. J. Fyer, "The Economic Burden of Anxiety Disorders in the 1990s," *J Clin Psychiatry* 60, no. 7 (July 1999): 427–35.

2. J. P. Lepine, "The Epidemiology of Anxiety Disorders: Prevalence and Societal Costs," *J Clin Psychiatry* 63, Suppl. 14 (2002): 4–8.

3. J. G. Barbee, "Mixed Symptoms and Syndromes of Anxiety and Depression: Diagnostic, Prognostic, and Etiologic Issues," *Ann Clin Psychiatry* 10, no. 1 (Mar. 1998): 15–29.

4. P. E. Cryer, "Symptoms of Hypoglycemia, Thresholds for Their Occurrence, and Hypoglycemia Unawareness," *Endocrinol Metab Clin North Am.* 28, no. 3 (Sept. 1999): 495–500, v–vi.

5. V. Rippere, "Can Hypoglycaemia Cause Obsessions and Ruminations?" *Med Hypotheses* 15, no. 1 (Sept. 1984): 3–13.

6. J. Rodriguez Jimenez, J. R. Rodriguez, and M. J. Gonzalez, "Indicators of Anxiety and Depression in Subjects with Gifferent Kinds of Diet: Vegetarians and Omnivores," *Bol Asoc Med P R.* 90, no. 4–6 (Apr.–June 1998): 58–68.

7. M. G. Monteiro, M. A. Schuckit, and M. Irwin, "Subjective Feelings of Anxiety in Young Men after Ethanol and Diazepam Infusions," *J Clin Psychiatry* 51, no. 1 (Jan. 1990): 12–16.

8. D. S. Charney, G. R. Heninger, and P. I. Jatlow, "Increased Anxiogenic Effects of Caffeine in Panic Disorders," *Arch Gen Psychiatry* 42, no. 3 (Mar. 1985): 233–43.

9. J. P. Boulenger, T. W. Uhde, E. A. Wolff 3rd, and R. M. Post, "Increased Sensitivity to Caffeine in Patients with Panic Disorders. Preliminary Evidence," *Arch Gen Psychiatry* 41, no. 11 (Nov. 1984): 1067–71.

10. M. S. Bruce and M. Lader, "Caffeine Abstention in the Management of Anxiety Disorders," *Psychol Med.* 19, no. 1 (Feb. 1989): 211–14.

11. H. Mohler, P. Polc, R. Cumin, L. Pieri, and R. Kettler, "Nicotinamide Is a Brain Constituent with Benzodiazepine-Like Actions," *Nature* 278, no. 5704 (Apr. 5, 1979): 563–65.

12. R. A. Akhundov, V. V. Rozhanets, T. A. Voronina, and A. V. Val'dman, "Mechanism of the Tranquilizing Action of Electron Structural Analogs of Nicotinamide," *Biull Eksp Biol Med.* 101, no. 3 (Mar. 1986): 329–31.

13. A. I. Fomenko, P. K. Parkhomets, S. P. Stepanenko, and G. V. Donchenko, "Participation of Benzodiazepine Receptors in the Mechanism of Action of Nicotinamide in Nerve Cells," *Ukr Biokhim Zh.* 66, no. 4 (July–Aug. 1994): 75–80.

14. M. F. McCarty, "High-Dose Pyridoxine as an 'Anti-Stress' Strategy," *Med Hypotheses* 54, no. 5 (May 2000): 803–7.

15. M. C. De Souza, A. F. Walker, P. A. Robinson, and K. Bolland, "A Synergistic Effect of a Daily Supplement for 1 Month of 200 mg Magnesium Plus 50 mg Vitamin B6 for the Relief of Anxiety-Related Premenstrual Symptoms: A Randomized, Double-Blind, Crossover Study," *J Women's Health Gend Based Med.* 9, no. 2 (Mar. 2000): 131–39.

16. M. S. Seelig, "Latent Tetany and Anxiety, Marginal Mg Deficit, and Normocalcemia," *Dis Nerv Syst.* 36 (1975): 461–65.

17. M. S. Seelig, A. R. Berger, and N. Spielholz, "Latent Tetany and Anxiety, Marginal Mg Deficit, and Normocalcemia," *Dis Nerv Syst.* 36 (1975): 461–65.

18. H. Kara, N. Sahin, V. Ulusan, and T. Aydogdu, "Magnesium Infusion Reduces Perioperative Pain," *Eur J Anaesthesiol.* 19, no. 1 (Jan. 2002): 52–56.

19. L. Landy, "Gallup Survey Finds Majority of American Diets Lack Sufficient Magnesium—at Potential Cost to Health," *Searle News*, Sept. 21, 1994.

20. M. Murray, N.D., and J. Pizzorno, N.D., *Encyclopedia of Natural Medicine* (Rocklin, CA: Prima Publishing, 1991), 159–60.

Autism

1. Based on prevalence statistics from the National Institutes of Health (2001) and the Centers for Disease Control and Prevention (2001); U.S. Department of Education,

"Twenty-First Annual Report to Congress on the Implementation of the Individuals with Disabilities Education Act" (1999).

2. S. E. Bryson, S. J. Rogers, and E. Fombonne, "Autism Spectrum Disorders: Early Detection, Intervention, Education, and Psychopharmacological Management," *Can J Psychiatry* 48, no. 8 (Sept. 2003): 506–16.

3. P. M. Kidd, "Autism: An Extreme Challenge to Integrative Medicine. Part 1: The Knowledge Base," *Altern Med Rev* 7 (2002): 292–316.

4. J. H. Clark, D. K. Rhoden, and D. S. Turner, "Symptomatic Vitamin A and D Deficiencies in an Eight-Year-Old with Autism," *JPEN J Parenter Enteral Nutr.* 17, no. 3 (May–June 1993): 284–86.

5. A. Vogelaar, "Studying the Effects of Essential Nutrients and Environmental Factors on Autistic Behavior" in *DAN! (Defeat Autism Now!) Think Tank* (San Diego, CA: Autism Research Institute, 2000).

6. J. B. Adams, L. Dinelli, R. Fabes, et al., *Effect of Vitamin/Mineral Supplements on Children with Autism* (Tempe, AZ: Arizona State University, College of Engineering and Applied Sciences, 2002).

7. B. Rimland, "Controversies in the Treatment of Autistic Children: Vitamin and Drug Therapy," *J Child Neurol* 3 (1988): S68–S72.

8. Autism Research Institute (ARI), "Treatment Effectiveness Survey" (San Diego, CA: Autism Research Institute, 2002). www.autism.com/treatrating.

9. M. C. Dolske, J. Spollen, S. McKay, E. Lancashire, and L. Tolbert, "A Preliminary Trial of Ascorbic Acid as Supplemental Therapy for Autism," *Prog Neuropsychopharmacol Biol Psychiatry* 17, no. 5 (Sept. 1993): 765–74.

10. J. Bradstreet and J. Kartzinel, "Biological Interventions in the Treatment of Autism and PDD," in *DAN! (Defeat Autism Now!) Fall 2001 Conference,* ed. B. Rimland (San Diego, CA: Autism Research Institute, 2001).

11. W. Walsh, "Metallothionein Promotion Therapy in Autism Spectrum Disorders," in *DAN! (Defeat Autism Now!) Spring 2002 Conference Practitioner Training,* ed. B. Rimland (San Diego, CA: Autism Research Institute, 2002).

12. B. H. Grahn, P. G. Paterson, K. T. Gottschall-Pass, and Z. Zhang, "Zinc and the Eye," *J Am Coll Nutr* 20 (2001): 106–18.

13. H. C. Freake, K. E. Govoni, K. Guda, et al., "Actions and Interactions of Thyroid Hormone and Zinc Status in Growing Rats," *J Nutr* 4 (2001): 1135–41; Food and Nutrition Board, Institute of Medicine, *Dietary Reference Intakes for Vitamin A, Vitamin K, Arsenic, Boron, Chromium, Copper, Iodine, Iron, Manganese, Molybdenum, Nickel, Silicon, Vanadium, and Zinc* (Washington, DC: National Academy Press, 2002). www.nap.edu/books/0309072794/html/.

14. D. G. Barceloux, "Zinc," *J Toxicol Clin Toxicol* 37 (1999): 279–92.

15. H. Tapiero, G. N. Ba, P. Couvreur, and K. D. Tew, "Polyunsaturated Fatty Acids (PUFA) and Eicosanoids in Human Health and Pathologies," *Biomed Pharmacother* 56 no. 5 (July 2002): 215–22.

16. P. Willatts and J. S. Forsyth, "The Role of Long-Chain Polyunsaturated Fatty Acids in Infant Cognitive Development," *Prostaglandins Leukot Essent Fatty Acids* 63 (2000): 95–100.

17. M. Makrides, M. Neumann, K. Simmer, J. Pater, and R. Gibson, "Are Long-Chain Polyunsaturated Fatty Acids Essential Nutrients in Infancy?" *Lancet* 345 (1995): 1463–68.

18. A. J. Richardson and M. A. Ross, "Fatty Acid Metabolism in Neurodevelopmental Disorder: A New Perspective on Associations Between Attention-Deficit/Hyperactivity

Disorder, Dyslexia, Dyspraxia and the Autistic Spectrum," *Prostaglandins Leukot Essent Fatty Acids* 63, no. 1–2 (July–Aug. 2000): 1–9.

19. S. Vancassel, G. Durand, C. Barthelemy, B. Lejeune, J. Martineau, D. Guilloteau, C. Andres, and S. Chalon, "Plasma Fatty Acid Levels in Autistic Children," *Prostaglandins Leukot Essent Fatty Acids* 65, no. 1 (July 2001): 1–7.

20. G. K. McKevoy, ed., *AHFS Drug Information* (Bethesda, MD: American Society of Health-System Pharmacists, 1998).

21. M. Shils, A. Olson, and M. Shike, *Modern Nutrition in Health and Disease*, 8th ed. (Philadelphia, PA: Lea and Febiger, 1994).

22. T. R. Covington et al., *Handbook of Nonprescription Drugs* (Washington, DC: Am Pharmaceutical Assn, 1996).

23. J. Martineau, C. Barthelemy, B. Garreau, and G. Lelord, "Vitamin B6, Magnesium, and Combined B6-Mg: Therapeutic Effects in Childhood Autism," *Biol Psychiatry* 20, no. 5 (May 1985): 467–78.

24. B. Rimland, E. Callaway, and P. Dreyfus, "The Effects of High Doses of Vitamin B6 on Autistic Children: A Double-Blind Crossover Study," *Am J Psychiatry* 135 (1978): 472–75.

25. B. Rimland, "The Use of Vitamin B6, Magnesium, and DMG in the Treatment of Autistic Children and Adults," in *Biological Treatments for Autism and PDD*, ed. W. Shaw (Lenexa, KS: The Great Plains Laboratory, 2002).

26. L. Galland, "Magnesium, Stress and Neuropsychiatric Disorders," *Magnes Trace Elem.* 10, no. 2–4 (1991–92): 287–301.

27. V. N. Herbert, "N,N-dimethylglycine for Epilepsy [letter]," *N Engl J Med* 308 (1983): 527–28.

28. I. Rapin and R. Katzman, "Neurobiology of Autism," *Autism Dev Disord* 27 (1997): 467–78.

29. J. K. Kern, V. S. Miller, P. L. Cauller, P. R. Kendall, P. J. Mehta, and M. Dodd, "Effectiveness of N,N-dimethylglycine in Autism and Pervasive Developmental Disorder," *J Child Neurol.* 16, no. 3 (Mar. 2001): 169–73.

Bipolar Disorder

1. W. E. Narrow, "One-Year Prevalence of Depressive Disorders Among Adults 18 and Over in the U.S.: NIMH ECA Prospective Data. Population Estimates Based on U.S. Census Estimated Residential Population age 18 and Over on July 1, 1998" (unpublished table).

2. D. A. Regier, W. E. Narrow, D. S. Rae, et al., "The De Facto Mental and Addictive Disorders Service System. Epidemiologic Catchment Area Prospective 1-Year Prevalence Rates of Disorders and Services," *Archives of General Psychiatry* 50, no. 2 (1993): 85–94.

3. American Psychiatric Association, *Diagnostic and Statistical Manual on Mental Disorders*, 4th ed. (*DSM-IV*) (Washington, DC: American Psychiatric Press, 1994).

4. L. N. Robins and D. A. Regier, eds., *Psychiatric Disorders in America: The Epidemiologic Catchment Area Study* (New York: The Free Press, 1991).

5. NIMH Genetics Workgroup, *Genetics and Mental Disorders*, NIH Publication No. 98–4268 (Rockville, MD: National Institute of Mental Health, 1998).

6. V. M. Durand and D. H. Barlow, *Abnormal Psychology: An Introduction* (Scarborough, Ontario: Wadsworth, 2000).

7. C. I. Hasanah, U. A. Khan, M. Musalmah, and S. M. Razali, "Reduced Red-Cell Folate in Mania," *Affect Disord.* 46, no. 2 (Nov. 1997): 95–99.

8. S. N. Young and A. M. Ghadirian, "Folic Acid and Psychopathology," *Prog Neuropsychopharmacol Biol Psychiatry* 13, no. 6 (1989): 841–63.

9. A. Coppen, C. Swade, S. A. Jones, R. A. Armstrong, J. A. Blair, and R. J. Leeming, "Depression and Tetrahydrobiopterin: The Folate Connection," *J Affect Disord.* 16, no. 2–3 (Mar.–June 1989): 103–7.

10. A. Coppen, S. Chaudhry, and C. Swade, "Folic Acid Enhances Lithium Prophylaxis," *J Affect Disord.* 10, no. 1 (Jan. –Feb. 1986): 9–13.

11. M. Hector and J. R. Burton, "What Are the Psychiatric Manifestations of Vitamin B12 Deficiency?" *J Am Geriatr Soc.* 36, no. 12 (Dec. 1988): 1105–12.

12. F. C. Goggans, "A Case of Mania Secondary to Vitamin B12 Deficiency," *Am J Psychiatry* 141 no. 2 (Feb. 1984): 300–301.

13. D. L. Evans, G. A. Edelsohn, and R. N. Golden, "Organic Psychosis without Anemia or Spinal Cord Symptoms in Patients with Vitamin B12 Deficiency," *Am J Psychiatry* 140, no. 2 (Feb. 1983): 218–21.

14. V. Lerner and M. Kanevsky, "Acute Dementia with Delirium Due to Vitamin B12 Deficiency: A Case Report," *Int J Psychiatry Med.* 32, no. 2 (2002): 215–20; S. D. Reid, "Pseudodementia in a Twenty-One-Year-Old with Bipolar Disorder and Vitamin B12 and Folate Deficiency," *West Indian Med J.* 49, no. 4 (Dec. 2000): 347–48; O. Kalayci, M. Cetin, B. Kirel, E. Ozdirim, S. Yetgin, S. Aysun, and A. Gurgey, "Neurologic Findings of Vitamin B12 Deficiency: Presentation of 7 Cases," *Turk J Pediatr.* 38, no. 1 (Jan.–Mar. 1996): 67–72.

15. W. C. Hawkes and L. Hornbostel, "Effects of Dietary Selenium on Mood in Healthy Men Living in a Metabolic Research Unit," *Biol Psychiatry* 39, no. 2 (Jan. 1996): 121–28.

16. D. Benton, "Selenium Intake, Mood and Other Aspects of Psychological Functioning," *Nutr Neurosci.* 5, no. 6 (Dec. 2002): 363–74.

17. Micromedex Healthcare Series. *AltMedDex® System: Comprehensive Referenced Data on Herbal Medicines and Dietary Supplements Covering Uses, Efficacy, Dosing, Toxicity, and More*" (Englewood, CO: MICROMEDEX Inc.).

18. G. J. Naylor, "Vanadium and Manic Depressive Psychosis," *Nutr Health* 3, no. 1–2 (1984): 79–85.

19. D. A. Dick, G. J. Naylor, and E. G. Dick, "Plasma Vanadium Concentration in Manic-Depressive Illness," *Psychol Med.* 12, no. 3 (Aug. 1982): 533–37.

20. G. J. Naylor and A. H. Smith, "Vanadium: A Possible Aetiological Factor in Manic Depressive Illness," *Psychol Med.* 11, no. 2 (May 1981): 249–56.

21. G. J. Naylor and A. H. Smith, "Defective Genetic Control of Sodium-Pump Density in Manic Depressive Psychosis," *Psychol Med.* 11, no. 2 (May 1981): 257–63.

22. "Vanadium, Vitamin C and Depression," *Nutr Rev.* 40, no. 10 (Oct. 1982): 293–95.

23. P. D. Leathwood, F. Chauffard, E. Heck, and R. Munoz-Box, "Aqueous Extract of Valerian Root (Valeriana Officinalis L.) Improves Sleep Quality in Man," *Pharmacol Biochem Behav.* 17, no. 1 (July 1982): 65–71.

24. P. J. Houghton. "The Scientific Basis for the Reputed Activity of Valerian," *J Pharm Pharmacol.* 51, no. 5 (May 1999): 505–12.

25. J. Kuhlmann, W. Berger, H. Podzuweit, and U. Schmidt, "The Influence of Valerian Treatment on 'Reaction Time, Alertness and Concentration' in Volunteers," *Pharmacopsychiatry* 32, no. 6 (1999): 235–41.

26. V. Schulz, R. Hansel, and V. E. Tyler, *Rational Phytotherapy: A Physician's Guide to Herbal Medicine*, 3rd ed., trans. Terry C. Telger (Berlin: Springer, 1998).

27. D. O. Kennedy, A. B. Scholey, N. T. Tildesley, E. K. Perry and K. A. Wesnes. "Modulation of Mood and Cognitive Performance Following Acute Administration of Melissa Officinalis (Lemon Balm)," *Pharmacol Biochem Behav* 72 (2002): 953–64.

28. A. Burns, J. Byrne, C. Ballard, and C. Holmes, "Sensory Stimulation in Dementia," *BMJ* 325 (2002): 1312–13.

29. A. Cerny and K. Shmid, "Tolerability and Efficacy of Valerian/Lemon Balm in Healthy Volunteers (A Double Blind, Placebo-Controlled, Multicentre Study)," *Fitoterapia* 70 (1999): 221–28.

30. B. J. Kaplan, J. S. Simpson, R. C. Ferre, C. P. Gorman, D. M. McMullen, and S. G. Crawford, "Effective Mood Stabilization with a Chelated Mineral Supplement: An Open-Label Trial in Bipolar Disorder," *J Clin Psychiatry* 62, no. 12 (Dec. 2001): 936–44.

Bulimia Nervosa

1. American Psychiatric Association, *Diagnostic and Statistical Manual on Mental Disorders*, 4th ed. (*DSM-IV*) (Washington, DC: American Psychiatric Press, 1994).

2. American Psychiatric Association Work Group on Eating Disorders, "Practice Guideline for the Treatment of Patients with Eating Disorders (revision)," *American Journal of Psychiatry* 157, Suppl. 1 (2000): 1–39.

3. "Bulimia." www.mamashealth.com/bulimia.as. Mamashealth.com™

4. L. S. Kortegaard, K. Hoerder, J. Joergensen, C. Gillberg, and K. O. Kyvik, "A Preliminary Population-Based Twin Study of Self-Reported Eating Disorder," *Psychol Med.* 31, no. 2 (Feb. 2001): 361–65.

5. C. M. Bulik, C. A. Prescott, and K. S. Kendler, "Features of Childhood Sexual Abuse and the Development of Psychiatric and Substance Use Disorders," *Br J Psychiatry* 179 (Nov. 2001): 444–49.

6. T. D. Wade, C. M. Bulik, K. S. Kendler, "Investigation of Quality of the Parental Relationship as a Risk Factor for Subclinical Bulimia Nervosa," *Int J Eat Disord.* 30, no. 4 (Dec. 2001): 389–400.

7. B. T. Walsh, E. Zimmerli, M. J. Devlin, J. Guss, and H. R. Kissileff, "A Disturbance of Gastric Function in Bulimia Nervosa," *Biol Psychiatry* 54, no. 9 (Nov. 1, 2003): 929–33.

8. B. E. Wolfe, E. Metzger, and D. C. Jimerson, "Research Update on Serotonin Function in Bulimia Nervosa and Anorexia Nervosa," *Psychopharmacol Bull.* 33, no. 3 (1997): 345–54.

9. T. D. Brewerton, "Toward a Unified Theory of Serotonin Dysregulation in Eating and Related Disorders," *Psychoneuroendocrinology* 20, no. 6 (1995): 561–90.

10. D. S. Goldbloom, P. E. Garfinkel, R. Katz, and G. M. Brown, "The Hormonal Response to Intravenous 5-Hydroxytryptophan in Bulimia Nervosa," *J Psychosom Res* 40 (1996): 289–97.

11. M. Mira and S. Abraham, "L-Tryptophan as an Adjunct to Treatment of Bulimia Nervosa," *Lancet* 2 (1989): 1162–63.

12. K. A. Smith, C. G. Fairburn, and P. J. Cowen, "Symptomatic Relapse in Bulimia Nervosa Following Acute Tryptophan Depletion," *Arch Gen Psychiatry* 56 (1999): 171–76.

13. D. Gelber, J. Levine, and R. H. Belmaker, "Effect of Inositol on Bulimia Nervosa and Binge Eating," *Int J Eat Disord*. 29, no. 3 (Apr. 2001): 345–48.

14. Fluoxetine Bulimia Nervosa Collaborative Study Group, "Fluoxetine in the Treatment of Bulimia Nervosa: A Multicenter, Placebo Controlled, Double-Blind Trial," *Arch Gen Psychiatry* 49 (1992): 139–47.

15. L. Patrick, "Eating Disorders: A Review of the Literature with Emphasis on Medical Complications and Clinical Nutrition," *Altern Med Rev*. 7, no, 3 (June 2002): 184–202.

16. B. H. Grahn, P. G. Paterson, K. T. Gottschall-Pass, and Z. Zhang, "Zinc and the Eye," *J Am Coll Nutr* 20 (2001): 106–18.

17. Food and Nutrition Board, Institute of Medicine, *Dietary Reference Intakes for Vitamin A, Vitamin K, Arsenic, Boron, Chromium, Copper, Iodine, Iron, Manganese, Molybdenum, Nickel, Silicon, Vanadium, and Zinc* (Washington, DC: National Academy Press, 2002). www.nap.edu/books/0309072794/html/.

18. L. Humphries, B. Vivian, M. Stuart, and C. J. McClain, "Zinc Deficiency and Eating Disorders," *Clin Psychiatry* 50, no. 12 (Dec. 1989): 456–59.

19. A. Schauss and C. Costin, "Zinc as a Nutrient in the Treatment of Eating Disorders," *Am J Nat Med* 4 (1997): 8–13.

20. C. L. Rock and S. Vasantharajan, "Vitamin Status of Eating Disorder Patients: Relationship to Clinical Indices and Effect of Treatment," *Int J Eat Disord*. 18, no. 3 (Nov. 1995): 257–62.

21. R. G. Laessle, P. J. Beumont, P. Butow, W. Lennerts, M. O'Connor, K. M. Pirke, S. W. Touyz, and S. Waadt, "A Comparison of Nutritional Management with Stress Management in the Treatment of Bulimia Nervosa," *Br J Psychiatry* 159 (Aug. 1991): 250–61.

22. J. E. Mitchell, R. L. Pyle, E. D. Eckert, D. Hatsukami, R. Lentz., et al., "Electrolyte and Other Physiological Abnormalities in Patients with Bulimia," *Psychol Med* 13 (1983): 273–78.

Dementia

1. Centers for Disease Control and Prevention, *Epidemiology of Traumatic Brain Injury in the United States* (Atlanta, GA: Centers for Disease Control and Prevention, 2000). (Note: Estimate includes all age groups and only those who have TBI-related disabilities. Estimates are based on provisional data.)

2. Federal Interagency Forum on Aging-Related Statistics, *Older Americans 2000: Key Indicators of Well-Being* (2000). www.agingstats.gov/default.htm.

3. Alzheimer's Disease and Related Disorders Association, *General Statistics/ Demographics* (Chicago: Alzheimer's Disease and Related Disorders Association, 2000).

4. M. Gonzalez-Gross, A. Marcos, and K. Pietrzik, "Nutrition and Cognitive Impairment in the Elderly," *Br J Nutr*. 86, no. 3 (Sept. 2001): 313–21.

5. J. Ma, M. J. Stampfer, E. Giovannucci, C. Artigas, D. J. Hunter, C. Fuchs, W. C. Willett, J. Jelhub, C. H. Hennekens, and R. Rozen, "Methylenetetrahydrofolate Reductase Polymorphism, Dietary Interactions, and Risk of Colorectal Cancer," *Cancer Res* 57 (1997): 1098–102.

6. R. F. Huang, Y. Ho, H. Lin, J. S. Wei, and T. Z. Liu, "Folate Deficiency Induces a Cell Cycle-Specific Apoptosis in HepG2 Cells," *J Nutr* 129 (1999): 25–31.

7. I. I. Kruman, T. S. Kumaravel, A. Lohani, W. A. Pedersen, R. G. Cutler, Y. Kruman, N. Haughey, J. Lee, M. Evans, and M. P. Mattson, "Folic Acid Deficiency and Homocysteine Impair DNA Repair in Hippocampal Neurons and Sensitize Them to Amyloid Toxicity in Experimental Models of Alzheimer's Disease," *J Neurosci.* 22, no. 5 (Mar. 1, 2002): 1752–62.

8. M. S. Morris, "Folate, Homocysteine, and Neurological Function," *Nutr Clin Care.* 5, no. 3 (May–June 2002): 124–32.

9. A. L. Miller, "The Methionine-Homocysteine Cycle and Its Effects on Cognitive Diseases," *Altern Med Rev.* 8, no. 1 (Feb. 2003): 7–19.

10. G. K. McKevoy, ed., *AHFS Drug Information* (Bethesda, MD: American Society of Health-System Pharmacists, 1998).

11. R. Carmel, R. Green, D.W. Jacobsen, K. Rasmussen, M. Florea, and C. Azen, "Serum Cobalamin, Homocysteine, and Methylmalonic Acid Concentrations in a Multiethnic Elderly Population: Ethnic and Sex Differences in Cobalamin and Metabolite Abnormalities," *Am J Clin Nutr* 70, no. 5 (1999): 904–10.

12. M. Lehmann, B. Regland, K. Blennow, and C. G. Gottfries, "Vitamin B12-B6-Folate Treatment Improves Blood-Brain Barrier Function in Patients with Hyper-homocysteinaemia and Mild Cognitive Impairment," *Dement Geriatr Cogn Disord.* 16, no. 3 (2003): 145–50.

13. E. M. Whyte, B. H. Mulsant, M. A. Butters, M. Qayyum, A. Towers, R. A. Sweet, W. Klunk, S. Wisniewski, S. T. DeKosky, "Cognitive and Behavioral Correlates of Low Vitamin B12 Levels in Elderly Patients with Progressive Dementia," *Am J Geriatr Psychiatry* 10, no. 3 (May–June 2002): 321–27.

14. V. Lerner and M. Kanevsky, "Acute Dementia with Delirium Due to Vitamin B12 Deficiency: A Case Report," *Int J Psychiatry Med.* 32, no. 2 (2002): 215–20.

15. I. J. Deary and A. E. Hendrickson, "Calcium and Alzheimer's Disease," *Lancet* 1, no. 8491 (May 24, 1986): 1219.

16. M. Yasui, K. Ota, and M. Yoshida, "Effects of Low Calcium and Magnesium Dietary Intake on the Central Nervous System Tissues of Rats and Calcium-Magnesium Related Disorders in the Amyotrophic Lateral Sclerosis Focus in the Kii Peninsula of Japan," *Magnes Res.* 10, no. 1 (Mar. 1997): 39–50.

17. M. Shils, A. Olson, and M. Shike, *Modern Nutrition in Health and Disease,* 8th ed. (Philadelphia, PA: Lea and Febiger, 1994).

18. T. R. Covington, et al., *Handbook of Nonprescription Drugs* (Washington, DC: Am Pharmaceutical Assn., 1996).

19. R. B. Costello and P. B. Moser-Veillon, "A Review of Magnesium Intake in the Elderly: A Cause for Concern?" *Magnes Res.* 5, no. 1 (Mar. 1992): 61–67; J. Durlach, "Magnesium Depletion and Pathogenesis of Alzheimer's Disease," *Magnes Res.* (Sept. 1990): 217–18.

20. J. L. Glick, "Dementias: The Role of Magnesium Deficiency and an Hypothesis Concerning the Pathogenesis of Alzheimer's Disease," *Med Hypotheses* 31, no. 3 (Mar. 1990): 211–25.

21. E. Andrasi, S. Igaz, Z. Molnar, and S. Mako, "Disturbances of Magnesium Concentrations in Various Brain Areas in Alzheimer's Disease," *Magnes Res.* 13, no. 3 (Sept. 2000): 189–96.

22. S. Douban, M. A. Brodsky, D. D. Whang, and R. Whang, "Significance of Magnesium in Congestive Heart Failure," *Am Heart J* 132, no. 3 (1996): 664–71.

23. M. Zimmermann, F. Colciaghi, F. Cattabeni, and M. Di Luca, "Ginkgo biloba Extract: From Molecular Mechanisms to the Treatment of Alzhelmer's Disease," *Cell Mol Biol* (*Noisy-le-grand*) 48, no. 6 (Sept. 2002): 613–23.

24. D. Loew, "Value of Ginkgo biloba in Treatment of Alzheimer Dementia," *Wien Med Wochenschr* 152, no. 15–16 (2002): 418–22.

25. J. Birks, E. V. Grimley, and M. Van Dongen, "Ginkgo biloba for Cognitive Impairment and Dementia," *Cochrane Database Syst Rev.* 4 (2002): CD003120.

26. E. K. Perry, A. T. Pickering, W. W. Wang, P. J. Houghton, and N. S. Perry, "Medicinal Plants and Alzheimer's Disease: From Ethnobotany to Phytotherapy," *J Pharm Pharmacol.* 51, no. 5 (May 1999): 527–34.

27. Kee Chang Huang, *The Pharmacology of Chinese Herbs*, 2nd ed. (Baca Raton, FL: CRC Press, 1999, 94.

28. B. Y. Lam, A. C. Lo, X. Sun, H. W. Luo, S. K. Chung, and N. J. Sucher, "Neuroprotective Effects of Tanshinones in Transient Focal Cerebral Ischemia in Mice," *Phytomedicine* 10, no. 4 (May 2003): 286–91.

29. Y. Nomura, T. Arima, T. Namba, M. Hattori, and S. Kadota, "Ameliorating Effects of Dan-Shen and Its Major Ingredient Calcium/Magnesium Lithospermate B on Cognitive Deficiencies in Senescence-Accelerated Mouse," *Nippon Yakurigaku Zasshi* 110, Suppl. 1 (Oct. 1997): 142P–47P.

30. L. Q. Min, L. Y. Dang, and W. Y. Ma, "Clinical Study on Effect and Therapeutical Mechanism of Composite Salvia Injection on Acute Cerebral Infarction," *Zhongguo Zhong Xi Yi Jie He Za Zhi* 22, no. 5 (May 2002): 353–55.

31. S. Budavari, ed., *The Merck Index*, 12th ed. (Whitehouse Station, NJ: Merck & Co., 1996).

32. X. C. Tang, P. De Sarno, K. Sugaya, and E. Giacobini, "Effect of Huperzine A, a New Cholinesterase Inhibitor, on the Central Cholinergic System of the Rat," *J Neurosci Res* 24, no. 2 (1989): 276–85.

33. J. Pepping, "Huperzine A," *Am J Health Syst Pharm* 57 (2000): 530–34.

34. D. H. Cheng, H. Ren H, and X. C. Tang, "Huperzine A, a Novel Promising Acetylcholinesterase Inhibitor," *Neuroreport* 8 (1996): 97–101.

35. A. A. Skolnick, "Old Chinese Herbal Medicine Used for Fever Yields Possible New Alzheimer Disease Therapy, *JAMA* 277 (1997): 776.

36. D. H. Cheng and X. C. Tang, Comparative Studies of Huperzine A, E2020, and Tacrine on Behavior and Cholinesterase Activities," *Pharmacol Biochem Behav* 60, no. 2 (1998): 377–86.

37. S. S. Xu, Z. X. Gao, Z. Weng, Z. M. Du, W. A. Xu, J. S. Wang, M. L. Zhang, Z. H. Tong, Y. S. Fang, and X. S. Chai, "Efficacy of Tablet Huperzine-A on Memory, Cognition, and Behavior in Alzheimer's Disease," *Zhongguo Yao Li Xue Bao* 16, no. 5 (1995): 391–95.

38. R. W. Zhang, X. C. Tang, Y. Y. Han, et al., "Drug Evaluation of Huperzine A in the Treatment of Senile Memory Disorders" [Article in Chinese] *Chung Kuo Yao Li Hsueh Pao* 12, no. 3 (1991): 250–52.

39. National Conference of State Legislature, "Pharmaceuticals" (2004). www.ncsl.org/programs/health/pharm.htm.

40. S. L. Gray, K. V. Lai, and E. B. Larson, "Drug-Induced Cognition Disorders in the Elderly: Incidence, Prevention and Management," *Drug Saf.* 21, no. 2 (Aug. 1999): 101–22.

Depression

1. D. A. Regier, W. E. Narrow, D. S. Rae, et al., "The De Facto Mental and Addictive Disorders Service System. Epidemiologic Catchment Area Prospective 1-Year Preva-

lence Rates of Disorders and Services," *Archives of General Psychiatry* 50, no. 2 (1993): 85–94.

2. W. E. Narrow, "One-year Prevalence of Depressive Disorders Among Adults 18 and Over in the U.S.: NIMH ECA Prospective Data." Population estimates based on U.S. Census estimated residential population age 18 and over on July 1, 1998. Unpublished table.

3. C.J.L. Murray and A. D. Lopez, eds., *Summary: The Global Burden of Disease: A Comprehensive Assessment of Mortality and Disability from Diseases, Injuries, and Risk Factors in 1990 and Projected to 2020* (Cambridge, MA: Harvard University Press, 1996). Published by the Harvard School of Public Health on behalf of the World Health Organization and the World Bank. www.who.int/msa/mnh/ems/dalys/intro.htm.

4. American Psychiatric Association, *Diagnostic and Statistical Manual on Mental Disorders*, 4th ed. (*DSM-IV*) (Washington, DC: American Psychiatric Press, 1994).

5. American Psychiatric Association, *Diagnostic and Statistical Manual on Mental Disorders*, 4th ed. (*DSM-IV*) (Washington, DC: American Psychiatric Press, 1994).

6. M. J. Taylor, S. Carney, J. Geddes, and G. Goodwin, "Folate for Depressive Disorders," *Cochrane Database Syst Rev.* 2 (2003): CD003390.

7. M. S. Morris, M. Fava, P. F. Jacques, J. Selhub, and I. H. Rosenberg, "Depression and Folate Status in the U.S. Population," *Psychother Psychosom.* 72, no. 2 (Mar.–Apr. 2003): 80–87.

8. J. E. Alpert and M. Fava, "Nutrition and Depression: The Role of Folate," *Nutr Rev.* 55, no. 5 (May 1997): 145–49.

9. A. Coppen and J. Bailey, "Enhancement of the Antidepressant Action of Fluoxetine by Folic Acid: A Randomized, Placebo-Controlled Trial," *J Affect Disord.* 60, no. 2 (Nov. 2000): 121–30.

10. M. T. Abou-Saleh and A. Coppen, "Serum and Red Blood Cell Folate in Depression," *Acta Psychiatr Scand.* 80, no. 1 (July 1989): 78–82.

11. G. K. McKevoy, ed., *AHFS Drug Information* (Bethesda, MD: American Society of Health-System Pharmacists, 1998).

12. R. Shiloh, A. Weizman, N. Weizer, P. Dorfman-Etrog, and H. Munitz, "Antidepressive Effect of Pyridoxine (Vitamin B6) in Neuroleptic-Treated Schizophrenic Patients with Co-Morbid Minor Depression—Preliminary Open-Label Trial," *Harefuah* 140, no. 5 (May 2001): 369–73, 456.

13. M. F. McCarty, "High-Dose Pyridoxine as an 'Anti-Stress' Strategy," *Med Hypotheses* 54, no. 5 (May 2000): 803–7.

14. T. Baldewicz, K. Goodkin, D. J. Feaster, N. T. Blaney, M. Kumar, A. Kumar, G. Shor-Posner, and M. Baum, "Plasma Pyridoxine Eficiency Is Related to Increased Psychological Distress in Recently Bereaved Homosexual Men," *Psychosom Med.* 60, no. 3 (May–June 1998): 297–308.

15. I. R. Bell, J. S. Edman, F. D. Morrow, D. W. Marby, S. Mirages, G. Perrone, H. L. Kayne, and J. O. Cole, "B Complex Vitamin Patterns in Geriatric and Young Adult Inpatients with Major Depression," *J Am Geriatr Soc.* 39, no. 3 (Mar. 1991): 252–57.

16. R. E. Hodges, J. Hood, J. E. Canham, H. E. Sauberlich, and E. M. Baker, "Clinical Manifestations of Ascorbic Acid Deficiency in Man," *Am J Clin Nutr.* 24, no. 4 (Apr. 1971): 432–43.

17. G. Milner, "Ascorbic Acid in Chronic Psychiatric Patients: A Controlled Trial," *Br J Psychiatry* 109 (1963): 294–99.

18. Z. A. Leitner and I. C. Church, "Nutritional Studies in a Mental Hospital," *Lancet* 1 (1956): 565–67.

19. M. Hector and J. R. Burton, "What Are the Psychiatric Manifestations of Vitamin B12 Deficiency?" *J Am Geriatr Soc.* 36, no. 12 (Dec. 1988): 1105–12.

20. D. Mischoulon, J. K. Burger, M. K. Spillmann, J. J. Worthington, M. Fava, and J. E. Alpert, "Anemia and Macrocytosis in the Prediction of Serum Folate and Vitamin B12 Status, and Treatment Outcome in Major Depression," *J Psychosom Res.* 49, no. 3 (Sept. 2000): 183–87.

21. J. Lindenbaum, E. B. Healton, D. G. Savage, J. C. Brust, T. J. Garrett, E. R. Podell, P. D. Marcell, S. P. Stabler, and R. H. Allen, "Neuropsychiatric Disorders Caused by Cobalamin Deficiency in the Absence of Anemia or Macrocytosis," *N Engl J Med* 318 (1988): 1720–28.

22. T. Bottiglieri, "Folate, Vitamin B12, and Neuropsychiatric Disorders," *Nutr Rev.* 54, no. 12 (Dec. 1996): 382–90.

23. B. W. Penninx, J. M. Guralnik, L. Ferrucci, L. P. Fried, R. H. Allen, and S. P. Stabler, "Vitamin B(12) Deficiency and Depression in Physically Disabled Older Women: Epidemiologic Evidence from the Women's Health and Aging Study," *Am J Psychiatry* 157, no. 5 (May 2000): 715–21.

24. S. Meyers, "Use of Neurotransmitter Precursors for Treatment of Depression," *Altern Med Rev.* 5, no. 1 (Feb. 2000): 64–71.

25. T. C. Birdsall, "5-Hydroxytryptophan: A Clinically-Effective Serotonin Precursor," *Altern Med Rev.* 3, no. 4 (Aug. 1998): 271–80.

26. A. L. Miller, "St. John's Wort (*Hypericum perforatum*): Clinical Effects on Depression and Other Conditions," *Altern Med Rev.* 3, no. 1 (1998).

27. E. Whiskey, U. Werneke, D. Taylor, "A Systematic Review and Meta-Analysis of Hypericum Perforatum in Depression: A Comprehensive Clinical Review," *Int Clin Psychopharmacol* 16, no. 5 (Sept. 2001): 239–52.

28. G. Laakmann, et al., "St. John's Wort in Mild to Moderate Depression: The Relevance of Hyperforin for the Clinical Efficacy," *Pharmacopsych* 31, Suppl. 1 (1998): 54–59.

29. V. Butterweck, "Mechanism of Action of St. John's Wort in Depression: What Is Known?" *CNS Drugs* 17, no. 8 (2003): 539–62.

30. W. E. Muller, "Current St. John's Wort Research from Mode of Action to Clinical Efficacy," *Pharmacol Res.* (Feb. 2003): 101–9.

31. Y. Lecrubier, G. Clerc, R. Didi, and M. Kieser, "Efficacy of St. John's Wort Extract WS 5570 in Major Depression: A Double-Blind, Placebo-Controlled Trial," *Am J Psychiatry* 159, no. 8 (Aug. 2002): 1361–66.

Hormonal Mental Health

1. E. W. Freeman, "Evaluation of a Unique Oral Contraceptive (Yasmin) in the Management of Premenstrual Dysphoric Disorder," *Eur J Contracept Reprod Health Care* 7, Suppl. 3 (Dec. 2002): 27–34; discussion 42–43.

2. J. W. Bailey and L. S. Cohen, "Prevalence of Mood and Anxiety Disorders in Women Who Seek Treatment for Premenstrual Syndrome," *J Women's Health Gend Based Med.* 8, no. 9 (Nov. 1999): 1181–84.

3. M. Murray, and J. Pizzorno, *The Encyclopedia of Natural Medicine* (Rocklin, CA: Prima Publishing, 1998).

4. P. Bermond, "Therapy of Side Effects of Oral Contraceptive Agents with Vitamin B6," *Acta Vitaminol Enzymol.* 4, no. 1–2 (1982): 45–54.

5. K. M. Wyatt, P. W. Dimmock, P. W. Jones, and P. M. Shaughn O'Brien, "Efficacy of Vitamin B-6 in the Treatment of Premenstrual Syndrome: Systematic Review," *BMJ* 318, no. 7195 (May 22, 1999): 1375–81.

6. M. S. Diegoli, A. M. da Fonseca, C. A. Diegoli, and J. A. Pinotti, "A Double-Blind Trial of Four Medications to Treat Severe Premenstrual Syndrome," *Int J Gynaecol Obstet.* 62, no. 1 (July 1998): 63–67.

7. A. F. Walker, M. C. De Souza, M. F. Vickers, S. Abeyasekera, M. I. Collins, and L. A. Trinca, "Magnesium Supplementation Alleviates Premenstrual Symptoms of Fluid Retention," *J Womens Health* 7, no. 9 (Nov. 1998): 1157–65.

8. D. L. Rosenstein, R. J. Elin, J. M. Hosseini, G. Grover, and D. R. Rubinow, "Magnesium Measures Across the Menstrual Cycle in Premenstrual Syndrome," *Biol Psychiatry* 35, no. 8 (Apr. 15, 1994): 557–61.

9. F. Facchinetti, P. Borella, G. Sances, L. Fioroni, R. E. Nappi, and A. R. Genazzani, "Oral Magnesium Successfully Relieves Premenstrual Mood Changes," *Obstet Gynecol.* 78, no. 2 (Aug. 1991): 177–81.

10. G. E. Abraham, "Nutritional Factors in the Etiology of the Premenstrual Tension Syndromes," *J Reprod Med.* 28, no. 7 (July 1983): 446–64.

11. M. C. De Souza, A. F. Walker, P. A. Robinson, and K. Bolland, "A Synergistic Effect of a Daily Supplement for 1 Month of 200 mg Magnesium Plus 50 mg Vitamin B6 for the Relief of Anxiety-Related Premenstrual Symptoms: A Randomized, Double-Blind, Crossover Study," *J Women's Health Gend Based Med.* 9, no. 2 (Mar. 2000): 131–39.

12. R. S. London, G. S. Sundaram, L. Murphy, and P. J. Goldstein, "The Effect of Alpha-tocopherol on Premenstrual Symptomatology: A Double-Blind Study," *J Am Coll Nutr.* 2, no. 2 (1983): 115–22; R. S. London, G. S. Sundaram, L. Murphy, and P. J. Goldstein, "Evaluation and Treatment of Breast Symptoms in Patients with the Premenstrual Syndrome," *J Reprod Med.* 28, no. 8 (Aug. 1983): 503–8.

13. R. S. London, G. Sundaram, S. Manimekalai, L. Murphy, M. Reynolds, and P. Goldstein, "The Effect of Alpha-Tocopherol on Premenstrual Symptomatology: A Double-Blind Study. II. Endocrine Correlates," *J Am Coll Nutr.* 3, no. 4 (1984): 351–56.

14. D. F. Horrobin, "The Role of Essential Fatty Acids and Prostaglandins in the Premenstrual Syndrome," *J Reprod Med.* 28, no. 7 (July 1983): 465–68.

15. J. Puolakka, L. Makarainen, L. Viinikka, and O. Ylikorkala, "Biochemical and Clinical Effects of Treating the Premenstrual Syndrome with Prostaglandin Synthesis Precursors," *J Reprod Med.* 30, no. 3 (Mar. 1985): 149–53.

16. C. J. Chuong and E. B. Dawson, "Zinc and Copper Levels in Premenstrual Syndrome," *Fertil Steril.* 62, no. 2 (Aug. 1994): 313–20.

17. C. Posaci, O. Erten, A. Uren, and B. Acar, "Plasma Copper, Zinc and Magnesium Levels in Patients with Premenstrual Tension Syndrome," *Acta Obstet Gynecol Scand.* 73, no. 6 (July 1994): 452–55.

18. E. Shlidge, "Essay on the Treatment of Premenstrual and Menopausal Mood Swing and Depressive States," *Rigelh Biol Umsch* 19, no. 2 (1964): 18–22.

19. E. Lehmann-Willenbrock and H. H. Riedel, "Clinical and Endocrinological Studies of the Treatment of Ovarian Insufficiency Manifestations Following Hysterectomy with Intact Adnexa" [Article in German], *Zentralbl Gynakol* 110 (1988): 611–18.

20. A. Milewicz, E. Gejdel, H. Sworen H, K. Sienkiewicz, J. Jedrzejak, T. Teucher, and H. Schmitz, "Vitex agnus Castus Extract in the Treatment of Luteal Phase Defects

Due to Latent Hyperprolactinemia: Results of a Randomized Placebo-Controlled Double-Blind Study" [Article in German], *Arzneimittelforschung* 43 (1993): 752–56.

21. J. Liu, J. E. Burdette, H. Xu, et al., "Evaluation of Estrogenic Activity of Plant Extracts for the Potential Treatment of Menopausal Symptoms," *J Agric Food Chem* 49 (2001): 2472–79.

22. A. Kumagai, K. Nishino, A. Shimomura, T. Kin, and Y. Yamamura, "Effect of Glycyrrhizin on Estrogen Action," *Endocrinol Jpn.* 14, no. 1 (Mar. 1967): 34–38.

23. K. Heldal and K. Midtvedt, "Licorice—Not Just Candy," *Tidsskr Nor Laegeforen* 122, no. 8 (Mar. 20, 2002): 774–76.

24. V. H. Guerrini, "Effect of Parenteral Antioxidants on Adrenal Pathobiology and Leukocytes in Hyperammonaemic Toxaemia," *Free Radic Res.* 22, no. 6 (June 1995): 545–53.

25. S. R. Bornstein, M. Yoshida-Hiroi, S. Sotiriou, M. Levine, H. G. Hartwig, R. L. Nussbaum, and G. Eisenhofer, "Impaired Adrenal Catecholamine System Function in Mice with Deficiency of the Ascorbic Acid Transporter (SVCT2)," *FASEB J.* 17, no. 13 (Oct. 2003): 1928–30. Epub Aug. 1, 2003.

26. T. Crook, W. Petrie, C. Wells, and D. C. Massari, "Effects of Phosphatidylserine in Alzheimer's Disease," *Psychopharmacol Bull* 28, no. 1 (1992): 61–66.

27. H. Y. Kim, M. Akbar, A. Lau, and L. Edsall, "Inhibition of Neuronal Aapoptosis by Docosahexaenoic Acid (22:6n-3). Role of Phosphatidylserine in Antiapoptotic Effect," *J Biol Chem* 275, no. 35 (2000): 215–23.

28. P. Monteleone, L. Beinat, C. Tanzillo, M. Maj, and D. Kemali, "Effects of Phosphatidylserine on the Neuroendocrine Response to Physical Stress in Humans," *Neuroendocrinology* 52 (1990): 243–48.

29. J. H. Koh, K. M. Kim, J. M. Kim, J. C. Song, and H. J. Suh, "Antifatigue and Antistress Effect of the Hot-Water Fraction from Mycelia of Cordyceps Sinensis," *Biol Pharm Bull.* 26, no. 5 (May 2003): 691–94.

Insomnia

1. T. Roehrs and T. Roth, "Alcohol-Induced Sleepiness and Memory Function," *Alcohol Health Res World* 19, no. 2 (1995): 130–35.

2. D. J. Kupfer and C. F. Reynolds, "Management of Insomnia," *N Engl J Med* 336, no. 5 (1997): 341–46.

3. K. L. Lichstein, N. M. Wilson, and C. T. Johnson, "Psychological Treatment of Secondary Insomnia," *Psychol Aging* 15, no. 2 (June 2000): 232–40.

4. H. P. Landolt, C. Roth, D. J. Dijk, and A. A. Borbely., "Late-Afternoon Ethanol Intake Affects Nocturnal Sleep and the Sleep EEG in Middle-Aged Men," *J Clin Psychopharmacol* 16, no. 6 (1996): 428–36.

5. M. V. Vitiello, "Sleep, Alcohol and Alcohol Abuse," *Addict Biol* 2 (1997): 151–58.

6. M. Scher, G. A. Richardson, P. A. Coble, N. L. Day, and D. S. Stoffer, "The Effects of Prenatal Alcohol and Marijuana Exposure: Disturbances in Neonatal Sleep Cycling and Arousal," *Pediatr Res* 24, no. 1 (1988): 101–5.

7. J. A. Mennella and C. J. Gerrish, "Effects of Exposure to Alcohol in Mothers' Milk on the Infants' Sleep and Activity Levels," *Pediatrics*, in press.

8. K. Takahashi, M. Okawa, M. Matsumoto, K. Mishima, H. Yamadera, M. Sasaki,

Y. Ishizuka, et al., "Double-Blind Test on the Efficacy of Methylcobalamin on Sleep-Wake Rhythm Disorders," *Psychiatry Clin Neurosci.* 53, no. 2 (Apr. 1999): 211–13.

9. M. Okawa, K. Mishima, T. Nanami, T. Shimizu, S. Iijima, Y. Hishikawa, and K. Takahashi, "Vitamin B12 Treatment for Sleep-Wake Rhythm Disorders," *Sleep* 13, no. 1 (Feb. 1990): 15–23.

10. H. Yamadera, K. Takahashi, and M. Okawa, "A Multicenter Study of Sleep-Wake Rhythm Disorders: Therapeutic Effects of Vitamin B12, Bright Light Therapy, Chronotherapy and Hypnotics," *Psychiatry Clin Neurosci.* 150, no. 4 (Aug. 1996):203–9.

11. M. Audebert, J. P. Gendre, and Y. Le Quintrec, "Folate and the Nervous System," *Sem Hop.* 55, no. 31–32 (Sept. 18–25, 1979): 1383–87.

12. K. A. Lee, M. E. Zaffke, and K. Baratte-Beebe, "Restless Legs Syndrome and Sleep Disturbance During Pregnancy: The Role of Folate and Iron," *J Women's Health Gend Based Med.* 10, no. 4 (May 2001): 335–41.

13. S. N. Young and A. M. Ghadirian, "Folic Acid and Psychopathology," *Prog Neuropsychopharmacol Biol Psychiatry* 13, no. 6 (1989): 841–63.

14. M. Shils, A. Olson, and M. Shike, *Modern Nutrition in Health and Disease,* 8th ed. (Philadelphia, PA: Lea and Febiger, 1994).

15. T. R. Covington, et al., *Handbook of Nonprescription Drugs* (Washington, DC: Am Pharmaceutical Assn., 1996).

16. R. P. Allen, "Should We Use Oral Magnesium Supplementation to Improve Sleep in the Elderly? Article reviewed: K. Held, I. A. Antonijevic, H. Kunzel, M. Uhr, T. C. Wetter, I. C. Golly, A. Steiger, and H. Murck, "Oral MG(2+) Supplementation Reverses Age-Related Neuroendocrine and Sleep EEG Changes in Humans," *Pharmacopsychiatry* 35 (2002): 135–43; *Sleep Med.* 4, no. 3 (May 2003): 263–64.

17. J. Durlach, N. Pages, P. Bac, M. Bara, A. Guiet-Bara, and C. Agrapart, "Chronopathological Forms of Magnesium Depletion with Hypofunction or with Hyperfunction of the Biological Clock," *Magnes Res.* 15, no. 3–4 (Dec. 2002): 263–68.

18. J. Durlach, N. Pages, P. Bac, M. Bara, and A. Guiet-Bara, "Biorhythms and Possible Central Regulation of Magnesium Status, Phototherapy, Darkness Therapy and Chronopathological Forms of Magnesium Depletion," *Magnes Res.* 15, no. 1–2 (Mar. 2002): 49–66.

19. H. R. Lieberman, S. Corkin, and B. J. Spring, "The Effects of Dietary Neurotransmitter Precursors on Human Behavior," *Am J Clin Nutr* 42 (1985): 366–70.

20. J. I. Hudson, H. G. Pope, S. R. Daniels, and R. I. Horwitz, "Eosinophilia-Myalgia Syndrome or Fibromyalgia with Eosinophilia?" *JAMA* 269 (1993): 3108–9.

21. A. M. Ghadirian, B. E. Murphy, and M. J. Gendron, "Efficacy of Light Versus Tryptophan Therapy in Seasonal Affective Disorder," *J Affect Disord* 50 (1998): 23–27.

22. J.E.F. Reynolds, *Martindale: The Extra Pharmacopea,* 31st ed. (London: The Royal Pharmaceutical Society of Great Britain, 1996), 336–37.

23. A. Soulairac and H. Lambinet, "The Effects of 5-Hydroxy-Tryptophan, a Precursor of Serotonin, on Sleep Disorder," *Annales Medico-Psychologiques* (1977): 792–97.

24. T. C. Birdsall, "5-Hydroxytryptophan: A Clinically-Effective Serotonin Precursor," *Altern Med Rev* 3, no. 4 (1998): 271–80.

25. A. Munoz-Hoyos, M. Sanchez-Forte, A. Molina-Carballo, G. Escames, E. Martin-Medina, R. J. Reiter, J. A. Molina-Font, and D. Acuna-Castroviejo, "Melatonin's Role as an Anticonvulsant and Neuronal Protector: Experimental and Clinical Evidence," *J Child Neurol* 13 (1998): 501–9.

26. A. Brzezinski, "Melatonin in Humans," *N Engl J Med* 336, no. 3 (1997): 186–95.

27. S. Carranza-Lira and F. Garcia Lopez, "Melatonin and Climactery," *Med Sci Monit.* 6, no. 6 (Nov.–Dec. 2000): 1209–12.

28. I. V. Zhdanova and V. Tucci, "Melatonin, Circadian Rhythms, and Sleep," *Curr Treat Options Neurol.* 5, no. 3 (May 2003): 225–29.

29. A. J. Lewy, S. Ahmed, J. M. Jackson, and R. L. Sack, "Melatonin Shifts Human Circadian Rhythms According to a Phase-Response Curve," *Chronobiol Int* 9 (1992): 380–92.

30. D. Garfinkel, et al., "Improvement of Sleep Quality in Elderly People by Controlled-Release Melatonin," *Lancet* 346, no. 8974 (Aug. 26, 1995): 541–44.

31. H. Niederhofer, W. Staffen, A. Mair, and K. Pittschieler, "Brief Report: Melatonin Facilitates Sleep in Individuals with Mental Retardation and Insomnia," *J Autism Dev Disord.* 33, no. 4 (Aug. 2003): 469–72.

32. E. J. Paavonen, T. Nieminen–von Wendt, R. Vanhala, E. T. Aronen, and L. von Wendt, "Effectiveness of Melatonin in the Treatment of Sleep Disturbances in Children with Asperger Disorder," *Child Adolesc Psychopharmacol.* 13, no. 1 (Spring 2003): 83–95.

33. M. G. Smits, H. F. van Stel, K. van der Heijden, A. M. Meijer, A. M. Coenen, and G. A. Kerkhof, "Melatonin Improves Health Status and Sleep in Children with Idiopathic Chronic Sleep-Onset Insomnia: A Randomized Placebo-Controlled Trial," *J Am Acad Child Adolesc Psychiatry* 42, no. 11 (Nov. 2003): 1286–93.

34. K. Dhawan, S. Kumar, and A. Sharma, "Anti-Anxiety Studies on Extracts of Passiflora Incarnata Linneaus," *J Ethnopharmacol* 78 (2001): 165–70.

35. K. Dhawan, S. Kumar, and A. Sharma, "Anxiolytic Activity of Aerial and Underground Parts of Passiflora Incarnata," *Fitoterapia* 72 (2001): 922–26.

36. J. B. Salgueiro, P. Ardenghi, M. Dias, et al., "Anxiolytic Natural and Synthetic Flavonoid Ligands of the Central Benzodiazepine Receptor Have No Effect on Memory Tasks in Rats," *Pharmacol Biochem Behav* 58 (1997): 887–91.

37. A. Y. Leung and S. Foster, *Encyclopedia of Common Natural Ingredients Used in Food, Drugs and Cosmetics*, 2nd ed. (New York: John Wiley & Sons, 1996).

38. L. Krenn, "Passion Flower (Passiflora incarnata L.)—A Reliable Herbal Sedative," *Wien Med Wochenschr.* 152, no. 15–16 (2002): 404–6.

39. T. B. Klepser and M. E. Klepser, "Unsafe and Potentially Safe Herbal Therapies," *Am J Health Syst Pharm* 56 (1999): 125–38.

40. P. J. Houghton, "The Scientific Basis for the Reputed Activity of Valerian," *J Pharm Pharmacol* 51, no. 5 (1999): 505–12.

41. P. D. Leathwood, F. Chauffard, E. Heck, and R. Munoz-Box, "Aqueous Extract of Valerian Root (Valeriana Officinalis L.) Improves Sleep Quality in Man," *Pharmacol Biochem Behav* 17 (1982): 65–71.

42. D. R. Poyares, C. Guilleminault, M. M. Ohayon, and S. Tufik, "Can Valerian Improve the Sleep of Insomniacs after Benzodiazepine Withdrawal?" *Prog Neuropsychopharmacol Biol Psychiatry* 26 (2002): 539–45.

43. Donath F, Quispe S, Diefenbach K, et al., "Critical evaluation of the effect of valerian extract on sleep structure and sleep quality," *Pharmacopsych* 33 (2000): 47–53.

44. C. Gyllenhaal, S. L. Merritt, S. D. Peterson, K. I. Block, and T. Gochenour, "Efficacy and Safety of Herbal Stimulants and Sedatives in Sleep Disorders," *Sleep Med Rev.* 4, no. 3 (June 2000): 229–51.

45. J. Gruenwald et al., *PDR for Herbal Medicines*, 1st ed. (Montvale, NJ: Medical Economics Company, 1998).

46. C. A. Newall, L. A. Anderson, and J. D. Philpson, *Herbal Medicine: A Guide for Healthcare Professionals* (London: The Pharmaceutical Press, 1996).

Learning Disability

1. Twenty-third Annual Report to Congress on the Implementation of IDEA, U.S. Department of Education, 2001.

2. H. Y. Kim, E. A. Frongillo, S. S. Han, S. Y. Oh, W. K. Kim, Y. A. Jang, H. S. Won, H. S. Lee, and S. H. Kim, "Academic Performance of Korean Children Is Associated with Dietary Behaviours and Physical Status," *Asia Pac J Clin Nutr.* 12, no. 2 (2003): 186–92.

3. R. E. Kleinman, S. Hall, H. Green, D. Korzec-Ramirez, K. Patton, M. E. Pagano, and J. M. Murphy, "Diet, Breakfast, and Academic Performance in Children," *Ann Nutr Metab.* 46, Suppl. 1 (2002): 24–30.

4. D. Gutierrez Sigler, J. Colomer Revuelta, C. Barona, P. Momparler, and C. Colomer Revuelta, "The Association Between Iron Deficiency and Learning Disorders in Preschoolers," *Gac Sanit.* 6, no. 32 (Sept.–Oct. 1992): 207–11.

5. A. G. Soemantri, E., Pollitt, and I. Kim, "Iron Deficiency Anemia and Educational Achievement," *Am J Clin Nutr.* 42, no. 6 (Dec. 1985): 1221–28.

6. B. Lozoff, "Iron and Learning Potential in Childhood," *Bull NY Acad Med.* 65, no. 10 (Dec. 1989): 1050–66; discussion 1085–88.

7. M. B. Youdim, D. Ben-Shachar, and S.Yehuda, "Putative Biological Mechanisms of the Effect of Iron Deficiency on Brain Biochemistry and Behavior," *Am J Clin Nutr.* 50, Suppl. 3 (Sept. 1989): 607–15; discussion 615–17.

8. J. Durlach, "Clinical Aspects of Chronic Magnesium Deficiency," in *Magnesium in Health and Disease*, ed. M. S. Seelig (New York: Spectrum Publication, 1980).

9. J. A. Cocores, R. K. Davies, P. S. Mueller, and M. S. Gold, "Cocaine Abuse and Adult Attention Deficit Disorder," *J Clin Psychiatry* 48, no. 9 (Sept. 1987): 376–77.

10. L. Galland, "Nutritional Supplementation for ADHD," in *Attention Deficit Hyperactivity Disorder: Causes and Possible Solutions*, ed. J. A. Bellanti, W. G. Crook, and R. E. Layton (Jackson, TN: International Health Foundation, 1999).

11. E. S. Halas, C. D. Hunt, and M. J. Eberhardt, "Learning and Memory Disabilities in Young Adult Rats from Mildly Zinc Deficient Dams," *Physiol Behav.* 37, no. 3 (1986): 451–58; A. Takeda, S. Takefuta, S. Okada, and N. Oku, "Relationship Between Brain Zinc and Transient Learning Impairment of Adult Rats Fed Zinc-Deficient Diet," *Brain Res.* 859, no. 2 (Mar. 24, 2000): 352–57.

12. A. L. Kubula and M. M. Katz, "Nutritional Factors in Psychological Test Behavior," *J Genet Psychol.* 96 (June 1960): 343–52.

13. Food and Nutrition Board, Institute of Medicine, *Dietary Reference Intakes for Vitamin A, Vitamin K, Arsenic, Boron, Chromium, Copper, Iodine, Iron, Manganese, Molybdenum, Nickel, Silicon, Vanadium, and Zinc* (Washington, DC: National Academy Press, 2002). www.nap.edu/books/0309072794/html/.

14. B. D. Tiwari, M. M. Godbole, N. Chattopadhyay, A. Mandal, and A. Mithal, "Learning Disabilities and Poor Motivation to Achieve Due to Prolonged Iodine Deficiency," *Am J Clin Nutr.* 63, no. 5 (May 1996): 782–86.

15. F. Vermiglio, M. Sidoti, M. D. Finocchiaro, S. Battiato, V. P. Lo Presti, S. Benvenga, and F. Trimarchi, "Defective Neuromotor and Cognitive Ability in Iodine-Deficient Schoolchildren of an Endemic Goiter Region in Sicily," *J Clin Endocrinol Metab.* 70, no. 2 (Feb. 1990): 379–84.

16. R. O. Pihl and M. Parkes, "Hair Element Content in Learning Disabled Children," *Science* 198, no. 4313 (Oct. 14, 1977): 204–6.

17. D. A. Cory-Slechta, "Relationships Between Lead-Induced Learning Impairments and Changes in Dopaminergic, Cholinergic, and Glutamatergic Neurotransmitter System Functions," *Annu Rev Pharmacol Toxicol.* 35 (1995): 391–415.

18. H. G. Preuss, "A Review of Persistent, Low-Grade Lead Challenge: Neurological and Cardiovascular Consequences," *J Am Coll Nutr.* 12, no. 3 (June 1993): 246–54.

19. P. E. Wainwright, "Dietary Essential Fatty Acids and Brain Function: A Developmental Perspective on Mechanisms," *Proc Nutr Soc.* 61, no. 1 (Feb. 2002): 61–69.

20. M. A. Crawford, "The Role of Essential Fatty Acids in Neural Development: Implications for Perinatal Nutrition," *Am J Clin Nutr.* 57, Suppl. 5 (May 1993): 703S–9S; discussion 709S–10S.

21. M. A. Crawford, W. Doyle, A. Leaf, M. Leighfield, K. Ghebremeskel, and A. Phylactos, "Nutrition and Neurodevelopmental Disorders," *Nutr Health* 9, no. 2 (1993): 81–97.

22. N. Salem Jr, T. Moriguchi, R. S. Greiner, K. McBride, A. Ahmad, J. N. Catalan, and B. Slotnick, "Alterations in Brain Function after Loss of Docosahexaenoate Due to Dietary Restriction of N-3 Fatty Acids," *J Mol Neurosci.* 16, no. 2–3 (Apr.–June 2001): 299–307; discussion 317–21.

23. M. E. Angelucci, M. A. Vital, C. Cesario, C. R. Zadusky, P. L. Rosalen, and C. Da Cunha, "The Effect of Caffeine in Animal Models of Learning and Memory," *Eur J Pharmacol.* 373, no. 2–3 (June 4, 1999): 135–40.

24. J. Sprafkin, K. D. Gadow, and P. Grayson, "Effects of Viewing Aggressive Cartoons on the Behavior of Learning Disabled Children," *J Child Psychol Psychiatry* 28, no. 3 (May 1987): 387–98.

Mental Fatigue

1. L. Jongman, and N. Taatgen, "An ACT-R Model of Individual Differences in Changes in Adaptivity Due to Mental Fatigue," in *Proceedings of the 21th Annual Conference of the Cognitive Science Society* (Hillsdale, NJ: Erlbaum, 1999).

2. D. H. Holding, "Fatigue," in *Stress and Fatigue in Human Performance*, ed. G.R.J. Hockey (New York: John Wiley & Sons, 1983).

3. R. L. West, "An Application of Prefrontal Cortex Function Theory to Cognitive Aging," *Psychol Bull.* 120, no. 2 (Sept. 1996): 272–92.

4. D. H. Bessesen, "The Role of Carbohydrates in Insulin Resistance," *J Nutr.* 131, no. 10 (Oct. 2001): 2782S–86S.

5. B. Spring, J. Chiodo, M. Harden, M. J. Bourgeois, J. D. Mason, and L. Lutherer, "Psychobiological Effects of Carbohydrates," *J Clin Psychiatry* Suppl. 50 (May 1989): 27–33; discussion 34.

6. H. M. Lloyd, P. J. Rogers, D. I. Hedderley, and A. F. Walker, "Acute Effects on Mood and Cognitive Performance of Breakfasts Differing in Fat and Carbohydrate Content," *Appetite* 27, no. 2 (Oct. 1996): 151–64.

7. W. L. Hasler, "Dumping Syndrome," *Curr Treat Options Gastroenterol.* 5, no. 2 (Apr. 2002): 139–45.

8. K. Fischer, P. C. Colombani, W. Langhans, and C. Wenk, "Cognitive Performance and Its Relationship with Postprandial Metabolic Changes after Ingestion of Different Macronutrients in the Morning," *Br J Nutr.* 85, no. 3 (Mar. 2001): 393–405.

9. D. Benton and P. Y. Parker, "Breakfast, Blood Glucose, and Cognition," *Am J Clin Nutr.* 67, no. 4 (Apr. 1998): 772S–78S.

10. T. M. Ortega, P. Andres, A. Lopez-Sobaler, A. Ortega, R. Redondo, A. Jimenez, and L. M. Jimenez, "The Role of Folates in the Diverse Biochemical Processes That Control Mental Function," *Nutr Hosp.* 9, no. 4 (July–Aug. 1994): 251–56.

11. V. Darbinyan, A. Kteyan, A. Panossian, E. Gabrielian, G. Wikman, and H. Wagner, "Rhodiola Rosea in Stress Induced Fatigue—A Double-Blind Cross-Over Study of a Standardized Extract SHR-5 with a Repeated Low-Dose Regimen on the Mental Performance of Healthy Physicians During Night Duty," *Phytomedicine* 7, no. 5 (2000): 365–71.

12. V. A. Shevtsov, B. I. Zholus, V. I. Shervarly, V. B. Vol'skij, Y. P. Korovin, M. P. Khristich, N. A. Roslyakova, and G. Wikman, "A Randomized Trial of Two Different Doses of a SHR-5 Rhodiola Rosea Extract Versus Placebo and Control of Capacity for Mental Work," *Phytomedicine* 10, no. 2–3 (Mar. 2003): 95–105.

13. V. Darbinyan, A. Kteyan, A. Panossian, E. Gabrielian, G. Wikman, and H. Wagner, "Rhodiola Rosea in Stress Induced Fatigue—A Double-Blind Cross-Over Study of a Standardized Extract SHR-5 with a Repeated Low-Dose Regimen on the Mental Performance of Healthy Physicians During Night Duty," *Phytomedicine* 7, no. 5 (Oct. 2000): 365–71.

14. A. A. Spasov, G. K. Wikman, V. B. Mandrikov, I. A. Mironova, and V. V. Neumoin, "A Double-Blind, Placebo-Controlled Pilot Study of the Stimulating and Adaptogenic Effect of Rhodiola Rosea SHR-5 Extract on the Fatigue of Students Caused by Stress During an Examination Period with a Repeated Low-Dose Regimen," *Phytomedicine* 7, no. 2 (Apr. 2000): 85–89.

15. D. O. Kennedy and A. B. Scholey, "Ginseng: Potential for the Enhancement of Cognitive Performance and Mood," *Pharmacol Biochem Behav.* 75, no. 3 (June 2003): 687–700.

16. M. Rudakewich, F. Ba, and C. G. Benishin, "Neurotrophic and Neuroprotective Actions of Ginsenosides Rb(1) and Rg(1)," *Planta Med.* 67, no. 6 (Aug. 2001): 533–37.

17. C. G. Benishin, R. Lee, L. C. Wang, and H. J. Liu, "Effects of Ginsenoside Rb1 on Central Cholinergic Metabolism," *Pharmacology* 42, no. 4 (1991): 223–29.

18. C. Stough, J. Clarke, J. Lloyd, and P. J. Nathan, "Neuropsychological Changes after 30-Day Ginkgo biloba Administration in Healthy Participants," *Int J Neuropsychopharmacol.* 4, no. 2 (June 2001): 131–44.

19. A. B. Scholey and D. O. Kennedy, "Acute, Dose-Dependent Cognitive Effects of Ginkgo biloba, Panax Ginseng and Their Combination in Healthy Young Volunteers: Differential Interactions with Cognitive Demand," *Hum Psychopharmacol.* 17, no. 1 (Jan. 2002): 35–44.

20. D. O. Kennedy, A. B. Scholey, and K. A. Wesnes, "Differential, Dose Dependent Changes in Cognitive Performance Following Acute Administration of a Ginkgo biloba/Panax Ginseng Combination to Healthy Young Volunteers," *Nutr Neurosci.* 4, no. 5 (2001): 399–412.

21. R. A. Anderson, M. M. Polansky, N. A. Bryden, S. J. Bhathena , and J. J. Canary. "Effects of Supplemental Chromium on Patients with Symptoms of Reactive Hypoglycemia," *Metabolism* 36 (1987): 351–55.

22. Micromedex Healthcare Series, Multiple Sclerosis, *AltMedDex® System: Comprehensive Referenced Data on Herbal Medicines and Dietary Supplements Covering Uses, Efficacy, Dosing, Toxicity, and More.* (Englewood, CO: MICROMEDEX Inc.).

Multiple Sclerosis

1. D. W. Anderson, J. H. Ellenberg, C. M. Leventhal, S. C. Reingold, M. Rodriguez, and D. H. Silberberg, "Revised Estimate of the Prevalence of Multiple Sclerosis in the United States," *Ann Neurol*. 31, no. 3 (Mar. 1992): 333–36.

2. *Multiple Sclerosis Information Sourcebook*, produced by the Information Resource Center and Library of the National Multiple Sclerosis Society. © 2003 The National Multiple Sclerosis Society. All rights reserved. www.nationalmssociety.org/Sourcebook-Epidemiology.asp

3. M. Victor and A. H. Ropper, "Multiple Sclerosis and Allied Demyelinative Diseases," in *Adams and Victor's Principles of Neurology*, 7th ed. (New York: McGraw-Hill, 2001), 954–82.

4. W. I. McDonald, A. Compston, G. Edan, D. Goodkin, H. P. Hartung, F. D. Lublin, and H. F. McFarland, "Recommended Diagnostic Criteria for Multiple Sclerosis: Guidelines from the International Panel on the Diagnosis of Multiple Sclerosis," *Annals of Neurology* 50 (2001): 121–27.

5. E. Granieri, I. Casetta, M. R. Tola, and P. Ferrante, "Multiple Sclerosis: Infectious Hypothesis," *Neurol Sci*. 22, no. 2 (Apr. 2001): 179–85.

6. C. E. Hayes, M. T. Cantorna, and H. F. DeLuca, "Vitamin D and Multiple Sclerosis," *Proc Soc Exp Biol Med*. 216, no. 1 (Oct. 1997): 21–27.

7. C. E. Hayes, "Vitamin D: A Natural Inhibitor of Multiple Sclerosis," *Proc Nutr Soc*. 59, no. 4 (Nov. 2000): 531–35.

8. E. Garcion, L. Sindji, S. Nataf, P. Brachet, F. Darcy, and C. N. Montero-Menei, "Treatment of Experimental Autoimmune Encephalomyelitis in Rat by 1,25-Dihydroxyvitamin D3 Leads to Early Effects within the Central Nervous System," *Acta Neuropathol (Berl)* 105, no. 5 (May 2003): 438–48. Epub Jan 31, 2003.

9. P. Goldberg, M. C. Fleming, and E. H. Picard, "Multiple Sclerosis: Decreased Relapse Rate Through Dietary Supplementation with Calcium, Magnesium and Vitamin D," *Med Hypotheses* 21, no. 2 (Oct. 1986): 193–200.

10. E. H. Reynolds, "Multiple Sclerosis and Vitamin B12 Metabolism," *J Neuroimmunol*. 40, no. 2–3 (Oct. 1992): 225–30.

11. L. F. Vasconcellos, R. B. Correa, L. Chimelli, F. Nascimento, A. B. Fonseca, J. Nagel, S. A. Novis, and M. Vincent, "Myelopathy Due to Vitamin B12 Deficiency Presenting as Transverse Myelitis," *Arq Neuropsiquiatr*. 60, no. 1 (Mar. 2002): 150–54.

12. E. H. Reynolds, T. Bottiglieri, M. Laundy, R. F. Crellin, and S. G. Kirker, "Vitamin B12 Metabolism in Multiple Sclerosis," *Arch Neurol*. 49, no. 6 (June 1992): 649–52.

13. J. Kira, S. Tobimatsu, and I. Goto, "Vitamin B12 Metabolism and Massive-Dose Methyl Vitamin B12 Therapy in Japanese Patients with Multiple Sclerosis," *Intern Med*. 33, no. 2 (Feb. 1994): 82–86.

14. R. Sandyk and G. I. Awerbuch, "Vitamin B12 and Its Relationship to Age of Onset of Multiple Sclerosis," *Int J Neurosci*. 71, no. 1–4 (July–Aug. 1993): 93–99.

15. D. Konig, K. H. Wagner, I. Elmadfa, and A. Berg, "Exercise and Ooxidative Stress: Significance of Antioxidants with Reference to Inflammatory, Muscular, and Systemic Stress," *Exerc Immunol Rev* 7 (2001): 108–33.

16. T. R. Golden, D. A. Hinerfeld, and S. Melov, "Oxidative Stress and Aging: Beyond Correlation," *Aging Cell* 1, no. 2 (Dec. 2002): 117–23.

17. H. T. Besler, S. Comoglu, and Z. Okcu, "Serum Levels of Antioxidant Vitamins and Lipid Peroxidation in Multiple Sclerosis," *Nutr Neurosci*. 5, no. 3 (June 2002): 215–20.

18. H. T. Besler and S. Comoglu, "Lipoprotein Oxidation, Plasma Total Antioxidant

Capacity and Homocysteine Level in Patients with Multiple Sclerosis," *Nutr Neurosci.* 6, no. 3 (June 2003): 189–96.

19. S. Gueguen, P. Pirollet, P. Leroy, J. C. Guilland, J. Arnaud, F. Paille, G. Siest, S. Visvikis, S. Hercberg, and B. Herbeth, "Changes in Serum Retinol, Alpha-Tocopherol, Vitamin C, Carotenoids, Zinc and Aelenium after Micronutrient Supplementation during Alcohol Rehabilitation," *J Am Coll Nutr.* 22, no. 4 (Aug. 2003): 303–10.

20. D. Bates, "Dietary Lipids and Multiple Sclerosis," *Ups J Med Sci Suppl.* 48 (1990): 173–87.

21. R. H. Dworkin, D. Bates, J. H. Millar, and D. W. Paty, "Linoleic Acid and Multiple Sclerosis: A Reanalysis of Three Double-Blind Trials," *Neurology* 34, no. 11 (Nov. 1984): 1441–45.

22. I. Nordvik, K. M. Myhr, H. Nyland, and K. S. Bjerve, "Effect of Dietary Advice and N-3 Supplementation in Newly Diagnosed MS Patients," *Acta Neurol Scand.* 102, no. 3 (Sept. 2000): 143–49.

23. R. L. Swank and B. B. Dugan, "Effect of Low Saturated Fat Diet in Early and Late Cases of Multiple Sclerosis," *Lancet* 336, no. 8706 (July 7, 1990): 37–39.

24. W. E. Barbeau, "Interactions Between Dietary Proteins and the Human System: Implications for Oral Tolerance and Food-Related Diseases," *Adv Exp Med Biol.* 415 (1997): 183–93.

25. A. K. Stuifbergen, "Physical Activity and Perceived Health Status in Persons with Multiple Sclerosis," *J Neurosci Nurs.* 29, no. 4 (Aug. 1997): 238–43.

26. J. H. Koh, K. M. Kim, J. M. Kim, J. C. Song, and H. J. Suh, "Antifatigue and Antistress Effect of the Hot-water Fraction from Mycelia of Cordyceps sinensis," *Biol Pharm Bull.* 26, no. 5 (May 2003): 691–94.

27. S. Hiai, H. Yokoyama, H. Oura, and S. Yano, "Stimulation of Pituitary-Adrenocortical System by Ginseng Saponin," *Endocrinol Jpn* 26 (1979): 661–65.

28. J. E. Robbers, M. K. Speedie, and V. E. Tyler, *Pharmacognosy and Pharmacobiotechnology* (Baltimore, MD: Williams & Wilkins, 1996).

Oppositional Defiant Disorder

1. Children with Oppositional Defiant Disorder (1999). Copyright © 2004 by the American Academy of Child and Adolescent Psychiatry. www.aacap.org/publications/factsfam/72.htm.

2. K. D. Dykman and R. A. Dykman, "Effect of Nutritional Supplements on Attentional-Deficit Hyperactivity Disorder," *Integr Physiol Behav Sci.* 33, no. 1 (Jan.–Mar., 1998): 49–60.

3. L. Galland, "Nutritional Supplementation for ADHD," in *Attention Deficit Hyperactivity Disorder: Causes and Possible Solutions*, ed. J. A. Bellanti, W. G. Crook, and R. E. Layton (Jackson, TN: International Health Foundation, 1999).

4. S. J. Schoenthaler, "Nutritional Deficiencies and Behavior," in *Attention Deficit Hyperactivity Disorder: Causes and Possible Solutions*, ed. J. A. Bellanti, W. G. Crook, and R. E. Layton (Jackson, TN: International Health Foundation, 1999).

5. P. Toren, S. Eldar, B. A. Sela, L. Wolmer, R. Weitz, D. Inbar, S. Koren, A. Reiss, R. Weizman, and N. Laor, "Zinc Deficiency in Attention-Deficit Hyperactivity Disorder," *Biol Psychiatry* 40 (1996): 1308–10.

6. J. A. Cocores, R. K. Davies, P. S. Mueller, and M. S. Gold, "Cocaine Abuse and Adult Attention Deficit Disorder," *J Clin Psychiatry* 48, no. 9 (Sept. 1987): 376–77.

7. B. Starobrat-Hermelin and T. Kozielec, "The Effects of Magnesium Physiological Supplementation on Hyperactivity in Children with Attention Deficit Hyperactivity Disorder (ADHD): Positive Response to Magnesium Oral Loading Test," *Magnes Res.* 10, no. 2 (June 1997): 149–56.

8. B. Starobrat-Hermelin, "The Effect of Deficiency of Selected Bioelements on Hyperactivity in Children with Certain Specified Mental Disorders," *Ann Acad Med Stetin.* 44 (1998): 297–314.

9. A. Blokland, W. Honig, F. Brouns, and J. Jolles, "Cognition-Enhancing Properties of Subchronic Phosphatidylserine (PS) Treatment in Middle-Aged Rats: Comparison of Bovine Cortex PS with Egg PS and Soybean PS," *Nutrition* 15 (1999): 778–83.

10. P. M. Kidd, "A Review of Five Nutrients and Botanicals in the Integrative Management of Cognitive Dysfunction," *Altern Med Rev* 4 (1999): 144–61.

11. P. M. Kidd, "Attention Deficit/Hyperactivity Disorder (ADHD) in Children: Rationale for Its Integrative Management," *Altern Med Rev.* 5, no. 5 (Oct. 2000): 402–28.

12. T. H. Crook et al., "Effects of Phosphatidylserine in Age-Associated Memory Impairment," *Neurology* 41, no. 5 (1991): 644–49.

Parkinson's Disease

1. National Institute of Neurological Disorders and Stroke, "Parkinson's Disease Backgrounder" (2001). www.ninds.nih.gov/health_and_medical/pubs/parkinson's_disease_backgrounder.htm.

2. P. Jenner, "Oxidative Mechanisms in Nigral Cell Death in Parkinson's Disease. *Mov Disord* 13 (1998): S24–S34.

3. M. R. Werbach, *Nutritional Influences on Illness* (Tarzana, CA: Third Line Press, 1993).

4. S. Fahn, "A Pilot Trial of High-Dose Alphatocopherol and Ascorbate in Early Parkinson's Disease," *Ann Neurol* 32 (1992): S128–S32.

5. W. Sacks and G. M. Simpson, "Ascorbic Acid in Levodopa Therapy," *Lancet* 1 (1975): 527.

6. M. W. Fariss and J. G. Zhang, "Vitamin E Therapy in Parkinson's Disease," *Toxicology* 189, no. 1–2 (July 15, 2003): 129–46.

7. J. Lokk, "Treatment with Levodopa Can Affect Latent Vitamin B 12 and Folic Acid Deficiency. Patients with Parkinson Disease Run the Risk of Elevated Homocysteine Levels," *Lakartidningen* 100, no. 35 (Aug. 28, 2003): 2674–77.

8. D. A. Bender, C. J. Earl, and A. J. Lees "Niacin Depletion in Parkinsonian Patients Treated with L-Dopa, Benserazide and Carbidopa," *Clin Sci* 56 (1979): 89–93.

9. M. J. Black, and R. B. Brandt, "Nicotinic Acid or N-Methyl Nicotinamide Prolongs Elevated Brain Dopa and Dopamine in L-Dopa Treatment," *Biochem Med Metab Biol* 36 (1986): 244–51.

10. A. B. Baker, "Treatment of *Paralysis Agitans* with Vitamin B6 (Pyridoxine Hydrochloride)," *JAMA* (May 31, 1941): 2484–88; M. A. Zeligs, "Use of Pyridoxine Hydrochloride (Vitamin B6) in Parkinsonism, *JAMA* (May 10, 1941): 2148–49.

11. M. F. Beal, "Mitochondria, Oxidative Damage, and Inflammation in Parkinson's Disease," *Ann N Y Acad Sci.* 991 (June 2003): 120–31.

12. V. Di Matteo and E. Esposito, "Biochemical and Therapeutic Effects of Anti-

oxidants in the Treatment of Alzheimer's Disease, Parkinson's Disease, and Amyotrophic Lateral Sclerosis," *Curr Drug Target CNS Neurol Disord.* 2, no. 2 (Apr. 2003): 95–107.

13. M. E. Anderson, "Glutathione: An Overview of Biosynthesis and Modulation," *Chem Biol Interact* 24, no. 111–12 (1998): 1–14.

14. B. M. Lomaestro and M. Malone, "Glutathione in Health and Disease: Pharmacotherapeutic Issues," *Ann Pharmacother* 29, no. 12 (1995): 1263–73.

15. P. Riederer, E. Sofic, W. Rausch, B. Schmidt, G. P. Reynolds, K. Jellinger, and M. B. Youdim, "Transition Metals, Ferritin, Glutathione, and Ascorbic Acid in Parkinsonian Brains," *J Neurochem* 52 (1989): 515–20.

16. P. M. Kidd, "Parkinson's Disease as Multifactorial Oxidative Neurodegeneration: Implications for Integrative Management," *Alt Med Review* 5, no. 6 (2000): 502–29.

17. G. Sechi, M. G. Deledda, G. Bua, W. M. Satta, G. A. Deiana, G. M. Pes, and G. Rosati, "Reduced Intravenous Glutathione in the Treatment of Early Parkinson's Disease," *Progr Neuropsychopharmacol Biol Psychiatry* 20 (1996): 1159–70.

18. S. Greenberg and W. H. Fishman, "Coenzyme Q10: A New Drug for Cardiovascular Disease," *J Clin Pharmacol* 30 (1990): 596–608.

19. T. Muller, T. Buttner, A. F. Gholipour, and W. Kuhn, "Coenzyme Q10 Supplementation Provides Mild Symptomatic Benefit in Patients with Parkinson's Disease," *Neurosci Lett.* 341, no. 3 (May 8, 2003): 201–4.

20. C. W. Shults, D. Oakes, K. Kieburtz, M. F. Beal, R. Haas, S. Plumb, J. L. Juncos, et al., "Parkinson Study Group. Effects of Coenzyme Q10 in Early Parkinson Disease: Evidence of Slowing of the Functional Decline," *Arch Neurol.* 59, no. 10 (Oct. 2002): 1541–50.

21. J. Wajsbort, "The 'Off-On' Phenomenon During Treatment of Parkinson's Disease with Levodopa," *J Neurol.* 215, no. 1 (Apr. 28, 1977): 59–66.

22. I. Mena I and G. C. Cotzias, "Protein Intake and Treatment of Parkinson's Disease with Levodopa," *New Engl J Med* 292 (1975): 181–84.

23. J. H. Carter, J. G. Nutt, W. R. Woodward, L. F. Hatcher, T. L. Trotman, "Amount and Distribution of Dietary Protein Affects Clinical Response to Levodopa in Parkinson's Disease," *Neurology* 39, no. 4 (Apr. 1989): 552–56.

24. J. K. Tsui, S. Ross, K. Poulin, J. Douglas, D. Postnikoff, S. Calne, W. Woodward, and D. B. Calne, "The Effect of Dietary Protein on the Efficacy of L-Dopa: A Double-Blind Study," *Neurology* 39 (1989): 549–52.

25. T. Yamaguchi, T. Nagatsu, T. Sugimoto, S. Matsuura, T. Kondo, R. Iizuka, and H. Narabayashi, "Effects of Tyrosine Administration on Serum Biopterin in Normal Controls and Patients with Parkinson's Disease," *Science* 219, no. 4580 (Jan. 7, 1983): 75–77.

26. P. Lemoine, N. Robelin, P. Sebert, and J. Mouret, "L-Tyrosine: A Long-Term Treatment of Parkinson's Disease," *C R Acad Sci III* 309, no. 2 (1989): 43–47.

27. B. Heller, E. Fischer, and R. Martin, "Therapeutic Action of D-Phenylalanine in Parkinson's Disease," *Arzneimittelforschung* 26, no. 4 (Apr. 1976): 577–79.

28. J. Lehmann, "Tryptophan Malabsorption in Levodopa-Treated Parkinsonian Patients: Effect of Tryptophan on Mental Disturbances," *Acta Med Scand.* 194, no. 3 (1973): 181–89.

29. J. Lehmann, "Levodopa and Depression in Parkinsonism," *Lancet* 1 (1971): 140.

30. A. Coppen, M. Metcalfe, J. D. Carroll, and J. G. Morris, "Levodopa and L-Tryptophan Therapy in Parkinsonism," *Lancet* 1, no. 7752 (Mar. 25, 1972): 654–58.

31. B. J. Diamond, S. C. Shiflett, N. Feiwel, R. J. Matheis, O. Noskin, J. A. Richards,

and N. E. Schoenberger, "Ginkgo biloba Extract: Mechanisms and Clinical Indications," *Arch Phys Med Rehabil* 81 (2000): 668–78.

32. R. Swain and B. Kaplan-Machlis, "Magnesium for the Next Millennium," *South Med J* 92 (1999): 1040–47.

Schizophrenia

1. Society for Neuroscience, "Advancing the Understanding of the Brain and Nervous System" (2004). http://web.sfn.org/.

2. S. N. Young and A. M. Ghadirian, "Folic Acid and Psychopathology," *Prog Neuro psychopharmacol Biol Psychiatry* 13 (1989): 841–63.

3. M. Audebert, J. P. Gendre, and Y. Le Quintrec, "Folate and the Nervous System," *Sem Hop* 55 (1979): 1383–87.

4. K. Quinn and T. K. Basu, "Folate and Vitamin B12 Status of the Elderly," *Eur J Clin Nutr* 50 (1996): 340–42.

5. A. Procter, "Enhancement of Recovery from Psychiatric Illness by Methylfolate," *Br J Psychiatry* 159 (Aug. 1991): 271–72.

6. F. M. Freeman, J. D. Finkelstein, and S. H. Mudd, "Folate-Responsive Homocystinuria and 'Schizophrenia': A Defect in Methylation Due to Deficient 5,10-Methylenetetrahydrofolate Reductase Activity," *N Engl J Med.* 292, no. 10 (Mar. 6, 1975): 491–96.

7. P. A. Berger, G. R. Elliott, E. Erdelyi, S. J. Watson, R. J. Wyatt, and J. D. Barchas, "Platelet Methylene Reductase Activity in Schizophrenia," *Arch Gen Psychiatry* 34, no. 7 (July 1977): 808–9.

8. V. Lerner, C. Miodownik, A. Kaptsan, H. Cohen, U. Loewenthal, and M. Kotler, "Vitamin B6 as Add-On Treatment in Chronic Schizophrenic and Schizoaffective Patients: A Double-Blind, Placebo-Controlled Study," *J Clin Psychiatry* 63, no. 1 (Jan. 2002): 54–58.

9. R. Shiloh, A. Weizman, N. Weizer, P. Dorfman-Etrog, and H. Munitz, "Antidepressive Effect of Pyridoxine (Vitamin B6) in Neuroleptic-Treated Schizophrenic Patients with Co-Morbid Minor Depression—Preliminary Open-Label Trial," *Harefuah* 140, no. 5 (May 2001): 369–73, 456.

10. R. Sandyk and R. Pardeshi, "Pyridoxine Improves Drug-Induced Parkinsonism and Psychosis in a Schizophrenic Patient," *Int J Neurosci.* 52, no. 3–4 (June 1990): 225–32.

11. K. Suboticanec, V. Folnegovic-Smalc, M. Korbar, B. Mestrovic, and R. Buzina, "Vitamin C Status in Chronic Schizophrenia," *Biol Psychiatry* 28, no. 11 (Dec. 1, 1990): 959–66.

12. K. Suboticanec, V. Folnegovic-Smalc, R. Turcin, B. Mestrovic, and R. Buzina, "Plasma Levels and Urinary Vitamin C Excretion in Schizophrenic Patients," *Hum Nutr Clin Nutr.* 40, no. 6 (Nov. 1986): 421–28.

13. R. Sandyk and J. D. Kanofsky, "Vitamin C in the Treatment of Schizophrenia," *Int J Neurosci.* 68, no. 1–2 (Jan. 1993): 67–71.

14. A. Hoffer, "Safety, Side Effects and Relative Lack of Toxicity of Nicotinic Acid and Nicotinamide," 1 *Schizophrenia* (1969): 78–87.

15. H. Mohler, P. Polc, R. Cumin, L. Pieri, and R. Kettler. "Nicotinamide Is a Brain Constituent with Benzodiazepine-Like Actions," *Nature* 278 (1979): 563–65.

16. D. F. Horrobin, "Schizophrenia as a Membrane Lipid Disorder Which Is Expressed Throughout the Body," *Prostaglandins Leukot Essent Fatty Acids* 55, no. 1–2 (Aug. 1996): 3–7.

17. M. Peet, "Eicosapentaenoic Acid in the Treatment of Schizophrenia and Depression: Rationale and Preliminary Double-Blind Clinical Trial Results," *Prostaglandins Leukot Essent Fatty Acids* 69, no. 6 (Dec. 2003): 477–85.

18. P. D. Skosnik and J. K. Yao, "From Membrane Phospholipid Defects to Altered Neurotransmission: Is Arachidonic Acid a Nexus in the Pathophysiology of Schizophrenia?" *Prostaglandins Leukot Essent Fatty Acids* 69, no. 6 (Dec. 2003): 367–84.

19. M. Arvindakshan, M. Ghate, P. K. Ranjekar, D. R. Evans, S. P. Mahadik, "Supplementation with a Combination of Omega-3 Fatty Acids and Antioxidants (Vitamins E and C) Improves the Outcome of Schizophrenia," *Schizophr Res*. no. 3 (Aug. 1, 2003): 195–204.

20. C. B. Joy, R. Mumby-Croft, and L. A. Joy, "Polyunsaturated Fatty Acid (Fish or Evening Primrose Oil) for Schizophrenia," *Cochrane Database Syst Rev.* 2 (2000): CD001257.

PART II: MOST COMMON BRAIN-TARGETED NUTRA-BOTANICALS

B-1

1. M. H. Beers and R. Berkow, *The Merck Manual of Diagnosis and Therapy,* 17th ed. (West Point, PA: Merck, 1999).

2. M. M. Murray, *Encyclopedia of Nutritional Supplements* (Rocklin, CA: Prima Publishing, 1996), 80–83.

3. M.W.P. Carner, "Vitamin Deficiency and Mental Symptoms," *Br J Psychiatr* 156 (1990): 878–82.

4. G. K. McKevoy, ed., *AHFS Drug Information* (Bethesda, MD: American Society of Health-System Pharmacists, 1998).

5. K. J. Meador, M. E. Nichols, P. Franke , M. W. Durkin, R. L. Oberzan, E. E. Moore, and D. W. Loring. "Evidence for a Central Cholinergic Effect of High Doses Thiamine," *Ann Neurol* 34 (1993): 724–26.

6. D. Benton, J. Fordy, and J. Haller, "The Impact of Long-Term Vitamin Supplementation on Cognitive Functioning," *Psychopharmacol* 117 (1995): 298–305.

7. M. I. Boetz, T. Botez, A. Ross-Chouinard, R. Lalonde, "Thiamine and Folate Treatment of Chronic Epileptic Patients: A Controlled Study with the Wechsler IQ Scale," *Epilepsy Res* 16 (1993): 157–63.

B-2

1. G. K. McKevoy, ed., *AHFS Drug Information* (Bethesda, MD: American Society of Halth-System Pharmacists, 1998).

2. Micromedex Healthcare Series, *AltMedDex® System: Comprehensive Referenced Data on Herbal Medicines and Dietary Supplements Covering Uses, Efficacy, Dosing, Toxicity, and More*" (Englewood, CO: MICROMEDEX Inc.).

3. S. M. Fishman, P. Christian, and K. P. West, "The Role of Vitamins in the Prevention and Control of Anemia," *Public Health Nutr* 3 (2000): 125–50.

4. J. Schoenen, M. Lenaerts, and E. Bastings, "High-Dose Riboflavin as a Prophylactic Treatment of Migraine: Results of an Open Pilot Study," *Cephalalgia* 14, no. 5 (1994): 328–29.

5. R. G. Cumming, P. Mitchell, and W. Smith, "Diet and Cataract: The Blue Mountains Eye Study," *Ophthalmology* 10 (2000): 450–56.

6. O. A. Ajayi, B. O. George, and T. Ipadeola, "Clinical Trial of Riboflavin in Sickle Cell Disease," *East Afr Med J.* 70, no. 7 (July 1993): 418–21.

7. M. Durusoy, E. Karagoz, and K. Ozturk, "Assessment of the Relationship Between the Antimutagenic Action of Riboflavin and Glutathione and the Levels of Antioxidant Enzymes," *J Nutr Biochem.* 13, no. 10 (Oct. 2002): 598–602.

8. J. Zempleni, J. R. Galloway, and D. B. McCormick, "Pharmacokinetics of Orally and Intravenously Administered Riboflavin in Healthy Humans," *Am J Clin Nutr.* 63, no. 1 (Jan. 1996): 54–66.

B-3

1. National Cholesterol Education Program, "Cholesterol Lowering in the Patient with Coronary Heart Disease." www.nhlbi.nih.gov/health/prof/heart/chol/chol_low.pdf.

2. G. K. McKevoy, ed., *AHFS Drug Information* (Bethesda, MD: American Society of Health-System Pharmacists, 1998).

3. Food and Nutrition Board, Institute of Medicine, *Dietary Reference Intakes for Thiamin, Riboflavin, Niacin, Vitamin B6, Folate, Vitamin B12, Pantothenic Acid, Biotin, and Choline* (Washington, DC: National Academy Press, 2000). http://books.nap.edu/books/0309065542/html/.

4. C. J. Hudson, A. Lin, S. Cogan, F. Cashman, and J. J. Warsh, "The Niacin Challenge Test: Clinical Manifestation of Altered Transmembrane Signal Transduction in Schizophrenia?" *Biol Psychiatry* 41 (1997): 507–13.

5. J. M. McKenney, J. D. Proctor, S. Harris, and V. M. Chinchili, "A Comparison of the Efficacy and Toxic Effects of Sustained- vs Immediate-Release Niacin in Hypercholesterolemic Patients," *JAMA* 271 (1994): 672–87.

6. H. Kolb and V. Burkart, "Nicotinamide in Type 1 Diabetes: Mechanism of Action Revisited," *Diabetes Care* 22 (1999): B16–B20.

7. E. A. Gale, "Theory and Practice of Nicotinamide Trials in Pre-Type 1 Diabetes," *J Pediatr Endocrinol Metab* 9 (1996): 375–79.

B-5

1. Micromedex Healthcare Series. *AltMedDex® System: Comprehensive Referenced Data on Herbal Medicines and Dietary Supplements Covering Uses, Efficacy, Dosing, Toxicity, and More* (Englewood, CO: MICROMEDEX Inc.).

2. A. Gaddi, G. C. Descovich, G. Noseda, C. Fragiacomo, L. Colombo, A. Craveri, G. Montanari, and C. R. Sirtori, "Controlled Evaluation of Pantethine, a Natural Hypolipidemic Compound, in Patients with Different Forms of Hyperlipoproteinemia," *Atherosclerosis* 50, no. 1 (Jan. 1984): 73–83.

3. G. Cighetti, M. Del Puppo, R. Paroni, E. Fiorica, and M. Galli Kienle, "Pantethine Inhibits Cholesterol and Fatty Acid Syntheses and Stimulates Carbon Dioxide Formation in Isolated Rat Hepatocytes," *J Lipid Res.* 28, no. 2 (Feb. 1987): 152–61.

4. L. Arsenio, P. Bodria, G. Magnati, A. Strata, and R. Trovato, "Effectiveness of Long-Term Treatment with Pantethine in Patients with Dyslipidemia," *Clin Ther.* 8, no. 5 (1986): 537–45.

5. P. C. Fry, H. M. Fox, and H. G. Tao, "Metabolic Response to a Pantothenic Acid Deficient Diet in Humans," *J Nutr Sci Vitaminol* (Tokyo) 22, no. 4 (1976): 339–46.

6. J. H. Cummings and G. Macfarlane, "Role of Intestinal Bacteria in Nutrient Metabolism," *J Parenter Enteral Nutr* 21, no. 6 (1997): 357–65.

7. E. C. Barton-Wright and W. A. Elliott, "The Pantothenic Acid Metabolism of Rheumatoid Arthritis," *Lancet* 38 (Oct. 26, 1963): 862–63.

B-6

1. G. K. McKevoy, ed., *AHFS Drug Information* (Bethesda, MD: American Society of Health-System Pharmacists, 1998).

2. E. L. Mayer, D. W. Jacobsen, K. Robinson, "Homocysteine and Coronary Atherosclerosis," *J Am Coll Cardiol* 27 (1996): 517–27.

3. V. Lerner, C. Miodownik, A. Kaptsan, H. Cohen, M. Matar, U. Loewenthal, and M. Kotler, "Vitamin B(6) in the Treatment of Tardive Dyskinesia: A Double-blind, Placebo-Controlled, Crossover Study," *Am J Psychiatry* 158 (2001): 1511–14.

4. A. S. Prasad, K. Y. Lei, K. S. Moghissi, J. C. Stryker, and D. Oberleas, "Effect of Oral Contraceptives on Nutrients. III. Vitamins B6, B12 and Folic Acid," *Am J Obstet Gynecol* 125 (1976): 1063–69.

5. R. Delport, J. B. Ubbink, W. J. Serfontein, P. J. Becker, and L. Walters, "Vitamin B6 Nutritional Status in Asthma: The Effect of Theophylline Therapy on Plasma Pyridoxal-5-Phosphate and Pyridoxal Levels," *Int J Vitam Nutr Res* 58 (1988): 67–72.

6. M. M. Murray, *Encyclopedia of Nutritional Supplements* (Rocklin, CA: Prima Publishing, 1996), 100–110.

7. S. Friso, P. F. Jacques, P. W. Wilson, et al., "Low Circulating Vitamin B(6) Is Associated with Elevation of the Inflammation Marker C-Reactive Protein Independently of Plasma Homocysteine Levels," *Circulation* 103 (2001): 2788–91.

8. S. I. Pfeiffer, J. Norton, L. Nelson, and S. Shott, "Efficacy of Vitamin B6 and Magnesium in the Treatment of Autism: A Methodology Review and Summary of Outcomes," *J Autism Dev Disord.* 25, no. 5 (Oct. 1995): 481–93.

9. B. T. Nobbs, "Pyridoxal Phosphate Status in Clinical Depression," *Lancet* 1, no. 7854 (Mar. 9, 1974): 405–6.

10. G. F. Crowell and E. S. Roach, "Pyridoxine-Dependent Seizures," *Am Fam Physician* 27, no. 3 (Mar. 19833): 183–87.

11. M. Coleman, G. Steinberg, J. Tippett, H. N. Bhagavan, D. B. Coursin, M. Gross, C. Lewis, L. DeVeau, "A Preliminary Study of the Effect of Pyridoxine Administration in a Subgroup of Hyperkinetic Children: A Double-Blind Crossover Comparison with Methylphenidate," *Biol Psych* 14 (1979): 741–51.

12. M. Cohen and A. Bendich, "Safety of Pyridoxine—A Review of Human and Animal Studies," *Toxicol Lett.* 34, no. 2–3 (Dec. 1986): 129–39.

B-12

1. G. K. McKevoy, ed., *AHFS Drug Information* (Bethesda, MD: American Society of Health-System Pharmacists, 1998).

2. A. M. Kuzminski, E. J. Del Giacco, R. H. Allen, S. P. Stabler, and J. Lindenbaum, "Effective Treatment of Cobalamin Deficiency with Oral Cobalamin," *Blood* 92 (1998): 1191–98.

3. J. Selhub, P. F. Jacques, P. W. Wilson, D. Rush, I. H. Rosenberg, "Vitamin Status and Intake as Primary Determinants of Homocysteinemia in an Elderly Population," *JAMA* 270, no. 22 (1993): 2693–98.

4. B. W. Penninx, J. M. Guralnik, L. Ferrucci, L. P. Fried, R. H. Allen, and S. P. Stabler, "Vitamin B(12) Deficiency and Depression in Physically Disabled Older Women: Epidemiologic Evidence From the Women's Health and Aging Study," *Am J Psychiatry* 157 (2000): 715–21.

5. R. Clarke, "Prevention of Vitamin B-12 Deficiency in Old Age," *Am J Clin Nutr.* 73 (2001): 151–52.

6. J. Lindenbaum, E. B. Healton, D. G. Savage, J. Lindenbaum, E. B. Healton, D. G. Savage, J. C. Brust, et al. "Neuropsychiatric Disorders Caused by Cobalamin Deficiency in the Absence of Anemia or Macrocytosis," *N Engl J Med.* 318 (1988): 1720–28.

7. R. Carmel, R. Green, D. W. Jacobsen, K. Rasmussen, M. Florea, C. Azen. "Serum Cobalamin, Homocysteine, and Methylmalonic Acid Concentrations in a Multiethnic Elderly Population: Ethnic and Sex Differences in Cobalamin and Metabolite Abnormalities," *Am J Clin Nutr* 70, no. 5 (1999): 904–10.

8. F. Abalan, G. Subra, M. Picard, and P. Boueilh, "Incidence of Vitamin B 12 and Folic Acid Deficiencies on Old Aged Psychiatric Patients," *Encephale.* 10, no. 1 (1984): 9–12.

9. M. M. Murray, *Encyclopedia of Nutritional Supplements* Prima Publishing, Rocklin, CA. 1996), P. 134.

10. R. J. Leeming, J. P. Harpey, S. M. Brown, and J. A. Blair, "Tetrahydrofolate and Hydroxocobolamin in the Management of Dihydropteridine Reductase Deficiency," *J Ment Defic Res.* 26, pt. 1 (Mar. 1982): 21–25.

Dimethylglycine (DMG)

1. W. J. Freed, "N,N-dimethylglycine, Betaine and Seizures," *Arch Neurol* 41 (1984): 1129–30.

2. E. A. Reap and J. W. Lawson, "Stimulation of the Immune Response by Dimethylglycine, a Nontoxic Metabolite," *J Lab Clin Med* 115, no. 4 (1990): 481–86.

3. E. S. Roach and L. Carlin, "N,N dimethylglycine for Epilepsy," *N Engl J Med* 307 (1982): 1081–82.

4. J. K. Kern, V. S. Miller, P. L. Cauller, P. R. Kendall, P. J. Mehta, and M. Dodd, "Effectiveness of N,N-dimethylglycine in Autism and Pervasive Developmental Disorder," *J Child Neurol.* 16, no. 3 (Mar. 2001): 169–73.

Docosahexaenoic Acid (DHA)

1. P. C. Calder, "N-3 Polyunsaturated Fatty acids, Inflammation and Immunity: Pouring Oil on Troubled Waters or Another Fishy Tale?" *Nutr Res* 21 (2001): 309–41.

2. J. A. Conquer and B. J. Holub, "Supplementation with an Algae Source of Docosahexaenoic Acid Increases (N-3) Fatty Acid Status and Alters Selected Risk Factors for Heart Disease in Vegetarian Subjects," *J Nutr* 126 (1996): 3032–39.

3. R. A. Gibson, "Long-Chain Polyunsaturated Fatty Acids and Infant Development," *Lancet* 354 (1999): 1919.

4. T. Moriguchi, R. S. Greiner, and N. Salem Jr., "Behavioral Deficits Associated with Dietary Induction of Decreased Brain Docosahexaenoic Acid Concentration," *J of Neurochem* 75 (2000): 2563–73.

5. S. Gamoh, M. Hashimoto, K. Sugioka, et al., "Chronic Administration of Docosa-

hexaenoic Acid Improves Reference Memory-Related Learning Ability in Young Rats," *Neuroscience* 93 (1999): 237–41.

6. P. Wainwright, "Nutrition and Behaviour: The Role of N-3 Fatty acids in Cognitive Function," *Br J Nutr* 83 (2000): 337–39.

7. J. J. Agren, O. Hanninen, A. Julkunen, L. Fogelholm, H. Vidgren, U. Schwab, O. Pynnonen, and M. Uusitupa, "Fish Diet, Fish Oil and Docosahexaenoic Acid Rich Oil LowerF and Postprandial Plasma Lipid Levels," *Eur J Clin Nutr* 50 (1996): 765–71.

8. T. A. Mori, V. Burke, I. B. Puddey, G. F. Watts, D. N. O'Neal, J. D. Best, and L. J. Eilin, "Purified Eicosapentaenoic and Docosahexaenoic Acids Have Differential Effects on Serum Lipids and Lipoproteins, LDL Particle Size, Glucose, and Insulin in Mildly Hyperlipidemic Men," *Am J Clin Nutr* 71 (2000): 1085–94.

9. G. J. Nelson, P. S. Schmidt, G. L. Bartolini, D. S. Kelley, and D. Kyle, "The Effect of Dietary Docosahexaenoic Acid on Platelet Function, Platelet Fatty Acid Composition, and Blood Coagulation in Humans," *Lipids* 32 (1997): 1129–36.

10. E. C. Van den Ham, A. C. vans Houwelingen, and G. Hornstra, "Evaluation of the Relation between N-3 and N-6 Fatty Acid Status and Parity in Nonpregnant Women from the Netherlands," *Am J Clin Nutr* 73 (2001): 622–27.

11. T. Hamazaki, S. Sawazaki, M. Itomura, E. Asaoka, Y. Nagao, N. Nishimura, K. Yazawa, T. Kuwamori, and M. Kobayashi, "The Effect of Docosahexaenoic Acid on Aggression in Young Adults: A Placebo-Controlled Double-Blind Study," *J Clin Invest* 97 (1996): 1129–33.

12. S. E. Carlson and S. H. Werkman, "A Randomized Trial of Visual Attention of Preterm Infants Fed Docosahexaenoic Acid Until Two Months," *Lipids* 31 (1996): 85–90.

13. B. J. Stordy, "Dark Adaptation, Motor Skills, Docosahexaenoic Acid, and Dyslexia," *Am J Clin Nutr* 71 (2000): 323S–26S.

14. R. A. Gibson, "Long-Chain Polyunsaturated Fatty Acids and Infant Development," *Lancet* 354 (1999): 1919.

15. A. T. Erkkila, S. Lehto, K. Pyorala, and M. I. Uusitupa, "N-3 Fatty Acids and 5-y Risks of Death and Cardiovascular Disease Events in Patients with Coronary Artery Disease," *Am J Clin Nutr* 78 (2003): 65–71.

Eicosapentaenoic Acid (EPA)

1. P. C. Calder, "N-3 Polyunsaturated Fatty Acids, Inflammation and Immunity: Pouring Oil on Troubled Waters or Another Fishy Tale?" *Nutr Res* 21 (2001): 309–41.

2. B. Nemets, Z. Stahl, and R. H. Belmaker, "Addition of Omega-3 Fatty Acid to Maintenance Medication Treatment for Recurrent Unipolar Depressive Disorder," *Am J Psychiatry* 159 (2002): 477–79.

3. T. A. Mori, V. Burke, I. B. Puddey, G. F. Watts, D. N. O'Neal, J. D. Best, and L. J. Beilin, "Purified Eicosapentaenoic and Docosahexaenoic Acids Have Differential Effects on Serum Lipids and Lipoproteins, LDL Particle Size, Glucose, and Insulin in Mildly Hyperlipidemic Men," *Am J Clin Nutr* 71 (2000): 1085–94.

4. R. J. Woodman, T. A. Mori, V. Burke, I. B. Puddey, G. F. Watts, and L. J. Beilin, "Effects of Purified Eicosapentaenoic and Docosahexaenoic Acids on Glycemic Control, Blood Pressure, and Serum Lipids in Type 2 Diabetic Patients with Treated Hypertension," *Am J Clin Nutr* 76 (2002): 1007–15.

5. T. Terano, A. Hirai, T. Hamazaki, S. Kobayashi, T. Fujita, Y. Tamura, and A.

Kumagai, "Effect of Oral Administration of Highly Purified Eicosapentaenoic Acid on Platelet Function, Blood Viscosity and Red Cell Deformability in Healthy Human Subjects," *Atherosclerosis* 46 (1983): 321–31.

6. M. C. Zanarini and F. R. Frankenburg, "Omega-3 Fatty Acid Treatment of Women with Borderline Personality Disorder: A Double-Blind, Placebo-Controlled Pilot Study," *Am J Psychiatry* 160 (2003): 167–69.

7. A. T. Erkkila, S. Lehto, K. Pyorala, and M. I. Uusitupa, "N-3 Fatty Acids and 5-y Risks of Death and Cardiovascular Disease Events in Patients with Coronary Artery Disease," *Am J Clin Nutr* 78 (2003): 65–71.

8. T. Pischon, S. E. Hankinson, G. S. Hotamisligil, N. Rifai, W. C. Willett, and E. B. Rimm, "Habitual Dietary Intake of N-3 and N-6 Fatty Acids in Relation to Inflammatory Markers among US Men and Women," *Circulation* 108, no. 2 (July 15, 2003): 155–60.

5-Hydroxytryptophan (5-HTP)

1. H. M. van Praag and C. Lemus, "Monoamine Precursors in the Treatment of Psychiatric Disorders," in *Nutrition and the Brain*, ed. R. J. Wurtman and J. J. Wurtman (New York: Raven Press; 1986), 89–139; J. A. den Boer and H. G. Westenberg, "Behavioral, Neuroendocrine, and Biochemical Effects of 5-hydroxytryptophan Administration in Panic Disorder," *Psychiatry Res* 31 (1990): 267–78; D. Chadwick, P. Jenner, R. Harris, et al., "Manipulation of Brain Serotonin in the Treatment of Myoclonus," *Lancet* 2 (1975): 434–35; C. Guilleminault, B. R. Tharp, and D. Cousin, "HVA and 5HIAA CSF Measurements and 5HTP Trials in Some Patients with Involuntary Movements, *J Neurol Sci* 18 (1973): 435–41.

2. M. G. Simic, M. al-Sheikhly, and S. V. Jovanovic, "Inhibition of Free Radical Processes by Antioxidants—Tryptophan and 5-hydroxytryptophan," *Bibl Nutr Dieta* 43 (1989): 288–96.

3. K. Shaw, J. Turner, and C. Del Mar, "Tryptophan and 5-hydroxytryptophan for Depression," *Cochrane Database Syst Rev* 1 (2002): CD003198.

4. T. C. Birdsall, "5-Hydroxytryptophan: A Clinically-Effective Serotonin Precursor," *Altern Med Rev* 3, no. 4 (1998): 271–80.

5. T. Nakajima, Y. Kudo, and Z. Kaneko, "Clinical Evaluation of 5-hydroxy-L-tryptophan as an Antidepressant Drug," *Folia Psychiatr Neurol Jpn* 32, no. 2 (1978): 223–30.

6. A. Coppen, P. C. Whybrow, R. Noguera, R. Magg, and A. J. Prange, Jr., "The Comparative Antidepressant Value of L-tryptophan and Imipramine With and Without Attempted Potentiation by Liothyronine," *Arch Gen Psychiatr* 26, no. 3 (1972): 234–41.

7. W. Poldinger, B. Calanchini, and W. Schwarz, "A Functional-Dimensional Approach to Depression: Serotonin Deficiency as a Target Syndrome in a Comparison of 5-hydroxytryptophan and Fluvoxamine," *Psychopathology* 24 (1991): 53–81.

Folate

1. C. W. Suitor and L. B. Bailey, "Dietary Folate Equivalents: Interpretation and Application," *J Am Diet Assoc* 100 (2000): 88–94.

2. J. Loscalzo, "Folate and Nitrate-Induced Endothelial Dysfunction: A Simple Treatment for a Complex Pathobiology," *Circulation* 104 (2001): 1086–88.

3. T. Bottiglieri, K. Hyland, and E. H. Reynolds, "The Clinical Potential of

Ademetionine (S-adenosylmethionine) in Neurological Disorders," *Drugs* 48 (1994): 137–52.

4. S. Voutilainen, T. A. Lakka, E. Porkkala-Sarataho, T. Rissanen, G. A. Kaplan, and J. T. Salonen, "Low Serum Folate Concentrations Are Associated with an Excess Incidence of Acute Coronary Events: The Kuopio Ischaemic Heart Disease Risk Factor Study," *Eur J Clin Nutr* 54 (2000): 424–28.

5. D. A. Snowdon, C. L. Tully, C. D. Smith, K. P. Riley, and W. R. Markesbery, "Serum Folate and the Severity of Atrophy of the Neocortex in Alzheimer Disease: Findings from the Nun Study," *Am J Clin Nutr* 71 (2000): 993–98.

6. A. D. Smith, "Homocysteine, B Vitamins, and Cognitive Deficit in the Elderly," *Am J Clin Nutr* 75 (2002): 785–86.

7. R. M. Ortega, L. R. Manas, P. Andres, M. J. Gaspar, F. R. Agudo, A. Jimenez, and T. Pascual, "Functional and Psychic Deterioration in Elderly People May Be Aggravated by Folate Deficiency," *J Nutr* 126 (1996): 1992–99.

8. H. Tiemeier, H. R. van Tuijl, A. Hofman, J. Meijer, A. J. Kiliaan, and M. M. Breteler, "Vitamin B12, Folate, and Homocysteine in Depression: The Rotterdam Study," *Am J Psychiatry* 159 (2002): 2099–101.

9. M. Alpert, R. R. Silva, and E. R. Pouget, "Prediction of Treatment Response in Geriatric Depression from Baseline Folate Level: Interaction with an SSRI or a Tricyclic Antidepressant," *J Clin Psychopharmacol* 23 (2003): 309–13.

10. M. S. Morris, M. Fava, P. F. Jacques, J. Selhub, and I. H. Rosenberg, "Depression and Folate Status in the U.S. Population," *Psychother Psychosom* 72 (2003): 80–87.

11. R. F. Huang, Y. Ho, H. Lin, J. S. Wei, and T. Z. Liu. "Folate Deficiency Induces a Cell Cycle-Specific Apoptosis in HepG2 Cells," *J Nutr* 129 (1999): 25–31.

12. L. B. Bailey, *Folate in Health and Disease* (New York: Marcel Dekker, 1995).

Ginkgo biloba

1. P. L. Le Bars, M. M. Katz, N. Berman, T. M. Itil, A. M. Freedman, and A. F. Schatzberg, "A Placebo-Controlled, Double-Blind, Randomized Trial of an Extract of Ginkgo biloba for Dementia," North American EGb Study Group. *JAMA* 278 (Oct. 22, 1997): 1327–32.

2. B. S. Oken, D. M. Storzbach, and J. A. Kaye, "The Efficacy of Ginkgo biloba on Cognitive Function in Alzheimer's Disease," *Arch Neurol* 55 (1998): 1409–15.

3. S. Logani, M. C. Chen, T. Tran, T. Le, and R. B. Raffa, "Actions of Ginkgo biloba Related to Potential Utility for the Treatment of Conditions Involving Cerebral Hypoxia," *Life Sciences* 67 (2000): 1389–96.

4. G. B. Kudolo, "The Effect of 3-Month Ingestion of Ginkgo biloba Extract on Pancreatic Beta-Cell Function in Response to Glucose Loading in Normal Glucose Tolerant Individuals," *J Clin Pharmacol* 40 (2000): 647–54.

5. S. Bastianetto, C. Ramassamy, S. Dore, Y. Christen, J. Poirier, and R. Quirion, "The Ginkgo biloba Extract (EGb 761) Protects Hippocampal Neurons Against Cell Death Induced by Beta-amyloid," *Eur J Neurosci* 12 (2000): 1882–90.

6. P. L. Le Bars, M. Kieser, and K. Z. Itil, "A 26-Week Analysis of a Double-Blind, Placebo-Controlled Trial of the Ginkgo biloba Extract EGb 761 in Dementia," *Dement Geriatr Cogn Disord* 11 (2000): 230–37.

7. S. Logani, M. C. Chen, T. Tran, T. Le, and R. B. Raffa, "Actions of Ginkgo biloba Related to Potential Utility for the Treatment of Conditions Involving Cerebral Hypoxia," *Life Sciences* 67 (2000): 1389–96.

8. S. Kanowski, W. M. Herrmann, K. Stephan, W. Wierich, and R. Horr, "Proof of Efficacy of the Ginkgo biloba Special Extract (EGb 761) in Outpatients Suffering from Mild to Moderate Primary Degenerative Dementia of the Alzheimer Type or Multi-Infarct Dementia," *Pharmacopsych* 29 (1996): 47–56.

9. M. R. Brautigam, F. A. Blommaert, and G. Verleye, "Treatment of Age-Related Memory Complaints with Ginkgo biloba Extract: A Randomized Double-Blind Placebo-Controlled Study," *Phytomedicine* 5 (1998): 425–34.

10. J. A. Mix and W. D. Crews, "A Double-Blind, Placebo-Controlled, Randomized Trial of Ginkgo biloba Extract EGb 761 in a Sample of Cognitively Intact Older Adults: Neuropsychological Findings," *Hum Psychopharmacol* 17 (2002): 267–77.

11. J. Schweizer and C. Hautmann, "Comparison of Two Dosages of Ginkgo biloba Extract Egb 761 in Patients with Peripheral Arterial Occlusive Disease Fontain's Stage llb: A Randomized, Double-Blind, Multicentric Clinical Ttrial," *Arzneimittelforschung* 49 (1999): 900–904.

12. K. A. Wesnes, T. Ward, A. McGinty, and O. Petrini, "The Memory Enhancing Effects of a Ginkgo biloba/Panax Ginseng Combination in Healthy Middle-Aged Volunteers," *Psychopharmacology* 152 (2000): 353–61.

Ginseng

1. A. Y. Leung and S. Foster, *Encyclopedia of Common Natural Ingredients Used in Food, Drugs and Cosmetics*, 2nd ed. (New York: John Wiley & Sons, 1996).

2. X. Wang, T. Sakuma, E. Asafu-Adjaye, and G. K. Shiu, "Determination of Ginsenosides in Plant Extracts from Panax Ginseng and Panax quinquefolius L. by LC/MS/MS," *Anal Chem* 71 (1999): 1579–84.

3. C. A. Newall, L. A. Anderson, and J. D. Philpson, *Herbal Medicine: A Guide for Healthcare Professionals* (London: The Pharmaceutical Press, 1996).

4. C. G. Benishin, R. Lee, L. C. Wang, and H. J. Liu, "Effects of Ginsenoside Rb1 on Central Cholinergic Metabolism," *Pharmacology* 42 (1991): 223–29.

5. P. Luo and L. Wang, "Peripheral Blood Mononuclear Cell Production of TNF-Alpha in Response to North American Ginseng Stimulation," *Alt Ther* 7 (2001): S21.

6. V. Vuksan, J. L. Sievenpiper, V. Y. Koo, T. Francis, U. Beljan-Zdravkovic, Z. Xu, and E. Vidgen, "American Ginseng (Panax quinquefolius L) Reduces Postprandial Glycemia in Nondiabetic Subjects and Subjects with Type 2 Diabetes Mellitus," *Arch Intern Med* 160 (2000): 1009–13.

7. M. R. Lyon, J. C. Cline, J. Totosy de Zepetnek, J. J. Shan, P. Pang, and C. Benishin, "Effect of the Herbal Extract Combination Panax quinquefolium and Ginkgo biloba on Attention-Deficit Hyperactivity Disorder: A Pilot Study," *J Psychiatry Neurosci* 26 (2001): 221–28.

8. A. Y. Leung and S. Foster, *Encyclopedia of Common Natural Ingredients Used in Food, Drugs and Cosmetics*, 2nd ed. (New York: John Wiley & Sons, 1996).

9. R. Lewis, G. Wake, G. Court, J. A. Court, A. T. Pickering, Y. C. Kim, and E. K. Perry, "Non-Ginsenoside Nicotinic Activity in Ginseng Species," *Phytother Res* 13 (1999): 59–64.

10. S. Hiai, H. Yokoyama, H. Oura, and S. Yano, "Stimulation of Pituitary-Adrenocortical System by Ginseng saponin," *Endocrinol Jpn* 26 (1979): 661–65.

11. T. Tode, Y. Kikuchi, J. Hirata, T. Kita, H. Nakata, and I. Nagata, "Effect of Ko-

rean Red Ginseng on Psychological Functions in Patients with Severe Climacteric Syndromes," *Int J Gynaecol Obstet* 67 (1999): 169–74.

12. H. Sorensen and J. Sonne, "A Double-Masked Study of the Effects of Ginseng on Cognitive Functions," *Curr Ther Res* 57 (1996): 959–68.

13. K. A. Wesnes, T. Ward, A. McGinty, and O. Petrini, "The Memory Enhancing Effects of a Ginkgo biloba/Panax ginseng Combination in Healthy Middle-Aged Volunteers," *Psychopharmacology* 152 (2000): 353–61.

14. E. A. Sotaniemi, E. Haapakoski, and A. Rautio, "Ginseng Therapy in Non-Insulin Dependent Diabetic Patients," *Diabetes Care* 18 (1995): 1373–75.

15. F. Scaglione, G. Cattaneo, M. Alessandria, and R. Cogo, "Efficacy and Safety of the Standardized Ginseng Extract G115 for Potentiating Vaccination Against the Influenza Syndrome and Protection Against the Common Cold," *Drugs Exp Clin Res* 22 (1996): 65–72.

16. M. Davydov and A. D. Krikorian, "Eleutherococcus Senticosus (Rupr. & Maxim.) Maxim. (Araliaceae) as an Adaptogen: A Closer Look," *J Ethnopharmacol* 72, no. 3 (2000): 345–93.

17. L. Han and D. Cai, "Clinical and Experimental Study on Treatment of Acute Cerebral Infarction with Acanthopanax Injection" [Article in Chinese], *Zhongguo Zhong Xi Yi Jie He Za Zhi* 18 (1998): 472–74.

18. P. J. Medon, P. W. Ferguson, and C. F. Watson, "Effects of Eleutherococcus Senticosus Extracts on Hexobarbital Metabolism In Vivo and In Vitro," *J Ethnopharmacol* 10 (1984): 235–41.

19. K. Winther, C. Ranlov, E. Rein E, and J. Mehlsen, "Russian Root (Siberian Ginseng) Improves Cognitive Functions in Middle-Aged People, Whereas Ginkgo biloba Seems Effective Only in the Elderly," *J Neurological Sci* 150 (1997): S90.

20. Z. Shi, C. Liu, and R. Li, "Effect of a Mixture of Acanthopanax senticosus and Elsholtzia splendens on Serum-Lipids in Patients with Hyperlipemia [Article in Chinese], *Zhong Xi Yi Jie He Za Zhi* 10 (1990): 155–56, 132.

21. L. Han and D. Cai, "Clinical and Experimental Study on Treatment of Acute Cerebral Infarction with Acanthopanax Injection" [Article in Chinese], *Zhongguo Zhong Xi Yi Jie He Za Zhi* 18 (1998): 472–74.

22. S. Y. Shang, Y. S. Ma, and S. S. Wang, "Effect of Eleutherosides on Ventricular Late Potential with Coronary Heart Disease and Myocarditis [Article in Chinese], *Zhong Xi Yi Jie He Za Zhi* 11 (1991): 280–81, 261.

Huperzine A

1. S. Budavari, ed., *The Merck Index*, 12th ed. (Whitehouse Station, NJ: Merck & Co., 1996).

2. X. C. Tang, P. De Sarno, K. Sugaya, and E. Giacobini, "Effect of Huperzine A, a New Cholinesterase Inhibitor, on the Central Cholinergic System of the Rat," *J Neurosci Res* 24, no. 2 (1989): 276–85.

3. J. W. Ye, J. X. Cai, L. M. Wang, and X. C. Tang, "Improving Effects of Huperzine A on Spatial Working Memory in Aged Monkeys and Young Adult Monkeys with Experimental Cognitive Impairment," *J Pharmacol Exp Ther* 288, no. 2 (1999): 814–19; D. H. Cheng and X. C. Tang, "Comparative Studies of Huperzine A, E2020, and Tacrine on Behavior and Cholinesterase Activities," *Pharmacol Biochem Behav* 60, no. 2 (1998):

377–86; Y. S. Cheng, C. Z. Lu, and Z. L. Ying, "128 Cases of Myasthenia Gravis Treated with Huperzine A," *New Drugs and Clinical Remedies* 5, no. 4 (1986): 197–99.

4. A. A. Skolnick, "Old Chinese Herbal Medicine Used for Fever Yields Possible New Alzheimer Disease Therapy," *JAMA* 277 (1997): 776.

5. J. Pepping, "Huperzine A," *Am J Health Syst Pharm* 57 (2000): 530–34.

6. S. S. Xu, Z. X. Gao, Z. Weng, Z. M. Du, W. A. Xu, J. S. Yang, M. L. Zhang, Z. H. Tong, Y. S. Fang, X. S. Chai, et al., "Efficacy of Tablet Huperzine-A on Memory, Cognition, and Behavior in Alzheimer's Disease," *Zhongguo Yao Li Xue Bao* 16, no. 5 (1995): 391–95.

7. R. W. Zhang, X. C. Tang, Y. Y. Han, G. W. Sang, Y. D. Zhang, Y. X. Ma, C. L. Zhang, and R. M. Yang, "Drug Evaluation of Huperzine A in the Treatment of Senile Memory Disorders," *Chung Kuo Yao Li Hsueh Pao* 12, no. 3 (1991): 250–52; S. S. Xu, Z. Y. Cai, Z. W. Qu, R. M. Yang, Y. L. Cai, G. Q. Wang, X. Q. Su, X. S. Zhong, R. Y. Cheng, W. A. Xu, J. X. Li, and B. Feng, "Huperzine-A in Capsules and Tablets for Treating Patients with Alzheimer Disease," *Zhongguo Yao Li Xue Bao* 20 (1999): 486–90.

8. Q. Q. Sun, S. S. Xu, J. L. Pan, H. M. Guo, and W. Q. Cao, "Huperzine-A Capsules Enhance Memory and Learning Performance in 34 Pairs of Matched Adolescent Students," *Chung Kuo Yao Li Hsueh Pao* 20 (1999): 601–3.

Magnesium

1. M. Shils, A. Olson, and M. Shike, *Modern Nutrition in Health and Disease*, 8th ed. (Philadelphia, PA: Lea and Febiger, 1994).

2. T. R. Covington et al., *Handbook of Nonprescription Drugs* (Washington, DC: Am Pharmaceutical Assn., 1996).

3. R. Swain and B. Kaplan-Machlis, "Magnesium for the Next Millennium," *South Med J* 92 (1999): 1040–47.

4. S. Douban, M. A. Brodsky, D. D. Whang, and R.Whang, "Significance of Magnesium in Congestive Heart Failure," *Am Heart J* 132, no. 3 (1996): 664–71.

5. B. T. Altura, Z. I. Memon, A. Zhang, T. P. Cheng, R. Silverman, R. Q. Cracco, and B. M. Altura, "Low Levels of Serum Ionized Magnesium Are Found in Patients Early After Stroke Which Result in Rapid Elevation in Cytosolic Free Calcium and Spasm in Cerebral Vascular Muscle Cells," *Neurosci Lett* 230 (1997): 37–40.

6. R. B. Costello, P. B. Moser-Veillon, and R. DiBianco, "Magnesium Supplementation in Patients with Congestive Heart Failure," *J Am Coll Nutr* 16, no. 1 (1997): 22–31.

7. A. Mauskop, B. T. Altura, R. Q. Cracco, and B. M. Altura. "Deficiency in Serum Ionized Magnesium But Not Total Magnesium in Patients with Migraines: Possible Role of ICa2+/IMg2+ Ratio," *Headache* 33, no. 3 (1993): 135–58.

8. K. A. Meyer, L. H. Kushi, D. R. Jacobs, J. Slavin, T. A. Sellers, and A. R. Folsom, "Carbohydrates, Dietary Fiber, and Incident Type 2 Diabetes in Older Women," *Am J Clin Nutr* 71 (2000): 921–30.

9. K. S. Moghissi, "Risks and Benefits of Nutritional Supplements During Pregnancy," *Obstet Gynecol*, 58, Suppl5. (Nov. 1981): 68S–78S.

10. M. M. Murray, *Encyclopedia of Nutritional Supplements* (Rocklin, CA: Prima Publishing, 1996), 159.

11. M. Sabatier, M. J. Arnaud, P. Kastenmayer, A. Rytz, and D. V. Barclay, "Meal Effect on Magnesium Bioavailability from Mineral Water in Healthy Women," *Am J Clin Nutr*

75, no. 1 (2002): 65–71; B. T. Altura, Z. I. Memon, A. Zhang, T. P. Cheng, R. Silverman, R. Q. Cracco, and B. M. Altura, "Low Levels of Serum Ionized Magnesium Are Found in Patients Early After Stroke Which Result in Rapid Elevation in Cytosolic Free Calcium and Spasm in Cerebral Vascular Muscle Cells," *Neurosci Lett* 230 (1997): 37–40; P. M. Suter, "The Effects of Potassium, Magnesium, Calcium, and Fiber on Risk of Stroke," *Nutr Rev* 57 (1999): 84–88; E. Whitney, C. B. Cataldo, and S. R. Rolfes, eds., *Understanding Normal and Clinical Nutrition* (Belmont, CA: Wadsworth, 1998).

N-Acetyl-Carnitine

1. J. W. Pettegrew, J. Levine, and R. J. McClure, "Acetyl-L-Carnitine Physical-Chemical, Metabolic, and Therapeutic Properties: Relevance for Its Mode of Action in Alzheimer's Disease and Geriatric Depression," *Mol Psychiatry* 5 (2000): 616–32.

2. R. Mayeux and M. Sano, "Treatment of Alzheimer's Disease," *N Engl J Med* 341, no. 22 (1999): 1670–79.

3. Micromedex Healthcare Series. *AltMedDex® System: Comprehensive Referenced Data on Herbal Medicines and Dietary Supplements Covering Uses, Efficacy, Dosing, Toxicity, and More*" (Englewood, CO: MICROMEDEX Inc.).

4. L. J. Thal, A. Carta, W. R. Clarke, S. H. Ferris, R. P. Friedland, R. C. Petersen, J. W. Pettegrew, E. Pfeiffer, M. A. Raskind, M. Sano, M. H. Tuszynski, and R. F. Woolson, "A 1-Year Multicenter Placebo-Controlled Study of Acetyl-L-Carnitine in Patients with Alzheimer's Disease," *Neurology* 47 (1996): 705–11.

5. D. Cucinotta, M. Passeri, and S. Ventura, "Multicenter Clinical Placebo-Controlled Study with Acetyl-L-Carnitine (ALC) in the Treatment of Mildly Demented Elderly Patients," *Drug Development Res* 14 (1988): 213–16.

6. P. M. Kidd, "A Review of Nutrients and Botanicals in the Integrative Management of Cognitive Dysfunction," *Alternative Medicine Review* 4 (1999): 144–61.

7. A. Postiglione, A. Soricelli, U. Cicerano, L. Mansi, S. De Chiara, G. Gallotta, G. Schettini, and M. Salvatore, "Effect of Acute Administration of L-Acetyl Carnitine on Cerebral Blood Flow in Patients with Chronic Cerebral Infarct," *Pharmacol Res* 23, no. 3 (1991): 241–46.

8. E. Tempesta, R. Troncon, L. Janiri, L. Colusso, P. Riscica, G. Saraceni, E. Gesmundo, M. Calvani, N. Benedetti, and P. Pola, "Role of Acetyl-L-Carnitine in the Treatment of Cognitive Deficit in Chronic Alcoholism," *Int J Clin Pharmacol Res* 10 no. 1–2 (1990): 101–7.

9. L. Di Marzio, S. Moretti, S. D'Alo, F. Zazzeroni, S. Marcellini, C. Smacchia, E. Alesse, M. G. Cifone, and C. De Simone, "Acetyl-L-Carnitine Administration Increases Insulin-Like Growth Factor 1 Levels in Asymptomatic HIV-1-Infected Subjects: Correlation with Its Suppressive Effect on Lymphocyte Apoptosis and Ceramide Generation," *Clin Immunol* 92, no. 1 (1999): 103–10.

10. G. Famularo, S. Moretti, S. Marcellini, V. Trinchieri, S. Tzantzoglou, G. Santini, A. Longo, and C. De Simone, "Acetyl-Carnitine Deficiency in AIDS Patients with Neurotoxicity on Treatment with Antiretroviral Nucleoside Analogues," *AIDS* 11, no. 2 (1997): 185–90.

11. L. J. Thal, A. Carta, W. R. Clarke, S. H. Ferris, R. P. Friedland, R. C. Petersen, J. W. Pettegrew, E. Pfeiffer, M. A. Raskind, M. Sano, M. H. Tuszynski, and R. F. Woolson. "A 1-Year Multicenter Placebo-Controlled Study of Acetyl-L-Carnitine in Patients with Alzheimer's Disease," *Neurology* 47 (1996): 705–11.

12. R. Golan, R. Weissenberg, and L. M. Lewin, "Carnitine and Acetylcarnitine in Motile and Immotile Human Spermatozoa," *Int J Androl* 7 (1984): 484–94.

Phosphatidylserine

1. J. Pepping, "Phosphatidylserine," *Am J Health-Syst Pharm* 56 (1999): 2038, 2043–44.

2. T. Crook, W. Petrie, C. Wells, and D. C. Massari. "Effects of Phosphatidylserine in Alzheimer's Disease," *Psychopharmacol Bull* 28, no. 1 (1992): 61–66; A. Blokland, W. Honig, F. Brouns, and J. Jolles, "Cognition-Enhancing Properties of Subchronic Phosphatidylserine (PS) Treatment in Middle-Aged Rats: Comparison of Bovine Cortex PS with Egg PS and Soybean PS," *Nutrition* 15 (1999): 778–83.

3. T. H. Crook, J. Tinklenberg, J. Yesavage, W. Petrie, M. G. Nunzi, and D. C. Massari, "Effects of Phosphatidylserine in Age-Associated Memory Impairment," *Neurology* 41 ,no. 5 (1991): 644–49.

4. H. Y. Kim, M. Akbar, A. Lau, and L. Edsall, "Inhibition of Neuronal Apoptosis by Docosahexaenoic Acid (22:6n-3): Role of Phosphatidylserine in Antiapoptotic Effect," *J Biol Chem* 275 (2000): 35215–23.

5. T. D. Fahey and M. S. Pearl, "The Hormonal and Perceptive Effects of Phosphatidylserine Administration During Two Weeks of Resistive Exercise-Induced Overtraining," *Biol Sport* 15 (1998): 135–44.

6. W. D. Heiss, J. Kessler, R. Mielke, B. Szelies, and K. Herholz, "Long-Term Effects of Phosphatidylserine, Pyritinol, and Cognitive Training in Alzheimer's Disease: A Neuropsychological, EEG, and PET Investigation," *Dementia* 5 (1994): 88–98; P. J. Delwaide, A. M. Gyselynck-Mambourg, A. Hurlet, and M. Ylieff, "Double-Blind, Randomized, Controlled Study of Phosphatidylserine in Senile Demented Patients," *Acta Neurol Scand* 73, no. 2 (1986): 136–40.

7. C. Villardita, S. Grioli, G. Salmeri, F. Nicoletti, and G. Pennisi, "Multicenter Clinical Trial of Brain Phosphatidylserine in Elderly Patients with Intellectual Deterioration," *Clin Trials J* 24 (1987): 84–93; T. Cenacchi, T. Bertoldin, C. Farina, M. G. Fiori, and G. Crepaldi, "Cognitive Decline in the Elderly: A Double-Blind, Placebo-Controlled Multicenter Study on Efficacy of Phosphatidylserine Administration," *Aging* (Milano) 5, no. 2 (1993): 123–33.

8. M. Maggioni, G. B. Picotti, G. P. Bondiolotti, A. Panerai, T. Cenacchi, P. Nobile, and F. Brambilla, "Effects of Phosphatidylserine Therapy in Geriatric Patients with Depressive Disorders," *Acta Psychiatr Scand* 81 (1990): 265–70.

9. P. Monteleone, L. Beinat, C. Tanzillo, M. Maj, and D. Kemali, "Effects of Phosphatidylserine on the Neuroendocrine Response to Physical Stress in Humans," *Neuroendocrinology* 52 (1990): 243–48.

10. M. M. Murray, *Encyclopedia of Nutritional Supplements* (Rocklin, CA: Prima Publishing, 1996), 356–58.

11. P. M. Kidd, "Attention Deficit/Hyperactivity Disorder (ADHD) in Children: Rationale for Its Integrative Management," *Altern Med Rev* 5 (2000): 402–28.

Vitamin C

1. M. Levine, S. C. Rumsey, R. Daruwala, J. B. Park, and Y. Wang, "Criteria and Recommendations for Vitamin C Intake," *JAMA* 281 (1999): 1415–23.

2. J. A. Simon and E. S. Hudes, "Serum Ascorbic Acid and Gallbladder Disease Prevalence Among U.S. Adults," *Arch Intern Med* 160 (2000): 931–36.

3. G. K. McKevoy, ed., *AHFS Drug Information* (Bethesda, MD: American Society of Health-System Pharmacists, 1998).

4. M. M. Murray, *Encyclopedia of Nutritional Supplements* (Rocklin, CA: Prima Publishing, 1996), 65–79.

5. C. S. Johnston and L. L. Thompson, "Vitamin C Status of an Outpatient Population," *J Am Coll Nutr* 17 (1998): 366–70.

6. S. J. Padayatty and M. Levine, "New Insights into the Physiology and Pharmacology of Vitamin C," *CMAJ* 164 (2001): 353–55.

7. R. M. Kasa, "Vitamin C: From Scurvy to the Common Cold," *Am J Med Technol* 49 (1983): 23–26.

Vitamin E

1. Food and Nutrition Board, Institute of Medicine, *Dietary Reference Intakes for Vitamin C, Vitamin E, Selenium, and Carotenoids* (Washington, DC: National Academy Press, 2000). www.nap.edu/books/0309069351/html/.

2. M. M. Murray, *Encyclopedia of Nutritional Supplements* (Rocklin, CA: Prima Publishing, 1996), 44–53.

3. G. K. McKevoy, ed., *AHFS Drug Information* (Bethesda, MD: American Society of Health-System Pharmacists, 1998).

Zinc

1. M. Spraycar, ed., *Stedman's Medical Dictionary*, 26th ed. (Baltimore, MD: Williams & Wilkins, 1995).

2. L. Sian, N. F. Krebs, J. E. Westcott, et al., "Zinc Homeostasis During Lactation in a Population with a Low Zinc Intake," *Am J Clin Nutr* 75 (2002): 99–103.

3. Food and Nutrition Board, Institute of Medicine, *Dietary Reference Intakes for Vitamin A, Vitamin K, Arsenic, Boron, Chromium, Copper, Iodine, Iron, Manganese, Molybdenum, Nickel, Silicon, Vanadium, and Zinc* (Washington, DC: National Academy Press, 2002). www.nap.edu/books/0309072794/html/.

4. D. G. Barceloux,. "Zinc," *J Toxicol Clin Toxicol* 37 (1999): 279–92.

5. E. Whitney, C. B. Cataldo, and S. R. Rolfes, eds., *Understanding Normal and Clinical Nutrition* (Belmont, CA: Wadsworth, 1998).

6. P. Toren, S. Eldar, B. A. Sela, L. Wolmer, R. Weitz, D. Inbar, S. Koren, A. Reiss, R. Weizman, and N. Laor, "Zinc Deficiency in Attention-Deficit Hyperactivity Disorder," *Biol Psychiatry* 40 (1996): 1308–10.

7. L. E. Arnold, N. A. Votolato, D. Kleykamp, G. B. Baker, and R. A. Bornstein, "Does Hair Zinc Predict Amphetamine Improvement of ADD/Hyperactivity?" *Int J Neurosci* 50 (1990): 103–7.

8. A. H. Shankar and A. S. Prasad, "Zinc and Immune Function: The Biological Basis of Altered Resistance to Infection," *Am J Clin Nutr* 68 (1998): 447S–63S.

9. A. S. Prasad, "Zinc and Immunity," *Mol Cell Biochem* 188 (1998): 63–69.

10. M. T. Murray, *Natural Alternatives to Over-the-Counter and Prescription Drugs* (New York: Quill, 1994).

11. M. M. Murray, *Encyclopedia of Nutritional Supplements* (Rocklin, CA: Prima Publishing, 1996), 181–89.

12. A. Peirce, *The Amer Pharmaceutical Assn Practical Guide to Natural Medicines* (New York: The Stonesong Press, 1999).

13. B. H. Grahn, P. G. Paterson, K. T. Gottschall-Pass, and Z. Zhang, "Zinc and the Eye," *J Am Coll Nutr* 20 (2001): 106–18.

14. H. C. Freake, K. E. Govoni, K. Guda, C. Huang, and S. A. Zinn, "Actions and Interactions of Thyroid Hormone and Zinc Status in Growing Rats," *J Nutr* 4 (2001): 1135.

Index

About the Series Editors and Advisors

MARGOT LONGENECKER, N.D., is Associate Series Editor. She is a Co-Director of the Integrative Medicine Center at Griffin Hospital and a member of the Clinical Faculty at the Naturopathic Medical College at the University of Bridgeport, both in Connecticut. Dr. Longenecker is also a member of the Board of Directors for the American Association of Naturopathic Physicians. She is in private practice in Guilford, Connecticut.

CHRIS D. MELETIS, N.D., is Senior Series Editor. He is Senior Science Officer and Associate Professor of Natural Pharmacology at the National College of Naturopathic Medicine. He was chosen for the Naturopathic Physician of the Year Award for 2003–2004 by the American Association of Naturopathic Physicians. He is an international lecturer, a radio personality, and an educator of medical doctors, nurses, pharmacists, and the allied healthcare fields. He has authored 9 books on natural health topics.

Advisor MARK NATHAN MILLER, M.D, N.D, is one of a small number of physicians in the United States who have been trained and board certified as both a medical doctor and a naturopath. After 13 years of practicing urgent care and internal medicine, he began his naturopathic education. Also a board member for the Oregon chapter of Physicians for Social Responsibility, he is a Clinical Instructor of Endocrinology at the National College of Naturopathic Medicine. He is also in private practice at the Legacy Urgent Care Clinic in St. Helen's, Oregon.

Advisor MICHAEL O'REILLY, M.D., is a surgeon and Chairperson of the Department of Obstetrics and Gynecology at Griffin Hospital, where he is also a Founding Member of the Integrative Medicine Center. He is a Diplomat of the

National Board of Medical Examiners, a guest lecturer at the University of Connecticut School of Medicine, and a Clinical Instructor at the University of Bridgeport Naturopathic Medical College.

Advisor GLEN ZIELINSKI, D.C., is a chiropractic physician and board certified chiropractic neurologist. He is a Diplomate of the American Chiropractic Neurology Board. Dr. Zielinski is an Assistant Professor of Clinical Neurology at the Carrick Institute in Oregon. He is also Director of Physical Medicine at the Pearl Clinic in Portland, Oregon. He lectures on neurology throughout the nation.

About the Authors

CHRIS D. MELETIS, N.D., is Senior Series Editor for the Praeger series, *Complementary and Alternative Medicine*. He is Senior Science Officer and Associate Professor of Natural Pharmacology at the National College of Naturopathic Medicine. He was chosen for the Naturopathic Physician of the Year Award for 2003–2004 by the American Association of Naturopathic Physicians. He is an international lecturer, a radio personality, and has authored 9 books on natural health topics.

JASON E. BARKER, N.D., is in private practice and has been Adjunct Professor of Naturopathy at the National College of Naturopathic Medicine, at Oregon Health Sciences University and at Southwest College of Naturopathic Medicine.